THE MANIC-DEPRESSIVE JUNKIE

PRESENTS:

LOGICAL

DEATH

By

Robert John Hanink
DSM IV BP CYCLOTHYMIC

ISBN 0-9719232-3-X

First printing: May 2002

Self-Published by:
Robert John Hanink
Manteno, IL 60950

"Illustrations used with permission of Jack Goodwin"

HEED THIS WARNING!!!

I thank you for purchasing my book. I hope that you find the content worthy of its cost.

It is the intent of this book to be of a practical value to any humans dealing with Bi-Polar friends, relatives, or patients although any interested human might enjoy the strangeness of it. The physical structure, language, sentence structure and poor grammar are of a revealing nature. My writing skills are as revealed - nothing more. My thoughts are as honest as words can describe. How can a "prim and properly edited book" maintain the honesty of thoughts felt by its author? It would then read as if the professional editor had improved or corrected the book into becoming what would be considered normal for all books. I thank my friends for their advice on the content of the book, and that is all there is to it. Fifteen years of taking notes, 7 years of research, 4 years of writing, sixteen months of editing, and this is what I have to offer to you.

This is not a guide for proper Manic-depressive behaviors. It must not be looked upon as a path to a better life for Bi-Polars. I do not seek becoming a role model for other Bi-Polars (or Bi-Polar want-a-be's), although I am sympathetic for their sufferings and proud of the courage they show every day, getting up, going to work, raising a family, or maybe only hanging-on everyday in desperation, but surviving nonetheless. Every one of them is a hero, every suicide a tragedy. Do not imitate my actions. Always follow your true self. Always look to friends and loved ones for help. Stay alive.

I offer you no hope

Presented

TO:

_____

_____

BY:

_____

_____

DATE: _____ 20____

Beware of false manics

This Certifies

THAT: _____

IS A REGESTERED: _____

[Ordinary human, Uni-polar, Bi-polar I, Bi-polar II, Cyclothymic]

BY: _____

ON: _____ 20 ___

AT: _____

> Death is the end of existence

Deaths

NAME, DATE, REASON

_____

_____

_____

_____

Suicides

NAME, DATE, METHOD

_____

_____

_____

_____

~~BOOK TOPICS~~

A Story

Somehow the humans came into existence on the planet with no name, along with the other living creatures of the natural world. The humans realized that they were a creature of many, and that they had dominion over all the other creatures of the earth by virtue of the human's ability to construct anything that needed constructing, or to kill anything that needed to be killed.

Now it came to pass that the humans began to speak and understand the many tongues of the many tribes of all the humans. As they became unified in thought, they believed that they were the divine life of the earth, and that because they all thought in unison, their thoughts must be common. They truly believed that every action that they did or committed or every idea that they thought; was acceptable and never un-ordinary in any way. Thus they became the ordinary humans and their numbers were great. They ruled with rules and always wished every human to behave within their set of rules of ordinariness.

It came to pass that among the ordinary humans, certain humans saw a vision - that vision was disturbing to see or know. These unique humans hid their abilities whilst among the ordinary humans out of fear of being anything but ordinary.

But they were discovered nonetheless and thus they became the topic of much concern by the ordinary humans.

"Who are these humans that are born to us?" the ordinary humans asked.

"Genetic misfits", proclaimed the doctors and the elite of the ordinary humans. They also added, "We must correct these misfits if they are going to live as happily as we do. This is our duty to them."

So rules and laws were made, and secret messages of behavioral correctness were invented and distributed and taught and put into effect legally.

"These un-ordinary humans are Bi-polar, manic-depressives, every one of them", stated the intellectuals of the ordinary humans. So the list of behavioral traits was to be published and distributed and it was to have appeared for you in this book, right here!

But something went wrong, and I must admit to you, my reader friend, that I am taking control of this book, and I am no ordinary human indeed. So relax and read-on while I lend you my eyes and my mind, and your world disintegrates about you. You will soon find that the view of the universe is not ordinary at all.

PREFATORY

VIII. I die and then I am born. An uneventful occurrence on another ordinary day on July 28th, 1951 c.e. the year of your Lord on a small nameless planet lost in the vastness of the Milky Way galaxy. An event that I don't remember but which is celebrated with unfaltering accuracy and persistence each earth year. My friends and family will always be constant reminders of my age progression through the physical life here on a planet with no name that the human's simply call; the earth. Of course, it is highly probable that in the future, certain humans will have the privilege of being reminded of their birthdays while living on another planet. However, that will not be my future. My future being unknown to me at birth, but was somewhat already decided by the date and geography of my birth, the genealogy of my parents, and the sequential arrangement of millions of four different types of DNA bases.

VII. My name was to be Robert John Hanink. Robert is copied from my grandfather, Robert Hanink, and can be seen on his tomb marker. I've only seen his tomb marker twice but I will not forget the coldness and permanence of my name chiseled into it. John is taken from John Felsecker my other grandfather. He is also dead - they are all dead, as is my dad. I have thoughts of them, but I fully understand that thoughts are only a meaningless waste of synaptic activity. Thoughts cannot change reality but they do define reality.

VI. By translation my name would mean "Bright fame" & "The Lord is gracious" Hanink. I suppose a name would have an effect on a child but my name did nothing for me and it means nothing to me now. Although deeþ within my brain, where twisted lies and þhables of false realities (having been taught to me throughout my childhood) are shoved into carefully concealed crevices, I want to hear a gentle voice calling my name to come into the light and warmth to receive an embrace of love; forever and beyond the infinite. But those are the thoughts that lead to a clearer vision of reality. A reality that when understood could lead even an ordinary human to suicide let alone a manic-deþressive as myself. Avoid the vision of reality and stay alive is what I now þrescribe.

V. Well, you bought this book (or received it as a gift, or stole it, or þerhaþs borrowed it with no intention of returning it; as is how I got my coþy) so let me get to the þoint. I am here to tell you about the existence of other realities; reasoning and reactions based on a logic that is different than most "ordinary human" þerceþtions can imagine. My goal for the þast three decades has been to find an understanding of the þhysical existence and to rationalize the ordinary human, better known as the *Homo sapiens sapiens*: another animal þigeonholed into scientific neologisms. To do this we must have a þarty. The guest list includes genes and memes, amoebae and cro-magnums, electrons and blackholes, time and infinity, and life and death themselves. I intend to define the basic building blocks required such that all of existence through time and sþace of the universe can be þredicted and understood to the extent in which it can be understood. I do this for my own understanding of it before I am comþelled to sleeþ with Kings and

Counselors, but why not share the path of logic dyslectic with you, my reader friend?

iv. The challenge in getting you this data comes in the way that the manic-depressive species, *Homo sapiens maniakos*, has the tendency to terminate its life when the vision of reality becomes too clear. Manic-depressive suicide is a matter of clear thinking and the understanding of the reality of the physical universe and a true feeling of time. Suicide is not always an irrational action. The manic-depressive human will be proven to possess a different genetic structure than that of the ordinary humans, and thus a different vision of reality and logic would be expected to be normal - as all humans are taught to operate under something called; "intelli-genetics". Intelli-genetics is the ability to control the thoughts that alter your actions demanded to be acted on by your human inherited genetics (chromosomes) as opposed to only behaving naturally as the beasts of fields.

iii. Race, as in human races (i.e. black, white, Asian, American Indian, etc.), exists in other forms. Should "race" be defined as a different sub-species or a variety of a specie due to genetic variation? Why aren't races defined by the categorizing of a human's perception of reality or the actual ability to see reality? We all don't see the same reality. I do not feel the ordinary human's reality. I study it and I try to rationalize it. I try to exist in it, but I live beyond it. I live in the isolated world of the manic-depressive.

ii. The year is the present year - the time is now. This is then the correct time to reveal the truth. A species lives among the ordinary humans that has been suppressed into submission and seclusion by psychological babble. A species that because of a greater sensitivity to human emotions has been channeled into the belief that they are inferior (due to being called "mentally ill") when in fact they are superior to all other human species. The *Homo sapiens sapiens* (i.e. ordinary humans) would call us: Manic-depressives. Within the English language the term is descriptive but of no significance. A name more appropriate for our species is the name *Homo sapiens maniakos* -the enhanced human. Now I propose that for the sake of a new beginning of our freedom, I will provide the taxonomy using a morphological subdivision of the human species. *Homo sapiens sapiens* is now the *Hosapiens:* the "ordinary human." *Homo sapiens maniakos* is now the *Homaniakos* [Best pronounced as; Ho-man-a-kos] - the "enhanced human" - the human with a clearer vision of reality; the ability to see beyond death.

i. For about 1% of human looking creatures along with myself, we live in a reality that only the enhanced human would understand. I do not want the ordinary humans cure and I can barely tolerate their world of falsehoods and delusions; thus I remain by via my own remaining free will, living day by day, as a Manic-Depressive Junkie. Please enjoy my story and perceptions of how I interpret the reality that surrounds me, written in various states of my mind (musically enhanced while being written) with full thought disorder, maximum self-esteem applied (giving the correct impression of supreme confidence or egoism), verbosity (resulting in long sentence structures), poverty of content of speech, distractible speech, derailment, incoherence, illogicality, circumstantially, and my favorite trait of clanging, all for the purpose of drawing you into my processes of logic.

CHAPTER
MANIC-DEPRESSION

The music that set the mood for writing this chapter was:
  "A Passion Play" CD by Jethro Tull.
  "Heart-Shaped Box" Song by Nirvana.

The *Homaniakos* (*Homo sapiens maniakos*)

1 . A calm me is hell. Manic-depressive characteristics do not usually form until about the human age of 15 to 25 standard earth years - or at least we and the ordinary humans do not suspect we are of a different species until that time in our life. Thus I had a normal and unremarkable childhood, adolescents, and early adulthood, but after living in the larva stage (believing to be an ordinary human), other manic-depressives and myself immerge into an alien world, the world of the ordinary human. It is as though we were not even born of this world. The world doesn't change, but our perceptions become enhanced and thus our understanding of the mechanisms of reality are changed and as we view strange sunsets of colors phantasm refracted, the feeling of loneliness sets in, and the darkness is strange to us also because depression is activated by the darkness as though the darkness looks at us deliberately. All of a sudden, we realize that what we perceive and our reaction to our perceptions are different than those humans that we know. The self-isolation begins – we don't reveal our thoughts to these humans around us, those humans are strange. How do we account for their thoughts or actions? The question we may ask of ourselves is: "I am different, but am I unique?" Since

we don't "self proclaim", as in some type of aversion therapy, we can only look and wonder about those humans around us - if any are also as us. Always looking into eyes unaware of us looking but looking for that revealing action that they recognize us as one of them. We hide too well, even from each other, and thus we bump into ourselves as though we are all blind and deaf and mute and as a dead man walking within a brilliant madness. Clues are there to be sensed by us only - not the ordinary humans, but we remain polite and do not ask of each other to reveal true identities or abilities. So now the loneliness continues and if you are not up to living in it, go ahead and kill yourself, it won't matter. We know that to be true.

2. As depression is such a negative feeling, it may appear more pronounced than the manic mood giving the impression of us being an emotionally different human. We may believe that we are only an intelligent energetic person with a depression problem, but for certain we are not. As this chapter will soon describe to you, manic-depression is taught to humans as though it is a mental illness. Manic-depression is rare enough, about 1% of the population (I am told), that most likely we will not receive our manic-depression cultural instructions from another manic-depressive. The ordinary humans will be our instructors and wardens as they try to pull us into their world with no understanding of our world at all - but we know that their reality is based on faulty logic. They have no vision. They will never understand our vision. The vision we the manic-depressives all see but may not understand yet. We perceive this vision as pain. It is pain, but it is also knowledge.

3. How can I lead other manic-depressives to see the knowledge that waits beyond the pain? We strive to know what are the true

understanding of reality and existence and the existence of death. I do have a þlan for us, and that þlan is this book. Although I exþect that both ordinary humans and us will read this book, the ordinary humans will not understand all of it, but the manic-deþressive will. The understanding of reality, existence, and the understanding of death will only be understood by a combination of the vision that all manic-deþressives share along with "The Most Basic Knowledge of the Physical Realm" and "The Most Basic Knowledge about the Human Animal". Only all three combined will bring an understanding of the reality of existence. I will start the outline of this knowledge for you, the reader, in CHAPTER CREATIVITY, and then reveal the missing data during the extent of this book. Each remaining chaþter will add þieces of knowledge for you to build your understanding of the reality of existence. Manic-deþressives must float down the stream of life and observe what occurs even if not þarticiþating. Being there becomes our goal. Being there means living one more day. As for me, before I close my eyes each morning I say, "I was alive to-day".

4a. Desþite the writing þrotocols of breaking toþics into þaragraþhs, as you might exþect to find in a þublished book, you must realize that many of us *Homaniakos'* will talk non-stoþ [*Pressured speech*]. So I set uþ my long sentences the same way, followed by my long and de-railed þaragraþhs as well, because my þaragraþhs are based on what þoint I wish to make, and how good it feels to write them as though I am sþeaking them to you - nothing more. If you should ever meet me, you would þroclaim, "Oh my Godd, it's true". Aside from *Gregg's* book or my *Idiot's Guide*, which [*that?*] I have been trying to master, I'll never get my "Infinitive Phrases" or "Plural Possessives" correct anyway. Besides, who found all those little " ' : ; , - ( ] * marks? If you can't hear it in the transmission of oral information, , , , , (more commas means a longer pause, I guess) then why have them? Oh well! I have misplaced about 3,000 commas or semi-colons throughout [sounds like "*threw out*"] this book anyway! I did add paragraphical numeration for your convenience, and why isn't that considered proper and mandatory[?] - because it is actually very useful to the function of the transmission of oral thoughts written read remembered.

4b. Getting back from paragraph number 3, what each *Homaniakos* will do with this understanding will be up to each individual. I do not believe there is any purpose for us to have this vision and knowledge, but we have it nonetheless. It is my intent only that manic-depressives take their true place of authority on this planet and that ordinary humans will no longer cause us to degrade ourselves by the actions of their faulty logic. I am that I am, and I will not apologize for my natural abilities. I will instead, look outward toward the infinity of space and time, and realize that we the *Homaniakos* are able to see what the *Hosapiens* will never see - the clearer vision of reality. Whereas there seems to be an endless variety of Manicism, not all manic-depressives exist within reality as easily as others do. I am one of the more fortunate ones, by chance of course, in that I became fully engaged at the end of my college years, and I was originally "episodic" at about 5-year intervals. Minor fluctuations occurred between depression and hypomanicism and I seemed to be more hypomanic than depressed. My sexual activities always followed the 6th and 7th protocols of manicism, but that doesn't seem to be that far outside of the ordinary humans' activity anyway. Living through haphazard suicide fantasies early in my life has brought better abilities later in life. I know that other manic-depressives developed too early in life (as human-children), or have more severe episodes or spend too much time depressed, or worst yet, they describe some type of non-existent evil creature that lives within their brain. Nothing good comes from an unrealistic understanding of your "true self" via creating fairy tales of invisible creatures or demons tormenting you at their will. That metaphor is the basis for the ordinary human's view that we are mentally ill. I don't wish to be associated with humans possessed of demons, real or not. I have no demons within my mind - that[*which?*] is for certain. However, I have compassion for my fellow *Homaniakos* whether they are borderline ordinary or extremely agitated and violent. Whether they have reached their journey's end of understanding their true self, or if they cry out for love from darkened, lonely rooms throughout the sleepless nights. There seems to be so many varieties of us, but actually what we end up with is maybe three or four basic types that then are combined within the variety of normal human personalities and beliefs. We may actually suffer from ordinary human's mental illnesses within our state of mind, and thus the confusion of what is our true self becomes complex to figure by us and the humans around us [*Order of words (consider revising)*]. As it took me approximately 10 earth years to figure the basics of what I am, it took another 13 earth years to gain control and fine-tune the knowledge of my species. The final knowledge came with the completion of this book. I am finished. What the ordinary humans don't realize is that the *Homaniakos* have a society separate from that of the *Hosapiens*. After most of the *Hosapiens* fall into their sleep, the *Homaniakos* take to the Internet until the early morning hours to find each other and offer life supporting conversation and data. The networks have been established and the matrix of electronic Internet communications will be our saviour [*British*]. We dominate the darkness hours with questions of support and survival, having been transformed from being ordinary humans into something the ordinary humans can't understand. But what all humans must remember is that for many of us, trying to exist within the framework of life and within some type of contrived culture, becomes a daily event of which I wish to be left alone with the task of it. We are guaranteed to fail when we attempt to put our lives within the structure of that of the ordinary humans.

5. My feeling of loneliness is as though I am trapped on this planet with no rescue ship to arrive. I will never live in a place that brings me a comfort, such as the feeling of being home, for where is my home? Although I have befriended many ordinary humans, it never ceases to amaze me at their lack of interest in reality. Something the human Alfred Hitchcock once said during a broadcasted taped interview comes to my mind, "*Reality is something that none of us can really stand, at anytime*". (Quote not confirmed with a source.). It makes me wonder if he was one of us and not one of them.

6. I suppose the first business at hand is to explain what constitutes a manic-depressive as a text book example of general traits. Every book we manic-depressive's write usually has to explain manic-depression in some type of specialized medical lingo within the contrived language of the *Hosapiens*. As you will find in my book, I can take this contrived language of the *Hosapiens* only so much as sometimes I feel so clever about my verb usage and other times I don't care about using words at all. How can I present my ideas to you without the use of a contrived language and thus not contradict half of my own opinions about contrived languages? I don't believe we should dwell on it because it's

starting to sound like that chicken and egg question and there will be no end of it. At any rate, data about manic-depressionism can also be found in many books and web sites but lets get on with it.

Manic-depression poorly defined

7. Manic-depressives go through various "moods", as the *Hosapiens* (*Homo sapiens sapiens*) would say, that has a marked effect on our behavior. In other words, we don't behave like them. By their faulty logic then, the *Hosapiens* say we have a mental illness.

8. *Normal.* Yes we can have behavior like the *Hosapiens,* but we can overcome it. We like good food, movies, parties, families, sex, etc. because we have all the human senses. We only don't like them as or when the *Hosapiens* do. The motivations to participate in those events are different than that of the *Hosapiens.* Sometimes tying to conform within the contrived unwritten rules of techciety (a technology-burdened society whereas technology is dominant over the social aspects of the organic life that created said technology as are the humans of the present U.S.A.) creates questions of "What the hell are they so concerned about?" during the events of ordinary importance.

9. *Hypomanic.* This is a good mood to be in and the creative manic-depressive is best served when feeling unbounded energy without drugs or even without sleeping but never being tired as though nature didn't devise sleep for us. Since I hate making lists in books because lists seem so unnatural as though you would find a list in nature (but I suppose someone will prove me wrong), so I don't give a damn about being perfectly correct as how correct can

a contrived language be anyway, and besides this book is written in the wrong **font** I've been told. There are seven identifiers that I constantly read about and in this poorly constructed paragraph (and stuck in number 9 no less) of nontraditionally ordered words will be all of them and you should have, I don't know, maybe four of them within some type of defined time period to make a full claim to be as me - so make your own determination and "list" if you must. As my thoughts are racing now and sometimes as quick as a blink I come up with a pun, often with a sexual note hidden in the words, it is only a natural trait of an unknown purpose. As far as fantastic self-esteem what could be wrong with that, especially the feeling of it within our minds to such an extreme? Those feelings lead to over achieving or the ordinary humans making remarks about where do you get the energy from[?], but it is within all humans I expect if everyone would only look for it. As these long sentences and illogical paragraphs that I won't remove from my edited book prove, speech can be constant and lengthy but nothing special will become of it so why should that be any different than the ordinary human's speech content? Leave my words alone, for who should know better what I want to write and how I wish to write it than me? Verbosity rules! During all this speaking we maintain short attention spans because we become inured to our distractions quickly and need more distractions even quickerly [*Word approximation*]. I'm at number seven now, but it's like trying to find the second set of ten commandments in the Bible I suppose, so we seek pleasure in ways that have a great potential for serious consequences within the *Hosapiens* laws. I would have the laws changed to accommodate us or maybe start my own church because at least there we could have strange sex while following some divine law. Otherwise watch your money because spending is not natural by any means and we haven't mastered money concepts - money is truly the *Hosapiens* contrivance.

10. *Manic.* The manic episode is the same as the hypomanic episode except that we may not be able to function in the *Hosapiens* world while manic. The *Hosapiens* around us will notice our genetic behavior differences. The best part of being manic is that we know that the sudden impact of depression lies ahead of us, but we don't have a remembrance of the pain of the depression or of the thoughts we will soon have or the vision of reality that will come into sight and bring with it the infinite despair driving logical suicide to within our arms reach. If I may throw in or out another topic, let me say [*write*] that states as in "states of mind" often mix themselves and you would need a score card to figure them out because in truth I don't believe mixed moods are chart-able even if they are closer to the norm than not, but the *Hosapiens* are driven to such pre-occupations of imagined importance such as charting what we do naturally and I will tell you that restlessness and excitement and writing beyond the comprehension of speech in a contrived language combined with motor retardation and short attention spans cause me to sometimes feel as thought I am sinning or that I am a sinner but without me even believing in a god of any type at that moment. But damn I have fun bouncing mixed emotions of fear and hate and anger at the world for messing with my normal state of mind (whatever "normal" would feel like?). All the while I'm naturally high as the arch of a great coaster about to make the plunge with silent screams and enhanced senses that smell life and touch infinity or seeing all of life's pleasures beyond reach but feeling them within my mind nonetheless and sometimes flicking or licking immoral thoughts with the tip of my tongue. The best part of all this

emotional stew is that I can cook it when I'm hungry or re-heat the leftovers for a quickie, and sometimes its like coming back from the dead being overjoyed that I am alive for another short moment knowing that I am a Manic-Depressive Junkie and few other humans are!

11. *Depressed.* Five or more of the following symptoms are present at the same time or during a brief time period is how the books are written in itemized format oh so nice and ordered but not in my book and as I am fully regnated (not a word, get used to it) and up to the thought fully disordered and will now write one very long and messed up paragraph with grammar tossed to the wind - you must realize that we might feel sad or tearful for no reason that the ordinary humans would notice. As we would try to express crying only in private to prevent the ordinary humans from exhibiting a normal and uncontrollable genetic reflex of no true concern, they wouldn't know what to say to us anyway because how can they know the unknown of rational thoughts? We are forced to hide our emotions and that is only faulty logic, as I would really like to cry my eyes out so that I may enjoy any type of an emotion, because I miss some of those emotions I used to have. Insomnia or sleep disorder to match my thought disorder are paired responses because the mind never sleeps and eyes closed see quite clearly even in the dark, for it is the mind that sees not the eyes as you might believe. I stay up until the morning searching the Internet for all the extremes and pretend to be whoever I would like to be because none of it is real and from what I can tell, those images suddenly appear on my screen as electrons deciphered logically for my pleasure. Planning for the trip - as in the final trip - causes us to think of death without fear, but as death is natural why not logical suicide as well? Eating can't be regular because

eating a fruit to a time schedule would be as a clockwork orange. Eating absorbs the pain of sex displaced or emotions lost or not received in big enough portions, but starving one's self is also an ability to be proud of. In case of thoughts of worthlessness you might wonder what is it anyone does that is worthwhile anyway? I search for distractions from reality and that has never been considered by me to be of any worth now or to the living human species a thousand years from now, so the need to attain pleasure in legal or moral or normal ways might be obscured or missing from my vision or thoughts, but what genetics are responsible anyway since there are so many technology contrivances to bring pleasure - thus pleasure becomes a consumer item for an income based techciety (technology & society). Who can concentrate on all this technology shit anyway because I should be hunting a rabbit and rutting a virgin, thus loss of thinking ability is probably only technology contrived proving our lack of an illness if you take the human's side, but because I rarely can hunt and rarely can rut, I get restless and caught in a circle with a loss of concentration applied. Last but not least I must cycle down thus low energy becomes real because the mind imagines it to be true. This puts me down for the count and getting out of it is none the easier either, as I would lie down for months if a child didn't sing or the doorbell ring. Cesare Pavese once remarked that suicide is within everyone's ability, but who the hell was he? There is nothing more exhilarating than a good manic suicide attempt episode where the confusion of mental pain and physical pain wouldn't even make sense to the ordinary humans. The attempt is a moment of maximum rationalization of mental and physical pain and thoughts disjointed but logically working toward a proper end hopefully with me in 51% control of what is occurring. The vision of reality beyond photon retinal sight is present at that time. The vision at that time cannot be described with words, but try we must by mentally compelling forces I guess.

12. Let me interrupt and add that I researched most of the scientific terms in this book, they do not sound from my tongue as a matter of fact, but the thought disorder is free of charge because it appears in the text in some fashion that I haven't detected. Do you color between the lines or do you realize in nature there are no lines? As of this moment, it is all said and done, and I am on to paragraph 13 and a new song is queuing up so don't get left behind.

Thought disorderly orderly

13. Although I might cover thought disorder in chapter whatever, I would like to mention a few thoughts on thought disorders in this chapter - since I feel like derailing on my present thoughts. In the coarse of a normal day, humans communicate by verbiage and physical motions as their communication methods whether it is mouth, eyes, and fingers that wiggle and lie, or arrangements of fly (wings), though office protocols are now beginning to favor E-mail (or E-diction, as I would call it for obvious reasons). If I may use a thought disorder of my so-called synaptic neologism machine, let me derail and mention that although you are not consciously thinking about it, eye contact and facial expressions are constantly used as subtle communicators because they are natural and have not been screwed by technology contrivances - especially when interacting within groups of humans. This silent but deadly killer allows verbal communication with one human while visually communicating with another even at a great distance. Sex is often initiated because

of the interpretation of facial expressions as opposed to suddenly saying out loud, "Lets rut" whereby your present life partner might overhear you. Thus I hope you buy into my very simple ideas of human procreation presented to you later in CHAPTER MANKIND AND WOMANTYPE. Of course, if your life partner is in the lines of sight of your adulterous facial say-so then you are out of luck anyway. Can you have a facial expression "thought disorder?" Spoken language that conjugates, verbalates, and nounates to be ended interrobangalated is not natural; it is contrived, but nobody has thought of that I guess. Therefore, the facial expressions remain relatively true because you are born to know and use them but smart doggies fake them also.

14. It is amazing that the *Hosapiens* will go to any lengths to prove we are, dare I say, mentally ill. Using thought disorders, many of which are actually traits of whether or not a human was successfully educated or has trouble speaking, because their father never allowed them to read comic books as a child, is really pulling at straws. All the while ordinary humans write songs and plays impersonating the best of us [the *Homaniakos*] to be as in a state of deep thought. But I grow tired of this topic now, not having accomplished the idea's I had hoped to convey to you my reader friend. Paragraph 15 will be started after a fifteen-minute break.

The reality of Manic-depression

15. We have moods that would be described as emotionless. The *Hosapiens* perceives this mood to be irritable. The truth is,

we can't stand being around so many ordinary humans with their moods.

1 6. Remember that mood characteristics mix themselves and that each manic-depressive is on an individual time schedule and level of intensity. We are not to be pigeonholed. We have traits that make us individuals within our own species. With electronic communications possible, we have our own society of isolated members based on hierarchies of intensities and abilities (not of power or wealth), with compassion applied for the survival of all.

1 7. It is unfortunate that a percentage of the *Homaniakos* are hyper-enhanced. Living with humans becomes very difficult for them and the clearer vision of reality can be overwhelming if they don't' learn or can't learn how to glance away. Life termination is the quickest way of ending the vision and the pain. One of my co-workers and friends from the 1970's described to me the reason for his son's suicide at about age 21. He told me his son could no longer live with the shortsighted, ignorant *Hosapiens*. He had seen the truth to reality and decided not to be an active part of it. Although he is dead, he remains a part of reality nonetheless, as I now release the thoughts of his life and death into a part of this book for all of its existence also. The *Homaniakos* also have the privilege of experiencing the anxiety attack or panic attack. There is no good description other than imagine you are bound and gagged and being lowered slowly into molten lava. Nothing helps the pain, you must ride it out, but even pain is a sensation that can be enjoyed if applied at the right time or if no other sensation is available at that time. If ever there were a living experience of death or vision of death or a feeling of hopelessness with no sensation omitted, the panic attack would be it. Thus heavy

breathing and take off fleeing is normal and expected. As a Manic-Depressive Junkie I know how to get these feelings when I need something exciting to feel because it's not like I can look forward to a night of making-out in the back seat of my automobile machine anymore. Whereas you have your manic-depressive humans that work at the mental control of suppressing thoughts and feelings and try to never go "there", if you are ever lucky enough to find a Manic-Depressive Junkie like me blending in very well, you're going to have to realize we like our roller coaster lives and learning to control the on and off of it is half of the fun, and as I have more than once stood upon a platform adjacent to an actual roller coaster, I have seen the vision of mathematical equations across the landscape defining every motion, rotation, translation, and displacement of the curved coaster rail. As certain that the minerals of the universe were properly arranged to produce such a treacherous path of inertia (as a metaphor of manic-depressive thoughts), so must the definition of the roller coaster's path via numbers in a contrived language also exist. So as I strap myself into my ride of inertial passion, and the cars appear to start forward with a load of unknown to me ride revelers, I realize that it is not the cars that move but the earth spins around me with what would appear to ordinary humans as an impossible motion of a planet so large. Backwards then down and up and twisting and turning and diving and looping the earth moves, and at the speed of light no less. With the equations of the motions defined, why would it be impossible to see and interpret the vision as anything other from my current vantage? And thus is my view of reality, I am at its vertex with reality spinning around me by predictable equations or some soon to be revealed axioms as I sit here wondering if anyone is in control?

18. For the benefit of all human species, we must learn to live with the *Hosapiens* and be courteous of their hospitality for sharing their resources with us. They are, after all, the dominant human species at least by numbers on this planet even if they are generally not very kind to us once they know what we are. By natural genetics, the *Hosapiens* will never learn to accept us. They must follow human genetic traits for the protection and survival of their species. Humans might talk of understanding and accepting each other and blah, blah, blah, but it will not happen, because it can only be brought about by memetic action. Memetic (see paragraph 19 below) action only masks what humans feel and is not expressed via their contrived language. Give up on the nonsense of a new age of understanding and acceptance. Besides, within the senses of reality, the *Homaniakos* are on top. By percentages alone, the *Homaniakos* dominate the creativity and intelligence on this planet, even if never fully acted on or revealed for profit.

19. Now I might interject that "meme" or "memes" or "memetic" are all the same and they are thoughts that live and they want to continue living by forcing you to convince your friends to believe in them also. Thus they live in your brain as thoughts only and can do your body good or harm, but more on them in another chapter I suppose. Otherwise be certain to read all the references at the rear of this book.

20. I do believe that depending on the mood cycle most of the *Homaniakos* can live through their enhancement, whether they use medical treatments or not. I plan on living through it. I have been following the "Rod Serling School of Manic-depression Live Till

To-morrow Plan" as follows: Patty Duke (also a *Homaniakos*) plays Holly Schaeffer a gossip columnist in a 1970/71 Night Gallery episode, receiving a diary that has the magic to write the next days events in itself. One day it no longer writes in the next day's events and the page is found blank. In a panic, Holly fills in the next page; otherwise she believes it will be the end of the world or whatever. She goes completely over the rainbow and spends the rest of her life in a padded room asking for the diary every day, so she can put the next day's events in it. The results shown are that she can live day by day via transferring her thoughts to the diary. This was actually a very up beat story for us.

21. Have a goal, have a plan, cover your suicide buttons, and stay out of mine fields. Talk all you like if it makes you happy. Avoid that movie, book, story, song, or person that will open the door between the imagined world in which the *Hosapiens* have created for themselves, and the world of a true understanding of existence and a clearer vision of reality, to which the *Homaniakos* has access. I suppose that one of my Axioms would fit nicely into this paragraph but the foreplay isn't over yet so you'll have to read the rest of this book - as is my plan for you.

22.   The *Homaniakos* must adjust their attitude right now. We have been told we are mentally ill but this is not the case. We are our own species for certain and if I can see that fact then why can't the scientists (see it)? Whereas ordinary humans run around blindly in "la-la" land, we are aware of our existence, of reality, and of the finite use of time. We cannot truly explain our perceptions with human words, only the thoughts truly exist. This is the source of our pain and anxiety. The use of drug treatment should be our choice. Our choice will be clearer when we realize that it will be us

in control. Drugs do not change us from a *Homaniakos* to a *Hosapiens*, but they are developed to make us imitate the feelings of the *Hosapiens*. They attempt to make us fit a 9 to 5 world when in actuality we would have never created the clock. This is all the *Hosapiens* can feel and understand with their limited vision. Because our species can suffer from ordinary human mental illnesses also or ordinary depression, the diagnosis of our true sense of unrest is difficult to determine. We must believe in the path we choose, take each step wisely and stay in control. Do minimal harm to others, find our true selves, accept our life, and live it. Be the best manic-depressive that you can be!

23. Now of clinical depressions, Bi-polar is the one to be. You get mania and depressive episodes. The mania helps us define the depression. Uni-polar, or depression only, ordinary humans, have no mania. They also lack all the enhanced abilities of the manic. Their senses are dull, as would be expected. They are easier to treat through drug therapies than manic-depressives. I believe they are a basically a depressed *Hosapiens* as opposed to the *Homaniakos* species - there is no genetic change to become a *Homaniakos* when a *Hosapiens* becomes depressed. It is unfortunate that these humans must undergo these depressed states but fortunate that drugs work relatively well with fewer side effects for them. The very fact that manic-depression is even classified from the same tree that also defines depressive disorders (like Uni-polar Affective Disorder), indicates that the *Hosapiens* are not yet ready to accept the fact that what they perceive as similarities in behavior are in fact based on their own genetic inclination to sort marbles by similar size with no regards to actual function. We are not them [they?]. The *Homaniakos* are genetically predisposed to their behavior as opposed to the

Hosapiens and their temporary depressions caused by a lack of understanding of the true nature of reality.

24. There are organizations full of ordinary humans that stick pins through our backs and would mount us as Zanti misfits in a 4-H project. Every one of us with a little tag under our morbid brains describing in some taxonomically regulated acronym as to why we are freaks to be sorted, diagrammed, and classified by statistical analysis. The *International Classification of Diseases* (ICD) is of course the worldwide source that classifies us as having (or suffering from) a psychiatric illness. The American Psychiatric Association (APA) has a *Diagnostic and Statistical Manual* (DSM) that also classifies us into some curiosity of Abby Normal. Naturally the two organizations can't agree on classifications of affective disorders. The fact that some mental illnesses have symptoms that mimic our normal behavior is what causes the confusion. As you read through their history of trying to classify us, you will see that they constantly change their diagnostic criteria. Their scientific test's for our discovery consists mainly of questionnaires borrowed from the warranty cards found inside the boxes of newly purchased durable goods such as toasters or VCR's of which the pro-phessionals are not even in agreement upon by they, themselves [*Sentence logic*]. They will never get it correct. We don't belong in their books.

25. What I would actually like to see is how those grandiose organizations classify the so-called "ordinary" humans; for I know I could fill a book with it (it is this book). Such as all the ordinary mentally stable humans that lead productive lives that I am suppose to strive to become, such as the ones I see on the evening news each day, via me using some perverse mind altering drugs.

There are so many types of ordinary humans I can hardly choose which one is my ideal and it's so exciting I might wet my undies only thinking about it. (And although words in a contrived language mean nothing to me, I understand that properly trained ordinary humans take their words seriously so let me tell you, my reader friend, that although it is only a slang phrase of this strange language that the ordinary humans created, somehow they feel that humans can be "screwed" but not as in the sense of that spiral removable fastener, but rather as the feeling of the fates having gone against them by either natural occurrences or by deliberate actions of another human.) Let's see, there's the "well adjusted and normal" humans that screw you out of your money when you buy a car, screw you out of your money to save your soul, screw with your children's minds while they're in government schools, screw you out of your money with excessive taxation without true representation, screw you out of your personal freedoms in the name of freedom, screw you when you try to do a simple legal transaction that always needs an attorney, screws with the truth during every news broadcast, screws with history to be politically correct, or screws you out of a job 15 minutes after giving a speech about how we are "one big family". Please help me, give me drugs, I want to be normal like them.

26. Manic-depression continues to exist down through the ages. What is its source of replication? It is a genotype? Is it a learned trait such as from implanting a meme? Or is it from a temporary or permanent alteration of brain functions due to a virus or bacterial infection? It would seem to favor genetic transmission or a change in the *Hosapiens* genetic structure at the correct moment, but for certain we are born to it thus it must be in our stem cells, don't you agree? The clever aspect is that mating should occur while the *Homaniakos* is in the larva stage, thus ensuring the successful continuance of my species. Death by suicide will ultimately occur after mating and the passage of the *Homaniakos* genes. We will exist into the future because of our revolutionary evolutionary procreationary plan. We are designed to continue into the future, this is no accident of nature.

27. I no longer believe that the function of the *Homaniakos* is to terminate the life, as in some type of ultimate fatal altruism of the host body that has been "infected" by some genetic defect. Rather what is happening is that the ability of an animal to understand true reality is too great a stress on its mental capacity. Thus destruction of the mind is the logical choice to stop the vision of the truth. It is the enhanced mental abilities that the *Homaniakos* typically have over the *Hosapiens* that account for the higher suicide rate of our species. At this level of intelligence and perception, suicide becomes logical and what thoughts and visions and feelings beyond death are possible by us also?

28. Now the *Hosapiens* (ordinary humans) would tell you that the *Homaniakos* only feel a heighten sense of oneness with the universe and an understanding of the grand plan of the mechanisms of nature, from creation to depletion and every interaction and every cause and effect of life, reality, and purpose. Because the *Hosapiens* don't have a clue with their limited vision causing faulty logic, they believe we can't have actual expanded knowledge. They are wrong. We are correct but there is little to do to convince them. We nod our heads as though we agree with them and they will let us go home. This makes them feel good and satisfies that strange trait ordinary humans have of being useful to the universe. It makes no difference to us; we know the ending of

the story. Thus with the *Homaniakos* enhancements of all of our senses as proved but rebuked as being a mental illness, we share a common vision, the clearer vision of reality, with answers that can't be explained in human words, as faulty as language has been proven to be, and yet we know the truth. We stand at the end of knowledge, of which the *Hosapiens* will never achieve.

Being ordinary

29. Getting back to the story, what ultimately worries me is the chemical masking of my natural genetic characteristics such that I will be forced to think and behave like a *Hosapiens*. I am afraid that I will loose myself to lithium or Prozac. You can research for yourself in books or on the web all the famous creative manic-depressives of recent times. In this list you will find the most creative names history has to offer. Many are writers. Many are unknown to us as they die along the wayside, touching private lives with bursts of energy and creativeness and visions of sorrow encapsulated within a very private loneliness. Creative writing, or the compulsion to write without skill, is one of the genetic traits of manic-depression. This also applies to music and the visual arts. Would you indiscriminately drug these individuals out of existence? Would you destroy my life because of an occasional uncommon desire? I fear life as a *Hosapiens*. It is unknown to me. What types of feelings would I have? What would I think or believe? What feelings would I loose? Would reality be hidden from my thoughts? Would I miss reality?

30. The *Hosapiens* are notorious for expecting that all-human species (and some other animals species too) behave as them. The *Hosapiens* believe the only way to be happy is for everyone

to be made equal. They carry this to an extreme even within their own species. The best example of course is the drugging of their own [*Reflexive pronoun use (consider revising)*] human-children. Any human-child that does not behave as expected compared to an invisible list of "ordinary traits" is given Ritalin to suppress any unwanted activity or creativity. With approximately 90% of the world's usage of Ritalin or equal in the USA alone, the ordinary humans will destroy future advances in their own techciety due to the suppression of individuality and creativity. With a greater amount of the creativity already possessed by the *Homaniakos*, I would think they wouldn't mess with their own species. But then again, they really don't know what is at stake here. Drug all your children, you *Hosapiens*, drug every one of them. Drug'm up and ship'm out another door! When they become adult pill popp'n zombies, they won't have a clue what to do without a red or a blue. They take pills till they're dead, or dead in the head, is what I've said. Their future is drug use for no reason at all, that someone might stare at them while passing in the hall. And then as with the mammals and the dinocreatures, we'll see which species makes it into the future. Manic-depressive Junkies will have a feast of the ordinary humans strung out on pills with no baseline of perceived reality. So drugs are used to "normalize" all humans, when the thinking is just ordinary at best. But I suppose it won't benefit ether of our species, so they must think about their human-children, not how their human-children interfere with their idealized or phable[*lized*] lifestyles. But then again, what do I care if they screw up their own species, look at what they would do to mine.

31. I sometimes watch humans at play and momentarily wonder what it would be like to not be aware of the impending end: not to know the infinity of darkness and the coldness of death. The

finality of being lowered into the ground, knowing beforehand that in a billion years, our sun will explode and destroy my grave and even the earth. When all is said and done sometime in the distant future, not even an alien race will know of the human's existence let alone of me, my passions, or my struggle to see the edge of the universe and infinite time. If you believe in a god then believe in him well, for it is true with gods or not, that all that you buy, love, or cherish on the earth will not bring you a warm loving hug a hundred years hence. And as now I find myself more often staring at human-children and myself drifting into waking dreams of my human-childhood lost forever, I want greatly to be as them again, because generally death is further from them, or at least they don't imagine it is coming so soon.

32. Being of a *Hosapiens* mind is not something that I remember well. My best description of it from my human-childhood would be to feel naive and fully distracted with hope for the future. I fell for every government school lie that nuclear energy would provide free and clean energy for my future, asbestos would end house fires and DDT would give us bountiful crops. Doctors would vaccinate us against every disease know to mankind and womantype, and cancer would be eliminated by the year 2k. I was to marry a dedicated woman and we would raise our children while we take yearly vacations to exciting places. Automobile machines would ride on a cushion of air down smooth highways. My children were to travel to the moon to live. Technology was to be every answer to every dream of happiness. I didn't give up until I was about 25 years old, but the future was never to arrive. What I have learned for certain as the truth to reality, is that the future only guarantees physical death. For if I am not dead to-day, then to-morrow I have a better chance of dying than on the day before.

33. What does comes to mind are those *Twilight Zone* episodes where þersons are forced into looking or behaving as everyone else. They were usually of a futuristic scenario of humans achieving the þerfect techciety. After the þerson's conversion, they are always haþþy as [*like*] everyone else. Why do you want me to behave like the rest of you anyway? Don't do me any favors.

34. What I would say to my sþecies is, unless you are inclined to, or of a mind to create harm to those around you, stay þure, search for your usefulness to our sþecies. By virtue of your exceþtional abilities you will be a hero of þerseverance to the *Hosapiens*, and they love that tyþe of thing. It's what talk shows are all about.

35. Let me entertain a different solution. Let's say that 99% of the humans of the earth were manic-deþressives and the 1% are [*is?*] as the *Hosapiens* are now. I would have a great time giving those ordinary humans drugs to induce random deþression and þanic attacks from Hell. All the while telling them they have a mental þroblem because of their continued þursuit of haþþiness and þreoccuþation with meaningless events. If it is by þercentages only, or by þoþular vote that you have determined what behavior is best for the human sþecies, then I would like another vote. Unfortunately for me, it is by the most basic genetic actions that the *Hosapiens* wish to þerform a mental castration of us. The *Hosapiens* have little mental control over their actions and most will never understand how genetically þredicable they are, as we are according to our sþecies þrotocols.

3 6. What would a world full of *Homaniakos* be like? Note pads and pens would be popular. After dinner everyone would go out and have an indiscriminate affair. The stock market would remain at an all time low due to a large percentage of bad business ventures. There would be more art galleries, movies, and novels than you can shake a stick at. Rhymes and puns would be normal. The news would be topped by exciting stories about the *Hosapiens* dying of natural causes. Movie theaters would have facial tissue dispensers at every seat. And the movie rating system would have categories of "Caution Free", "No depressed persons allow unless accompanied by a Hypomanic", and "Suicidal: Lithium users only".

3 7. Being a *Hosapiens* has its weird side also. Do you believe it is easy living with all of them? I might as well be living on a planet occupied by Martians. In fact, I would say before ordinary humans think of drugging us, they should look at what they consider normal. They have allowed themselves to propagate thousands of special interest group memes. Each one heading in some bazaar direction in an abuse of logic, but still following a genetic actuator. Remember that no meme can be created unless it is a reaction to a genetic trait. Otherwise humans would have creative thoughts.

3 8. The basic problem with all the information about the *Homaniakos* is that *WE* are described as the mentally ill species. As a Manic-Depressive Junkie, I would describe the *Hosapiens* as: "Lacking in a full range of emotions with poor perceptional abilities. An inferior species that memes fairy tales to fill in the gaps created by faulty logic, and they can't perceive the difference. Preoccupied with trivial events all the while believing they are the most significant creature on the earth or in the universe. The *Hosapiens* believe they have been ordained the ultimate caretakers of all animals, plants, and ecological systems of the earth by some god. No two humans can agree on the characteristics of this god, or what divine doctrines this god has set forth. Belief in this god has resulted in more hate, abuse, and murder than the abuse of sex, money, or power could ever do. The *Hosapiens* believe that by raising their arm and directing their index finger toward the sky, they are pointing 'up'. Thus they create a reality based on the perceptions of their immediate position and situation". They need to see with their minds eyes - there is no "up".

When we know what we are

39. The phrase: "...you can help your family member, or a friend return to a normal and productive life" implies that the *Hosapiens* believe being normal is so great, with normal thoughts and normal senses, and that all humans must be productive for humankind. It's kind of an ant colony mentality. I ask you, what do they think all these manic-depressive actors, writers, artists, and plan Manic-Depressive Junkies like me are doing? Rotting in a hole of self-pity and self-indulgence? Don't fall for the scam. The *Homaniakos* need to free their minds and emerge the dominant species on this planet. One difference between a *Homaniakos* and a *Hosapiens* is that a *Homaniakos* sits frozen in a depressed state, knowing that they are not able to be involved in reality at that moment, while the *Hosapiens* feel great and fulfilled having spent the same amount of time in front of a TV memorizing script from *Steinfeld* reruns.

40. Manic-depressives necessarily do not suffer from an affective disorder or mood disorder if you could see it through my eyes. While depression is a disorder that any human may have on a temporary basis, even manic-depressives can have ordinary human depression, but ordinary humans can't see the difference. While the *Hosapiens* may enjoy being depressed occasionally, they will never have the full abilities of a manic-depressive lifestyle, thus creating the confusion of offering "treatment" to manic-depressives in order to push them into an ordinary human lifestyle.

41. I am falling prey to using a list because I make lists for a living, so I'll try not to use another one like it in my book but the big "treatment" scam goes as follows:

> **#1** *Telling manic-depressives that they are mentally ill.* This is done to degrade us, and make us submissive to treatment and dependant on paying cash to a consoler for life.

> **#2** *Telling manic-depressives that they should behave as the rest of the ordinary humans (the Hosapiens) if they every wish to be happy again.* For us there will never be happiness, we must be happy without it. (The apparent contradiction of the words happiness and happy with respect to paragraph 295 are not so. I am really mostly concerned with the sound of the words in my book and what the hell does the logic matter when I actually believe ordinary humans have faulty logic anyway? I rather live my life in self-induced delusions to avoid seeing reality and thus stories and music and movies become a world not real but that I can feel, thus look for the quotes and titles hidden within the text like one of those Television machine

game shows and enjoy yourself because if you're alive now, you'll be dead later, and what will any of this matter?)

#3 *Telling manic-depressives that drugs and therapy will make them lead a more normal life.* Since when are drugs and therapy normal? All the drug side effects are part of a normal life also? Normal to me, is what my life is now. Why do ordinary humans believe that drugs, in place of natural lifestyles, are the better [*betters?*] of the two therapies? The sexualness of hypomanic protocol #7 should tell them that physical contact with a mate is the best natural therapy.

#4 The *Hosapiens* species created a set of federal & state laws that prevent proper support of manic-depressives by recognizing only doctors trained in the *Hosapiens* methods of treating manic-depression as a mental illness. If you are unfortunate enough such that you can't afford a doctor, one will be assigned to you whether they are helpful or not. Doctors in institutions have free reign over our mind and body and our treatment and our opinion doesn't always matter because what could we possibly know about ourselves?

42. Although this paragraph contains no deep thought, the *Hosapiens* are by genetics a species that causes them to want to make us mimic them, not that we will truly ever be them, but only that we mimic them properly. Once we mimic them, we are OK and everyone goes home happy. Remember this is the same creature (the *Hosapiens*) that puts clothing on dogs, buys furniture for cats, and believes that they can teach apes to speak in sign language. They pet dolphins and call them intelligent. They put pictures of deer and rabbits on poster boards for VBS and advertise that Jesus loves you and the sinner within me. When

actually, millions of bacteria are waiting to get into your body to kill you, a lion would eat your human-child, and most animals are disgusting casual defecators, lick their anus, stink, and want nothing to do with you. The *Hosapiens* see what they believe because they don't see what the *Homaniakos* are capable of seeing or feeling. The *Hosapiens* believe - keep them busy and you keep them happy when in fact you're not living, you're just keeping time.

43. I would never suggest that you approach a manic-depressive and say: "You are special and Godd made you special for a reason".

44. In a technology driven techciety, the social aspect of humans is restricted from fulfilling its natural intentions. We cannot act on instincts for survival - we cannot protect our life, family or property how we see fit. Despite what you may believe, countries like the United States do not have an advanced society. They have rudimentary traits that a society had once existed. I hear humans make statements about our great techciety, but they don't know what possibilities exist for them or for that matter, for all of us. Governments set up the *Hosapiens* laws based on the *Hosapiens* logic. That logic is flawed. Genetics do not fit these laws, and the logic defies explanation. If we, the *Homaniakos*, are to survive, we must learn to live in the flawed world because the *Hosapiens* strive to have technology correct technology with no regards for the genetic needs of the body and mind. The *Hosapiens* sit in undersized cubicles isolated from physical contact and comfort for most of the day like calves being primed for a veal entrée (and they gave me a cubicle all my own). The ordinary humans are amazed at the misfits displayed on the

10 o'clock who cares, but all of humanity is becoming misfits, freaks of nature striving to have technology improve their lives. Atmospheric controlled, luminance on a switch, plastic under your fingertips, to satisfy the "hunt" and the "kill" or the needs of the clan. These are technology substitutions that create a twisted nerve of your genetics and restrain you from reaching out to grasp your true function. Humans have gone too far to stop, too far to turn back. I cry for the simplicity of life, a vista without straight lines, but I too was caught, and I will die on the drug of contrivances.

Madness within madness

45. It is amazing that some "ordinary humans" believe that they don't have problems and that all the *Homaniakos* do have problems. They feel so sorry for us. When I look at many of them, what I see is mostly miserable humans whose lives are busy never reaching that imaginary happiness, and that supposedly I can attain that imaginary happiness under their care and their drugs and in their limited vision of reality. What they can't feel, thus know, is to be manic or hypomanic is true satisfaction that is unbounded in scope. The *Hosapiens* always work at stopping those feelings of the *Homaniakos* species, but their efforts are mostly futile. They wish to insult us into their life of the limited view of reality and their delusional goals. As ordinary humans their lives are mostly screwed up in every dimension and direction. To find their happiness they become drug addicts, alcoholics, spouse abusers, and ill tempered at work. Frustrated they destroy family relationships in order to rush their kids to practices and games of soccer, band practice, cheerleading, football, etc. etc. and then they must get family memberships at their

psychotherapist. They stand at the sidelines and insult the coaches, the other team, or their children for not "putting out" 100% of what their fat ass could never do in the first place. No more family talks, meals together, nights around the fire reading and family interaction game playing. They're all fattening up on fast food eaten out of paper feed bags strapped on highway driving faces to get from here to there to do this or that, while listening to that radio device shouting survey results of what the "other" ordinary humans are doing or should be doing in order to straighten-out their screwed-up lives. I will gladly take the down side of the clearer vision of reality if I can avoid living as ordinary humans do, but how can I live my true life within their world and their laws, their morals, their 24 hour clocks, their money techciety, etc.? All of us are trapped in the only true perpetual motion machine of technological advancement fueled by societal degradation. Technology consumes society and once consumed there is no replenishing it, because it is lost from within the human mind.

Suicide

46. There are many institutions, societies, networks, and "Will you tell me how you feel?" organizations that are set up for suicide prevention. All suicide attempts or suicides are not the same. Humans, whales, apes, and maybe a few other species get depressed for various reasons - captivity usually. Depression and manic-depression are very different. Humans live their life as a manic-depressive or they kill themselves. Humans get over ordinary depression or they kill their family, their friends, and then themselves. Ordinary humans never get an opportunity to get used to only depression, and they are more likely to respond

inappropriately by killing their family members, etc. Ordinary depression (as in uni-polar) does not allow an ordinary human (a *Hosapiens*) to see the clearer vision of reality, so they remain as delusional as always about life, but depressed also. Those thoughts can't be cognized. Usually an ordinary human gets ordinary depression over a divorce, loss of job, loss of a loved one, a stock market crash or something that the screwed-up world forces upon them. When they are finally over their temporary depression, they are fine. All their delusions are back in place, and there's nothing to worry about. Ordinary humans claim that they suffer from that type of depression all the time in order to account for their poor judgement of murdering their family members at an inappropriate time. Bad press from those humans harms our image as manic-depressives. All depression is generally "clumped" into one big category by the media thus how can ordinary humans know the difference? I cannot address the ordinary human's depression and suicides, that is an issue alien to my thoughts. I am incapable of those thoughts or feelings.

47. Some ordinary human may choose to write their own book to describe ordinary depressions but for manic-depression I have a message for you – a very sad message! The start of the treatment is with the "discovery" (usually during or after a suicide attempt), doctors prescribing drugs and telling the patient they have a mental illness, followed by, "You will need to see me every week". Then all the mom's and wives cry a lot and try to maintain a certain appropriate behavior around the "mentally ill" family member. Usually relatives of the "discovered" *Homaniakos* spend their time looking for symptoms found on the "10 signs of suicide" card they got from the doctor. That card also has at least one acronym on it to make the ordinary humans feel better. Also a lot

of Fon (sounds like "on") calls are made after the discovery of a manic-depressive family member so the mom's and wives may cry and express their worries. From my observations it would seem that's why mankind stumbled on the Fon mechanism - to relieve women's tensions.

48. It is eight rotations later, as I came to my senses, in a *Homaniakos* fashion, I have chopped the next four pages and replaced the word sequence with the following arrangement of the same words as my mood is now of a different mind. When words are rearranged but are the same words, the interpretation changes. This remains a mystery to most humans but then language is only a contrivance and not natural, therefore how are we to figure it?

49. I have never called, as in "dialed on a Fon", a suicide Hotline for many reasons, but then again I have someone to find my body and make the call for me in retrospect. During the planning phase of suicide, as opposed to the panic attack type of fast suicide, there is calmness. Plans are made into great detail - time and place, what method to use, music to play, and the verbalized note becomes a record to leave for the living fools who couldn't understand the signals you gave them for months and months, so thus you will now do it and they will learn their lesson well after seeing your dead body. How many times I have planned is more than attempts, but music was always to be there because music can take me there without pain or bring me back depending upon the tune I select. My standardized suicide note was always to be the same two words and only eight letters at that, because simplicity avoids misinterpretation. I had always envisioned that whoever found my body would scream and cry and rush to dial 911 on that

Fon mechanism and then count the seconds until the save-your-life technology gang and all their relatives arrive to push everyone I love aside from my dead or dying body. In that brief moment of their disbelief will actually be a true reaction of genetic behavior, and it illustrates the complexity of understanding life and death as temporarily the viewers are primitive and not believing in their perceived reality due to a lack of understanding of how physical truths defy cognition or a contrived language. The truth be known that when I die, for whatever reason, a simple hug and hold my hand for a quiet moment until I am gone, would serve me fine and I expect that my fellow *Homaniakos* would want the same.

50. During the thoughts of the escape, the suicide attempt as ordinary humans would call it, but it is really a suicidal fantasy, what stops me? A distraction, maybe a bird fly's by the window, where is it going? I heard it chirp, but my life is still silent. I look around the room, being able to see beyond thoughts again, and I notice a piece of birthday cake sitting on the table, all nicely wrapped in that Saran Wrap material. "Who is it for, I don't remember? There is no happiness in that cake remaining after the party and the party guests have left - it's only sugar and chocolate. Do ordinary humans fall for the ploy that sugar in their food makes them happy?" The rationalization process speeds up; everything is so clear so logical coming back from the edge of reality, why don't the ordinary humans see it? "Are they so gullible that sugared food with primary colors added brings about happiness? They are so primitive compared to us, the only visionaries. I think that to be only ordinary has blocked their ability to reason clearly - to see the truth of physical existence. They fall for this gilded cage of sensations, false front emotions, all the while telling each other that they have a meaningful life. They believe they will all

become somebody someday, or that they are needed somehow. Oh, excuse me for not being interested but you're as dead as I am before long and life will drive by both our grave markers at 60 miles per hour and not give us a first glance". I take a deep breath and the play begins again as they see me quite normally and fitting so nicely into their world – smiling through the thick of it as though it meets with my approval. Would you believe we have come to visit you in peace and with goodwill?

51. I am told that only the living, those that are "left behind", suffer as if the dead and deceased were going somewhere great without them. Now that overwhelms me, completely overwhelms me. So a thousand deaths the living suffer as if they have survivor rights to suffering as every Christmas and birthday filled with contrived artifacts of trophies and pictures and jewelry reminds them of the human they miss, but never a thought by them that suicide is a means to an end, and that the end was well thought out and worth it at least at one moment in time for the person now dead, or how can you rationalize the extreme of it?

52. Maybe ordinary depression is salvageable but how well can you dope-up a manic-depressive? Pills to cure become pills to kill and even lawsuits after the fact don't resolve the truth, for the only truth is in the death already occurred. What does it matter how we pick our end game? We are all going to die; can't you realize that fact? I suspect that the *Hosapiens* with their natural delusionary ideas really can't foresee death or feel the reality of it prior to it, but you my reader friend, must give the *Homaniakos* more credit than that. For what is felt as pain is real and so is the vision of the real, and the reality of all thoughts ends in death.

53. Of quilts quilted and ribbons of some color, whatever that color would be for suicide þinned on laþels, and acronyms galore can't sþan the gaþ when you aim a gun too high. Meetings and schedules and events for þublic awareness are all held by the living still remaining, for the best volunteer has a dead loved one to motivate time senselessly sþent. Everyone þroclaims, "To save another life" but they only want the love of their life back so eyes closing at night can count the security of sleeþing children safe for one more day. Do you measure your reality on the feeling of beating hearts and restless sounds from bedrooms down the hallway in the night, or are your hallways quiet with only the sounds of the floor cracking from drying lumber, waking you uþ from a lucid dream quickly into the reality of loneliness?

54. Everyday we view the walking dead, smiling and laughing, making þlans and telling jokes and stories about friends and families. We shake their hands and buy them gifts and tell them they look good, losing all that weight. No one knows when he or she is going to die, exactly. Most humans never see or susþect it's coming only a minute or two away. First you are here, then you are gone or you wouldn't show uþ for the event, I supþose. Without suicide you wouldn't have a clue about your demise or its method. Crossing a street, driving a car, climbing too high, or swimming too far, you don't þlan it but it haþþens anyway - to everyone's surþrise. All of a sudden the living are dead, but we analyze the method or intention and that is how grief or sorrow or joy is aþþlied to the event, using a contrived language sþoken within your mind.

55. Þhysical life is a drug machine þroducing, consuming, and sometimes altering nature by intentional digestion of any drug it finds amusing or þleasing. The most basic rule is that humans take the easy road to satisfaction or distraction from þerceived realities or þain in general, so drug'm uþ and shiþ'm out. Our lives are filled with drug use of every kind imagined, but why not since your body oþerates only on drugs þroduced via some tyþe of gene to þrotein or enzyme or who knows what? So take asþirins or Valiums or LSD and coffee while its still legal. Isn't it the laws that determine how much fun you can have by yourself, at the exþense of your own self?

56. When drugs are illegal you can still get your fill, simþly claim you are deþressed or mentally ill. Then what about humans that don't act like the rest, but are doing their best only to walk around unnoticed without any harm? It is human nature to level the þlaying field by surrounding itself with only what aþþears normal, whether it truly is or not, because ordinary humans can't know otherwise exceþt from the metaþhors of þoets. So the world of the ordinary human is exactly as *Logan's Run* or *The Matrix* or so many other stories, because the stories are all science fiction and we would never exþect reality to be exþressed as anything other than what we see.

57. Now let me be forthright at this time and tell you that I have nothing against the *Homaniakos* using þrescribed drugs to alter their clearer vision of reality. And in some unfortunate circumstances drugs seem to be mandatory. The first and þrimary reason a *Homaniakos* should use drugs is to survive. But þlease,

do not combine your medication with other drugs because we have all seen the results of drug induced shooting sprees and unnatural suicides (poorly planned, that is). I want to see our species rise to be the dominant human species on this planet. This will not occur if we continue to self terminate and loose our ability to control intellectual and creative media's (or if we continue to hide). Not all of us can learn to avert the clearer vision of realty. We are all not good at creating constant distractions of our ability to create a mental pit deep enough too physically fall into and not escape from. Not all manic-depressives are up to remaining pure of body and thus (while under the control of drug therapy) they won't trespass on the moral sins created by mankind and womantype in the name of some type of dead or non-existent god. As a Manic-Depressive Junkie I'll think what I want and isn't depression a feeling to be felt when there are no other feelings left? Besides, as distractions become inured and I push the mental envelope, I'll risk what I'll risk and that's all that's needed be said, but what a dangerous life as a game we all play - drugs or not.

58. Some of us by the nature of our species spend an excess of time depressed or an excess of time as manic. It is absolutely no different than the *Hosapiens* that have their greatly varied behaviors. For the *Hosapiens* you have persons driven to excess in sports, work, sex, gambling, or politics. All of those topics I have mentioned have destroyed many ordinary human lives and the lives of their family's. This is all for some abnormal pursuit of a goal of imagined importance or imagined happiness. Personally, those ordinary humans need drug treatment and maybe a slap in the face to say: "Wake-up, the world does not revolve around you putting a sphere in a hole, keeping some company out of the hole, putting a

penis in a hole, putting your finances in the hole, or being an ass-
hole (same order as previous mentioned topics)".

59. Manic-depression is not an easy mechanism to alter. The
Homaniakos have different traits that are very difficult to put into
categories. Perhaps ordinary humans can be put into categories
also, but they all look the same to me, wouldn't you agree?
Getting back at it, when you try to alter with drug usage a
personality that you can't define, you are doomed to a lot of
failures. Drugs do not cure manic-depressives; they only alter our
thoughts. After some time, the body adjusts to the drugs or it
changes and doesn't accept the conditioning of the drugs or is
poisoned by the drugs or we overdose on the drugs out of
frustration. I suppose its like coloring your hair, bleach then tint,
anti-depressant then mood stabilize. It's as noticeable also,
because the roots always show.

60. Manic-depressives lie to their licensed therapists so that
they either *won't* alter, or *will* alter their dosages. This must be
done because the manic-depressive is not at this time allowed
control over their own *[Reflexive pronoun use]* drug treatment or
over their own *[Reflexive pronoun use]* life once "found out". But
there is always a search for Heath-Food cures. Manic-
depressives combine controlled substances with their treatment or
use controlled substances in place of their treatment in order to
have more control over their lives, and from this you can end up on
the 6 p.m. network news and not as an honored guess either.

61. I should say at this time, to make the lawyers satisfied,
"Consult your physician" concerning medication and treatment,

this book is not giving medical advice or possibly even sound advice – as if a book can give you something.

62. It gets confusing how the drug combinations are used to alter each variety of depression, manias, cycle time, etc. Drug reaction time can be weeks long from what I read. Since mental control can override drug reactions, it is possible that you might cycle during drug use. Basically, the *Homaniakos* are looking for a change that they are not able to bring about by pure mental control. They wish to have the clearer vision of reality reduced, reduce the up and down of it, or they wish to reduce the depression time. Getting rid of those panic attacks would be another objective of drug therapy, and possibly the only reason that I would resort to drug usage. The panic attacks are not considered fun or enjoyable or even desirable when you are a *Homaniakos*, and possibly not at all much fun even if you are a *Hosapiens* that receives them on occasion, but I wouldn't know about those *Hosapiens* feelings. Although I am way off the topic of paragraph 62, I really don't care and you must realize that the onset of a panic attack for a Manic-Depressive Junkie as myself is actually quite thrilling as all of my perceptions of reality transmigrates (metempsychosis) initially with a fantastic feeling throughout my body as my mind can't keep up with the emotions on the lamb. Running and hiding with eyes bulged and heavy breathing occur as I hang on to something physical (as if the event had anything to do with physics), or I clutch my chest for dear life while all the pieces of the delusional universe fall out of place only to reveal the true reality. Shapes and forms become disjointed as the clearer vision of reality sets into place and optical vision is no longer required to see clearly, as perception becomes a thinking thing only. Usually about 4 minutes into it, I realize it's going to be

another past life regression with no end in sight and nothing short of drugs or death will bring its finish. But panic attacks always pass, because I've lived through enough of them, but during them the senses do not allow you to see the happy ending. Nobody gets used to a panic attack I suppose. I know there are drugs to alleviate the panic attacks, but *are* (my computer states "*am*") there drugs that can induce them for the ordinary humans to enjoy? But getting back on track from sentence number 7 without a change in paragraphs as would be expected or required, the pure intention of mind altering drugs for the *Homaniakos* is to allow the mind to be more susceptible to delusions, and thus reducing depression brought on by the understanding of reality. This fact alone should be enough to convince you, my fine reader friend, that the ordinary humans, the *Hosapiens,* are by birth delusional and they haven't a chance to figure it out, for how can we drug them out of their delusions?

63. Going off of drugs can be like starting over with your *Homaniakos* emotions. This can lead to suicide. Taking drugs can lead to suicide. As a Manic-Depressive Junkie, I prefer to stay how I am. Don't ever say to me, "Why don't you drug yourself into the ordinary human's reality?" I am willing to take the sometimes bad, for the sometimes fantastic. As an aspiring artist (Aren't we all?) I do not want to lose the creativeness that the *Homaniakos* has over ordinary humans. Besides, I do believe in the battered spouse theory of survival. That is, when you are close to your threat, you can see and feel its moods. You can even control them a bit. You see the abuse coming. If you move out (emotionally), you lose the ability to somewhat control the threat and you certainly won't see it coming. Of course, it's not the ideal life either but then what the hell is? Where is it written or spoken or implied by mouth interrobangs that all humans should have the ideal life? The quest for the ideal life is much of the *Hosapiens* problem, anyway.

64. For the entertainment of the ordinary humans, if I were to review all the possible drugs for their various uses, I would come up with a list of side effects that reads as follows: Diarrhea, weight gain, nausea, dizziness, confusion, reduce sexual drive, tremor, induced rapid cycling, dry mouth, anxiety, sores in mouth, insomnia, high blood pressure, stroke, heart attack, death (imagine death is only a side effect of a helpful drug), severe headaches, seizures, involuntary movements, and slow speech. Of course suicidal fantasies are also a side effect of these drugs.

65. Some of these drugs will interact with common over the counter medications so you must be careful. These drugs interact with alcohol and party drugs and sometimes end up creating murderous combinations. Some of these drugs interact with ordinary foods so you must be careful, again. You must wear a medical alert bracelet, which along with your wrist scars will make a nice after dinner conversation topic at parties.

66. You must remember that this whole process is like drugging a cat into believing that it's a fish and then using therapy to convince the cat that it naturally lives underwater but it should come up for air once a week. Drugs also have a toxicity that after prolonged use or too high a dosage may cause the following; confusion, convulsions, the shakes, and blurred vision. Of course, you can take all your pills at once if things get too confusing. The music is finished and so am I, so please advance to the conclusion of the confusions.

67. Now so you, my reader friend, know where you stand, sit, or place the immortal soles of your feet, ordinary humans don't want us for a house þet to show off to their friends. If you are a human of the ordinary type, a *Hosapiens* that is, you might be making your þarty "A" list and want all those so interesting þeoþle on it for the entertainment of your very dear guests. We may find you somewhat tolerable for awhile and þossibly even useful at times, but you are in the way of our þreferred genetics, and thus we blend in whenever required and simþly do what we must when you aren't looking. Muellerian mimicry is real, whether you know that þhrase it matters not. Your laws simþly caþtivate us and your moralities get in the way of our constant sought after and needed distractions. As with all those ordinary humans that believe keeþing an 8 foot þython for a þet is an easy way to acquire a þersonality without actually having one, sooner or later it – well you find out that it was behaving naturally and you should have known better. You can't see it, you can't feel it, and you will never understand it, but take our reality serious.

68. You have now comþleted CHAþTER MANIC-DEþRESSION, þlease turn the þage and þroceed to CHAþTER MYSELF. Do not mark in your book and þlease visit, at your convenience, our reference þages at the rear of the book.

CHAPTER
MYSELF

The music that set the mood for writing this chapter was:
    "Glorias RV 588 & 589" CD by Vivaldi.
    "Devil without a cause" CD tracks 1, 2, 3, & 4 by Kid Rock

What, me worry?

69. Where is everybody? For me a chapter will be given in its entirety but actually it is of all the *Homaniakos* that I write. Me, my favorite subject, my name, the best sound in the world [*Fragment sentence*]. I hear my name and I know I am alive. What words of yours can describe the world of me, thought disordered of course? What have I been driven driving to write by preservation compulsion over and beyond the past 25 standard earth years? If 25 years of cycling (as in cycles of manic, depression and every feeling of reality in between) could be explained in human words in an unremarkable chapter of contrived words describing the emotional states of mind, reality perceived from my eyes, here it is for your entertainment tonight and complemented by the beauty of Vivaldi's *Glorias*.

70. I need control. I need to control my thoughts, the inputs of sound, vision, and touch, but most importantly the perception of the true reality. As you might have already surmised (if you were ahead of thinking about it) this control is going to be a failure. Thus I must reduce my life to that which can be controlled via a clear understanding of the reason for existence. As with any of the human's mechanical devices, such as automobiles, losing

control can result in losing one's life. Ordinary humans do not need to worry about excessive sensory input because their brains cannot analyze the standard sensory inputs completely - thus they remain delusional about reality and life's compliments of faulty logic. But the manic in me keeps me believing that if I run fast enough I will fly over the walls of the knowledge that imprisons me. Run, run away in a mental way from the thoughts of the ordinary humans that pull at my feet with skeletal hands. "Don't leave us", they shout with eyes wide shut not understanding where I go when I am where I am now. Suicide becomes logical. Clang, here's one for the angels, what a fucking way to earn your wings.

71 . I want to run naked down a tropical beach under green trees with blue sky's and clear warm water. Is this the most basic of version 1.0 genetic feelings that my body craves for? To be as I was intended to be by some cosmoillogical action when molecule meets molycule? Will the most simplistic of actions, void of technology, clothology, and data dependant oddities create a feeling of my true belonging in and with the universe even if only for 3 minutes? After 3 minutes of walking distance my mind catches up to the intentional distractional and I begin to realize it is only a point on a sidebar keeping me from the fact that I, along with 1% of the human population, know the fate of our existence. There is no escape clause, we will all die and be dead, deader than the lonely hearts of love lost widows staring at their abnormal husbands (suicided). Hug me for an infinity of eternities when I have stopped time - which the ordinary humans can't do. There is time enough at last before the dripping blood energizes the tongues have muted gnats - my spell checker states my words have slant. Clang. Confused about language protocols I hope? Have you succumbed to ordinary conventions and thus you find my

numerical paragraphing and non-numerical chapter naming disturbing? Transitive dependency relationships rule my written tongue and everyone will be smiling through the thick of it as though it meets with their approval.

72. Bury my skeletal corpse under a green palm tree in the silica where it never gets cold as hell and the sun is shinning every day. Where pornographic children run naked, laughing and splashing in the primordial waters of life. Laughing is a natural sound. I want the energy of laughter to penetrate my cadaver as the last energy to enter my dead meat before I become fossilized. "Perchance to dream" Shakespeare would say, but what a stupid dolt was he. Mathematics would have done him some good. Divide zero by infinity for your logical death without dreams I hope. Don't put me in cold concrete in some government controlled, trade union laborized, memetic reactionized, profitized by death and lies, created by man for eyes, with synthetic emotions that sympathize, hole in the ground for worms and flies.

73. The Lord is my Shepherd, I shall not love. He maketh me take my life. He leadeth me besides a clearer vision of reality. He hath giveth me no soul. He leadeth me in the paths of Hell for his creation's sake. Yea, though I live in the valley of despair, I understand no love, for thou have forsaken me. Thy rod curses me. Thou preparest a place in the infinity of loneliness for me. My mind runneth over with thoughts. No mercy has been shown to me. I appoint myself the keeper of my life. I will look outward forever toward the loneliness of the infinity of space and time. Fuck life.

74. I have sympathy for those ordinary humans that even if they were manic-depressives would be weak-minded and feeble. Falling for every verbiage of lies to become infinity-man on judgement night. Crawling like humans to a bloody fairy tale corpse on a tree, "Save me, save me from the clearer vision of reality" to live forever as a happy human in the light of some type of never-to-exist universe of out-of-body experiences. And when the sky was opened, worms fell to purge the earth of human flesh. Your destroyer crawls under your feet every living day you walk and dream of what you need - but you never get it. Godd, Jesus, the most holy of ghosts, and me will be all that is within my thoughts at that most critical, inspirational moment of my exit. The four of us are dying, all at once, repeated forty thousand times a day. To be second from the son but third from the sun makes no sense when you say it, but it is the way we pray it for the elegy of our lamentations.

75. I shouldn't talk down about the *Hosapiens* (ordinary humans) but when you start looking at what is out there, its like a mirror image world of cognition from us. Of course, they can't even begin to rationalize as us. Look at all of them, walking around like there is a to-morrow. People are alike all over, they plan events, trips, and gatherings. Constantly filling the voids of time in their lives with an activity but with no thought to it at all. To what purpose is this waste? Ants in chimpanzee body's, all of them. I worked so hard to stay human, as we all did, but we can't win. How am I to remember the wonder of thoughts as a human-child? The *Hosapiens* world is a nice place to visit but we can't live there, with them. It is in our genes to become a *Homaniakos*. And when you realize it, you will not be late for your own execution, or learn to live

as described in this chapter. If you learn to live as a þrim and proþer *Homaniakos*, you might still kill yourself with not much thought to it at all. You acceþt the fact that for our species, in *our* reality, suicide is logical. After all, they shoot horses, don't they?

76. What beauty and innocence I have seen. I see forbidden angels that þlay on the earth. Smiles that have never known the þain or loneliness that waits for all of us. I will look through your body into the heart of your soul for what is truly you. I can see the hell that you squeezed into a black hole waiting to suck your love of life away when your aging universe falls aþart as a universe loosing its gravity. You cannot hide your þain from us, we see beyond visionary hiddenary actions of denial. Slowly everyday it sliþs away, but you don't notice it until life is out of reach and þain fills every movement. The sound of laughter, the warmth of the human touch, to gaze into the clearest of clearest eyes of youthful hoþe that knows not the end of time and has not learned of eternal þain. But deeþ they must go if they will find what remains of a human love lost within the mind of someone who is no longer human as I [*Comparisons*]. I am as a criþþled child watching my friends run and þlay and believing that when I wakeuþ to-morrow I will do the same. I can barely shut my eyes anymore for the nightmare as a child continues to þush forward out of my brain and stare at me through conceþtual eyes. Sleeþ is a hell of its own creation. The vision remains, it waits for me, it hides in every object of possible haþþiness. A vision of worms eating the beauty of the flesh, blood flows, a scream in the darkness that goes unanswered by human love. Emþtiness divided by forever is successfully þerformed. Another death, the þain ends. Suicide becomes logical.

77. Sleep is different for the *Homaniakos* than ordinary humans. We are aware of the state of sleep. We plan our sleep. We think about our sleep as though it is a trip that must be completed successfully. I enter sleep and I exit sleep. I wakeup aware that I have arrived at the other end of my journey. To be deprived of sleep is to loose the conscious ability to control your mind from looking directly at the clearer vision of reality. I will not take of the man in the bottle; the ordinary humans cure for all that appears different in the eye of the beholder. Thoughts run more freely when we are tired, but sleep and tiredness are not the same. When depressed or only existing with time stopped in an emotionless state of mind, we appear to need sleep, but we really don't. We become lethargic because of the emotionless sensations. It is us drifting from the ordinary humans imagined reality. We have stopped but the world hasn't. We know it, but we succumb to the feeling. We sit down, lay down, we fall down without energy into a mass of metabolizing flesh with no mind to move. We don't move we only blink. Our mind screams at our body to get up, wake up, time is stopped for us but not for the world. Get back into the world, it is moving closer to its end. Be ready in a nick of time for the end. Finish your tasks, kiss one more lover, and touch one last beating heart. For when you are dead, even the memory of it is lost. They all think we're napping. Let them think what they want, the *Hosapiens* always see what they believe and can't imagine anything other.

78. Getting off the bed, couch, or floor after succumbing to the cycle change of mental states via the ninth configuration is similar to pulling yourself out of almost hard concrete. I am the chick in

the egg that doesn't want to be born again and again and again every day the same nightmare over and over same time and þlace and feeling the infinite of it. My memory of it does me no good; I must exþerience it new each day no learning curves allowed. Once standing, find out the time, year, and where the hell am I? I get in my car to get a small fleeing rush watching humans in their technology world of steel structures þainted, faded, light þoles with sunlight shinning out of magic wand tiþs, cars þumþing fuel into mesmerized humans at gas station drive through þaþer bag food disþensers for hunter-gathers on the drug of button þushing þleasures. What have we done to our lives? Smooth þaved mechanical traveling þast long-legged girls on synthetic roller wheels with short shorts flashing by at unnatural sþeeds and unnatural thoughts disaþþearing in closer than they aþþear mirrors. Everything is aligned, in-line, and digitized no static sounds, click click click on the mouse, George Jetson never had such a good life - if you love þlastic þlease won't someone hold my hand in an un-virtual reality way? All of this must occur so that I may shut my eyes for 30 minutes a day. I wonder how the ordinary humans do it?

79. I attack sleeþ. I will not loose control in my sleeþ even in the lateness of the hour. Never wakeuþ in the darkness - alone. Never oþen my eyes, staring into an emþty þillow surrounded by coldness and darkness and loneliness and no human touch. Do not look back there where I have learned never to look even in the lightness of the new day. If I stare at my þillow in the darkness I will see through it then through the earth and into the infinity of static, timeless sþace. Not a trick but only we can do it. Get uþ; run for your very life! The þrime mover becomes our imþending death. Suicide is always within the reach of our logical thoughts.

80. "Are you OK", she asked? "Yes" I replied, changing positions so that I am sitting up on the edge of the bed. It's 3:00 a.m. two hours into sleep; "I must have come to bed too early", I stated. Bad sleep. When a dream gets control of your mind and drives your thoughts in aimless directions, sooner or later the pinball will end up in the dead zone. My last peaceful moment of sleep this morning was abruptly ended when in a moment of a clearer vision of reality I felt the true existence of infinite pain for infinite time, while experiencing with the ultimate of reality that my mind could present to me, my dead self within my coffin staring at the red hellish numerals of a digital clock counting the seconds into infinity never to escape the darkness or the confinement of the tomb or the total loneliness of isolation from love and my beloved children. I get up and walk around with thoughts of logical suicide. Deep breaths and despair fill the darkness. The experience is now a permanent record in my mind. This is why the *Homaniakos* die. The reality of zero divided by infinity, emptiness divided by forever, comes close to claiming another member of our species on another otherwise unremarkable moment in the universe. The sunlight will arrive and a new day will be here whether I see it or not - what does it matter to the thing you call "existence?"

81. I have evolved a method of sleep that I tell my friends is "fast sleep". I do not lie down to sleep until I can't even sit up and stay awake [*Negation use (no suggestions)*]. If I lay down too soon or when not really sleepy, I knowingly pass from conscious to subconscious states of mind. That trip is a hellish 3-D version of an extrasensory percepted real ultraviolence horrorshow confabulation. The mind's journey always reaches the id's end as it should but you would never want to feel the sight of it. It takes two seconds, of which the universe doesn't feel the þain of anymore, but lasts a lifetime of a minds life. It is the arrival of sleeþ that is a slice of time and existence, which I þerceive as real and you my ordinary human brother could never feel, not even in a hynagogic state. My mind creates a thought of ultimate desþair that I can't cogitate [*cognize?*] logically þast as I feel it coming as a blade þushing quickly into my harnessed skull. I see an image of someone I love fall into the þit of forever loneliness (The þit that I know exists at the end of þhysical time and the beginning of our encaþsulated death). They always call my name to save them, but they are out of reach, in the grave of living eternal loneliness. Seþaration, human-wise, of that naturally worthless emotion of love that is at the bottom of all this, and at the toþ of almighty Godd's fucking þlan for you and I. I jumþ uþ, breathe heavily and þush another nightmare of the clearer vision of reality into a secret crevice of my conscious thoughts. One after another the visions accumulate. I remember each vision. Visions that drive suicide to the surface of logical actions with a reality that exceeds the ordinary senses. It is these two seconds that will bring my death, I know it, to its aþþointed time, but death will be lonely as all death is for suicide because "they" can't imagine it. Don't sleeþ.

8 2. Now a naþ in the sunlight is a different story. Lying in the full sunlight, the fresh breeze þushing on the tiny nerve cells of my skins sensory inþuts of micro-sized molecules of invisible catalysts. Listening to the children þlay and laugh in the distance, þeaceful thoughts that for a moment no one is in the þit of infinite deþth and desþair. It's a good life I tell myself. Light, warmth, and youth forever and forever, far from the end of time where the truth will be revealed as a curtain of infinite height is drawn aside to reveal your true and undeserved fate, by natural þrovidence I guess. Give me rest with sounds of waves touching the shore - motions of infinite life. Timelessness, and no pain to be rationalized, but even in a nap I've gone through states of critical paranoia as complex as most near death experiences.

Onward

83. The *Homaniakos* can hallucinate, but we know when we are hallucinating until we become schizophrenic at least in the prodromal or residual phase. I would say this is one of the more fun aspects of being a manic-depressive. I don't believe that all of us do hallucinate but I don't mind that I am one of the few, except for that motion out of the corner of my eye, whatever the name of that condition is called, does spook me now and then. What the mind perceives as real, is real. Hallucinations add a whole dimension to our lives beyond that of the *Hosapiens*. My reality is not your reality, ever. My best hallucination was seeing an old, nicely dressed man walking into the room. He started to become transparent. I looked through him to focus on the distant wall, and then back at him, but he became more transparent until he evaporated completely. It was a great hallucination but so fake and thus understanding reality defines how we divide reality from illusions – the *Hosapiens* have difficulties with this principle as in a backward manner they create hallucinations from reality. But at any rate I could see through him, but I couldn't see guts or even the other side of his clothing. This is because the mind cannot construct the unimaginable – please remember that thought. I can't say that even in the greatest of 3-D daymares, that I would be able to construct at the speed of movement a walking talking transparent see-their-guts human. This is the secret to a hallucination. You must understand that you can't imagine what

you cannot know in your senses or even out of them. While most of my hallucinations seem to occur after the lights are out and I am between waking and sleeping, I have never had the urge to act on what I have seen because I know that what I see can't exist. Hallucinations must be logictized [A metonym] in order to avoid them causing harmful effects in your daily activities. Once you are beyond the logic, you are lost and everyone around you will know it. This is where the Homaniakos have an advantage over the Hosapiens with regards to seeing a clearer vision of reality. Our enhanced senses enable us to feel more, thus we imagine more than ordinary humans do. Even to the point of what ordinary humans can only wonder about, we can feel as reality. What unknown sights are here! Why should we be unable to preserve a remembrance of them? The result of seeing this reality often leads to death. Humans were not evolved to see reality. Humans evolved were to be mentally as apes, chimpanzees, or pheromonal ants but somehow nature or Godd did not anticipate the Homaniakos species.

84. The Hosapiens are delusional as opposed to being hallucinogenic. Being delusional is why the Hosapiens don't understand that they are given the short end of the stick with regards to sensual perceptions and thus "understanding" in general. Ordinary humans will believe absolutely anything, and they will prefer the un-provable in place of what they can touch with their own hands. So many of the Christians I know are hoping the Rapture comes at any moment. Every time some fortuitous alignment of the planets or some significant numbers on the human made calendar arrives, they are off to some mountaintop or taking cyanide Kool-Aid reciting once upon a time fairy tales of a better life than this. Some of the favorite

delusions I have been told of are of my parents telling me that my Grandparents will be "whole" in heaven. They were both deaf from childhood and mostly mute by choice. I don't know why so many humans believe we will metabolize in heaven? How will that work? Who of you can understand the science to the violence of the Son?

85. It is said that the human Godd (the Christian type) is our father. Most religions of the world believe something similar to that. He is omni-powerful and omni-present. What parent would treat their children, as a god would see fit to do? When my grandmother was hospitalized, deaf, mute, blind, and basically on the negative side of sensory perception, if you are getting the painted metaphor, where was her father the god of the humans? Was this the test that every pathetic human believes s/he is going through by Godd's will to avoid actually rationalizing their own life, or can't ordinary humans ever see past the delusions? Was this how she earned her way to heaven via the world of the earthly netherland of lost love? Does Godd for all his power, wisdom, and love believe this is a proper way of treating his prized guinea pigs? To send an old lady to a fleshly hell of silence and darkness while she prays in her functioning mind, "How will I know that I am not alone when I die?" I am sure she wondered about death but how could we have ever known her last thoughts? We are all doomed to become pseudo-Jobs in our jerked-off techciety of the discarded aged. All death does is make me one more pallbearer wearing a dead man's shoe. The *Hosapiens* are too delusional for us to tolerate. The father of my best childhood playmate waits for his own death in order to be reunited with his dead son. It's very sad, but ultimately they will both be dead, and you too someday, only dead, and the earth won't stop spinning for

you. Humans will curse your funeral procession for holding up traffic as person or persons unknown clog the freeways with energy wasted lights on for you. Next time it will be someone else at the changing of the guard as you literally drop off the face of the earth, trials and tribulations lost and forgotten. Your existence soon to be never realized only categorized by whatever government is in control at the moment to be used for statistical payments of insurance benefits given to the greedy living. Who will visit your grave in 2 generations? But won't they all take your money?

86. I walk through graveyards, past gravestones of unknown loves, youthful beauty lost, Saturday night romances embracing the last day of summer, and tales of bold young studs using luring words to persuade adolescent girls into swallowing their first lie - and I loved every one of them in the past of my now present future. Of what conquests and trials have these long since gone and forgotten humans endured to land them dead? With tales of brave Ulysses on the airways of technology memories, it did them no good to become immortal via human standards with cultural changes dropping them from the top 40 every week.

87. This is what a clearer vision of reality brings to me: Ordinary humans are not mentally equipped to deal with religions or gods. This is evident by the number of religions, the religious wars, hatred based on religion, and how every religion changes with each generation but each generation can't perceive the change. "Oh you're really walking in the footsteps of that Jesus boy", your mother says. Humans apply concept dress to cover up their physical embarrassments and run off to some church building each week and pretend to keep their genes in line for an hour and 3 minutes, then its þut away the religious memes and its back to every young man's fancy in short skirts and bursting buttoned tight toþ daydreams. They have no þerceþtion of their reality as opþosed to the reality we the *Homaniakos* þerceive. We terminate ourselves when the reality becomes too clear and we have not yet learned by logic or trial and error not to cut too deeþ while staring at a knife blade þointed in the direction of infinite absoluteness sharþened on the next decision we would make. To the *Hosaþiens* delusions are natural, but the *Homaniakos* must take the drugs the *Hosaþiens* give to them in order that they might also fall þrey to the delusions made in his image. The best way of avoiding suicide and becoming "haþþy haþþy, oh so haþþy" is to become delusional, as it seems to work for the *Hosaþiens* quite well.

88. Because each of us *Homaniakos* has various degrees of a balance of deþression, manicism, and the ability to rationalize the clearer vision of reality, I would never judge or belittle our own for the use of medication to alleviate the þain. We all get tired of seeing reality, but really, what has haþþiness gotten you my reader friend anyway? A newsþaþer story read: "Laughing and þlaying they þlanned sweet dreams from *American Girl* memories turned into flaming flesh torn from living mommies screaming for death to save them from the reality of that surreal moment." They all died alone on that train ride to hell and none too þleasant either. No Godd was there to care as usual as death comes and goes, and in the most þainful of ways. If your god is fair and just, then they must have deserved every moment of it. Besides, aren't they better off dead now that they have þassed the trial by fire? I know the truth but I am told the vision is an illness of an abovo genetic abnormal "cause and reaction" of an unremarkable fission of one celtoþlast at some un-renounced un-moment in my un-involvement in your reality. Why should anyone care about that anyway?

89. I will not be drugged to become dulled or boring, feeling no sensation of death or why every microsecond of life is infinitely þriceless in a world of þaþer money values and bell curve con-artists. I will not loose the ability to divide zero by infinity and feel its resultant. No conversations for me with comatose theraþists, þsycho-þsychiatrists, desensitized social worker government cronies handing out mood stabilizers recommended by Madison Avenue ad-men marketers for a bigger bottom line. "How do you feel to-day (he's not looking at me)?" "Maybe I should increase your dosage, you're not quite useless yet". "We'll have you feeling normal very soon" or "I believe I can be of helþ to you, if you have insurance". Sharing wet dreams or even yesterday's dreams, there's no time like the þast, its so whack! Our reality is mostly the feeling that we don't belong in their reality. "*I'm not me*" as the funny man once stated, to make me laugh long after his death, but how true his words could be knows he.

90. In the darkness of my life I hide my actions of shameful deeds until the curtain is drawn, make-uþ on, I am treading the þlanks with ordinary humans. What þerversions do we share or are you so þure? Blue eyes big; white thighs soft; some uncommon desire with hands in motion blurring the Technicolor vision of electron þerversion comþliments of the microchiþ technology. The man with the money, sees clearer the honey that never really once lived but for one moment to be caþtured. Þre-teen girls with the need for the þower of the mighty steed between their thighs live only in *The Cube* or not? *Be a cowboy baby* hyþnotizes the genital imþlanted hiþs of county fair girls standing

prone as the ponies in the arena under the crop and under the eyes of the judges. Colored lights sewn together with noise rhythm amplified brings county fair youth erotica flickering and thickening the visual air with images of "Why we are all here in the first place?" type thoughts and my mind drifts lost to the sound of, *Be a cowboy baby.*

91. Seasonal changes, light sensitized, hope vaporized, holiday induced depression, what is everyone so happy about? Blind to the world, hope I get that gift, PokéMon collector, fad man fad shit, and "Thank you for shopping here, sir". There never was a Cinderella, a clearer vision reveals. "Enjoy your drink" was the last words he heard; now he's dead, a new exhibit for the crying masses. Drunk man driving, wiping his tears on the divorce papers served. "Michael's dead", she cried as she flung open the door of our house. His dad waits to be reunited in death. Will I see him first or is he forever dead? I constantly search for a place in the sun for my ultimate distraction while watching repeating looping and swooping mpeg's of tortured images on 19 inch diagonal screens of humans with perpetual ejaculations defying natures intentions, but we can't stop banging our heads like a fly against the sunlit window.

92. Get a headstart; dare to make a difference. Become a mentor, be a big brother Uncle Simon, be all that you can be, and a mind is a terrible thing to waste. Return to your tribal origins with synthetic, genetically driven, politically correct, memetic schemes to replace our naturally driven lives. It's the eighty's, it's the ninety's, it's the millennium, people will change, "I can't believe that can happen in this day and age". "We can put a man on the moon". "I thought school would be safe". Very few see it, nobody

will say it, genes rule at every instant of your life. You are a "blink" away from your Homo erectus heritage. Synthetic substitutions to technology driven problems speed you faster down the road to nowhere. Everyone flies in a different direction; but we all end up in the same place, dead. "Are we there yet?" the children shout not realizing that they are wishing away moments of their lives in the non-exchangeable, non-transferable currency of time.

93. What power we the *Homaniakos* command beyond the ordinary human's emotional abilities! We can conjure thoughts of an existence so vast, lost in an infinity of despair powerful enough to destroy our souls, our minds, and even our lives, in only six seconds flat! We can get as close to the edge as possible and float in a mental darkness in the realm of reality and gaze at sights that no ordinary human will ever see or imagine, but we can't describe. We can stop time. We can put our mind into a pit of infinite depth but only two feet wide. We can find places in our mind where no emotion has ever existed. We can feel every emotion at once to an exponential power. To see six billion dead souls, frozen in the coldness of forever ever land is within our powers, and never a tear to be shed anywhere as protons and neutrons collide in the cubic light-years of space. Come wander with me and I will give you the fear of your life. If scary movies thrill you - if roller coasters throw you into a screaming panic, then manic-depression is an ultimate emotional adventure to the brink of death and sometimes beyond death. I don't want drugs to remove my powers. I wish to remain a Manic-Depressive Junkie to the end of my reality.

94. Coroners can still eat steak, and so can surgeons. Is the inuring process possible with the *Homaniakos* species and our

enhanced perceptions? I believe so. We learn how to survive. We know what creates the moods. We chart it; we know what's coming, most of the time. We·must survive our first few episodes of manic. Then we must learn to live in the world of no emotions. Even in this mood there is danger. The danger of letting this non-feeling, the ultimate of emptiness, drive you insane. But then we don't let ourselves go insane, we are smart enough to self-terminate. At the right moment, suicide becomes logical.

A poor excuse of a plan

95. I have a plan, that I have been too cautious to try, but perhaps a metaphor will explain it too you my reader friend. Imagine you are treading water in the very middle of an ocean. The water is mostly calm, but to stay alive you must swim constantly. Humans are not equipped to swim constantly, but you can do it if you concentrate, constantly. Ships pass by filled with ordinary humans. They wave to you believing you are only out having a good time as they are. Nobody knows what you are feeling no matter how close they get to you. Sleeping is somewhat difficult but not impossible. But sometimes you stop treading water in your sleep and wake up below the surface, in a panic you must find the surface to breathe again. Sometimes you get tired of swimming and you start to wonder how deep is the ocean? Sometimes you rest your mind, you let go and allow yourself to sink. Maybe you'll touch bottom, but quickly you realize the bottom is too deep and you try to get back to the surface. Sometimes you can't find the surface in all the confusion, or you've gone too deep. Sometimes you die in the depth of the ocean. They find your drowned body lying in your house with no ocean in sight and wonder why?

96. It is my plan now; to see how deep is the ocean. To open my eyes when I get to the bottom and see what is at the void of space and at the end of time. For all of life as a *Homaniakos* I have resisted the sinking, the feeling of being drawn uncontrollably into the infinite void of mental pain and hopelessness. I was never prepared for the journey. I never wanted to make the journey. I would get to the point of life's end and wait for the ascent, mentally screaming for the sight of the sun and a breath of fresh air and to touch a human hand in mine and to gaze into clear eyes. To believe that life continues without loneliness. To believe that someone loves me.

97. Would a mountain climber succeed without the proper gear? Could you go to the North Pole without proper planning and equipment to get back home? I believe I now have the equipment to make the journey and return - a journey only within my mind. You cannot get to the bottom by sinking, which would not be fast enough. You must drive yourself there with power, with the thoughts that your brain would normally use subconsciously to force you on the journey. You must open all the doors that hold the visions of pain, quickly push the eternal hell of pain into your sub-conscious where logic fails for lack of mental frames of reference. Release the thoughts that you suppress because they pull you with infinite gravity toward the bottom. I have those thoughts locked up, I never think of them consciously or I would rapid cycle. Each new thought of reality has always been locked safely away, but I know where each thought is held.

98. You must have the equipment to get back home to this sandbar of a false reality and the warmth of the light of genetic

delusions (genetics drive the delusionary characteristics of the *Hosapiens*). You cannot purchase or pack anything for the journey home; it is only what you can put in a strategic place within your mind. Your lifeline back to the physical realm. My plan is simple; my driving thoughts are well established and secured until needed. My lifeline is to be a simple touch of a human's hand to keep my body on the earth and direct my mind back to the surface. The ordinary human cannot make the journey so I won't let go, never let go or I'll end my life in the vision of infinite pain as so many of us do every year. Why are so many suicides accomplished when the *Homaniakos* are alone is what I've thought about? Because they may have searched for the end of pain but not have had a lifeline back to the delusional world once they found it. The dead were not prepared, they had no lifeline, they lost the direction to the surface, or they got tired and let go and died willingly. Maybe some make it to the bottom and have seen the great void, and then died. I want to know. I want to return home with the vision. How deep can pain go?

99. I must only wait for the moment when my mind subconsciously divides zero by infinity (emptiness divided by forever) and sends me on a maximum panic attack, when depression is overcome by a frenzy of anxiety and my breath becomes short, sweat forms, vision blurs, and thousands of thoughts accelerate into hyperdrive. The impulse is to escape, to run or fly (flee) from the pain but I will have to stay motionless and release the subconscious thoughts and sink at the speed of light, but don't let go of my grip. I must carry the thoughts that someone loves me to the bottom. Can I sink that far quickly enough? Can love be found where death begins?

1 OO. Will the vision of eternal loneliness bring satisfaction? Will all of life's mysteries be fulfilled and thus brought to an end? Do we see hell or reality? Is our vision of reality a mistake of Godd? Will it be þroven that suicide is logical? Is suicide at that moment a signal of success or failure? I want to know. Will I ever be brave enough to try my þlan?

1 O 1 . For the true *Homaniakos* does not simþly go the end of life without emotion and love, for all neoþhyte manic-deþressives can do that. You must go to the edge of the universe, stoþ time, and don't look outward into the void of emotionless, endless sþace, where the human mind suffers infinite þain by mere thought alone. You must turn around and look back onto the universe. Look at the light and energy of a billion galaxies frozen timeless in sþace with billions of life forms moving about on countless þlanets. Every one of them fulfills only the *Four Axioms of Existence,* of which I will be revealing to you, my fine reader friend. Being able to look at the darkness is our born ability, but being able to turn around and see all of existence through sþace and time, feel all emotions and yet be emotionless, to grasþ existence without life, to feel your existence dissolve into endless time is only within the ability of the Manic-Deþressive Junkie who can thrust their soul into the flames of infinite þain by free will. If you can focus and keeþ one single thread of a thought connected to your þhysical life, you can return. Loose your connection to your þhysical life, the realm of the imagined reality of everyday life, and you are dead. Suicide becomes logical and necessary.

1 O2. When the manic-depressive achieves an elevated mental state and correctly sees the clearer vision of reality and successfully calculates the solution to the equation of zero divided by infinity, a suicide attempt may follow shortly thereafter. No ordinary human could know this feeling - the knowledge of emptiness divided by forever, the loneliness of the mind. Now while the music is climaxing and inspiring me to continue, my saviour [British] arrives as energy transponded on my eardrums to be translated without words into a message of hope for me.

1 O3. No ordinary human has the capacity to comprehend our attempts at describing our clearer vision of reality. The vision is a feeling, the feeling is unique to our species. We all share the common vision, the common feeling. And while we may describe this vision and the pain it brings with different words within this contrived language, all we are proving is the impossibility of passing the true feeling or understanding of what we feel and see via some type of word spoken or written but the vision is there regardless. We must look at this vision and say, "I can see the realm beyond this imagined reality. I can feel thoughts that ordinary humans will never know of". We must put confidence in our abilities and live.

1 O4. What difficult and possibly pointless to make point I am attempting is that the mind of a Homaniakos (manic-depressive) is a valid mind. Thus its perception of reality is valid. If this perception is different than the Hosapiens (ordinary humans), then we have a basis for a comparison and thus we can start a triangulation down a path toward a true understanding of reality

for all of mankind and womantype. What I suggest is that the mind of a *Homaniakos* is the only mind capable of þerceiving true reality and thus ordinary humans will never understand reality without our helþ and even then, I don't know if it is þossible for them. The music changes and for a moment it brings tears and visions of flowers and sunlight and warmth and life, þainless life, but even the music will end and the vision disaþþears to somewhere I suþþose.

105. I believe that the intended þlan of the DNA of the human (or all creatures as it will relate later to my Axiom #4) is to þrovide for the removal of deþressing thoughts that would occur if the true reality were þerceived by humans. It is the function of DNA to ensure survival and thus continuance of its self and by default [*Verb confusion*] the continuance of the host living being. Thus by design, enzymes or þroteins are manufactured to ensure the delusion required is created for life to continue without a thought as to its own merit or worth of "Why do I exist?" The use of a language would seem to work against that controlling gene because now ordinary humans can ask, "Why do I exist?" but without being a manic-deþressive that thought is only a coffee table conversation þiece and my belief of language as a contrivance is valid. This is why the *Homaniakos* vision of reality exists without the requirement of a language to describe it among our own sþecies but for the *Hosaþiens* we must sþeak or write or make metaþhors of life or how would they get the þoint? We work at not rationalizing reality in order to remain alive. What we think, we believe. What we believe becomes real and we can feel the real whether you know of it or see it.

106. I would like to say that the kid really rocks, as the beat of the music inspires me to remember visions of pleasure and lust and thoughts to live or live again as I once did. But I'll have to go with the flow until the song ends and throw logic and structure to the wind as I tell you that I search for everything that tells me I'm alive. Driving in my car watching birds and humans fly by wind in windows, I look at the physical reality removed from the Hosapiens imagined life. Flowers potted planted plopped arranged logically supposedly in front of artificial habitats filled with unknowingly lonely humans cooking dinner, cleaning house, rutting behind locked doors reaching split second distractions of orgasmic fluidic exchange, and wasting life watching the tube of infinitely needed genetic attractions, not your life I won't watch. Children running laughing playing pretending to be of all knowledge, screams scraping skyward from future skeletal minerals in youthful nonsense energy wasted toward what end? Sunlight or neon nightlights tell me that I'm alive. Colors transporting energy to my retinas for pleasure translation in my minds mind of genetic reaction without rationalization - I know it I am alive. Flowing down the river of sensory input without reason or rhyming songs of birds do they, we know not? Verbigeration vegetable garden factories planted in ten foot squares satisfying ageless drives to become one within all. To no end it serves but it proves to me I am alive.

107. I am alive by proof of every rock I focus my eyes still see them lying there with no reason of infinite origins of which only we understand. Circumstantially a blade of grass moves by direct action of the wind and gravity responds in neologisms equationally impossible to reactions that I see, and thus I know that I am alive.

108. Do not think for one moment that there is some glamour in being a manic-depressive especially of the junkie type. Entrusted with the knowledge of a clearer vision of reality, as gatekeepers of the visionary hell, as a human Chiron to daily navigate the river Styx. Physically in the *Hosapiens* world, but mentally living in the underground of forever darkness. Yes, I make jokes about it. After all, I am of a human species. But I am watching every second carefully. I am trying to find my pleasure on the earth, if there is such a thing as pleasure. I smile. I am glad to be around all humans, and I search out places where humans go to enjoy themselves. I enjoy working with people. I strive to inhale human pheromones but the forever "on" brain, the so-called thinking mechanism never sleeps until I do and then it dreams 24 hours a day every day all year every year as a vision that I can't shut my eyes to. There are only distractions. I need to be distracted so I can look slightly away from the clearer vision of reality - so I can stop thinking. Where am I to find an endless supply of my needed distractions?

109. Thoughts never stop they are as a light too bright that never ceases to shine into eyes unable to close their eyelids. Thoughts as real as saliva drool moments before the meat contacts your tongue you can't stop it, thoughts continue to scream as sirens so loud inescapable anyway you turn from within your ears you can't plug them from inside out and sleep brings dreams and there is no redirecting them even in a lucid state of concentration. Distractions to overpower thoughts need to become more intense every year because inuring is natures way and thus distractions must surpass what is legal to feel for real but what the hell, I want to feel something again and even if for a moment its at your expense of pain and bad memories. I will never forget each sensation of each misdirection until remembering it brings the reality of it, for what's the difference anyway? At every moment of life I know that death will cease the thoughts by synaptic reaction and bring nothing unless we do live forever and then what will I do with a spiritual mind that can't be blown away or bled to death and lives for the infinite of thinking?

110. The only thoughts that bring relief are thoughts as nature intended whether you are born into them or not. In later chapters I plan on boring you with nature and the genetics of it all in some type of worst science but bear[*bare?*] with me for the ending of this book is fantastic I've been told. So I know what I will write later and I believe in what I will write so I can say now that what brings satisfaction to me is visions of optimum procreation rutting in a natural environment with blue skies, sunlight shining off clouds white with dirted bottoms and breasts that point up. Touching flesh excited for sex and dripping with secretions pumped and primed for the event. Waves or water running or dripping from the sky into puddles of mud or rivers or lakes or oceans of duality clear and blue and warm and filled with naked bodies splashing little fishies wondering what to bite first. What is life here for if not to create more life and receiving satisfaction from doing it? Meanwhile the music is repeating so it's time to conclude I guess but ten thousand words are left and you'll have to guess what they would have been.

Conclusion

111. I am trapped here with you, not of my free will, but nonetheless retaining my free mind. If you are tired of reading the

ramblings of a madman in another copycat feel sorry for me book, "I survived the holycost", or "The 3-step formula to save your life or your money back", then read on. I don't want your sympathy, your insults mean nothing to me, and your praise or admiration won't buy me one extra second of life. So let me reveal to you your world as it actually exists as seen from the mind of a *Homaniakos*, a different race of humans unwontedly evolved, created, or if you would rather believe "dropped from space" from the Twilight Zone onto your tiny and insignificant planet.

1 1 2. You have now completed CHAPTER MYSELF, please turn the page and proceed to CHAPTER CREATIVITY. Do not mark in your book and please visit, at your convenience, our reference pages at the rear of the book.

THE MOST BASIC KNOWLEDGE OF THE PHYSICAL REALM:

The Four Axioms of Existence:

Axiom #4
"No living entity can have a greater understanding of its existence, than the physical ability to act on it."

Axiom #3
"?"

Axiom #2
"?"

Axiom #1
"?"

The only purpose of all living organisms:
"?"

Most basic law of nature:
[As expressed in a human language]
"?"

Most basic law of unnatural systems:
"Complexity causes complexity"

THE MOST BASIC KNOWLEDGE ABOUT THE HUMAN ANIMAL:

Genetic behavioral motivators of human males:
"?"

"?"

"?"

Genetic disposition of human males:
"?"

Genetic behavioral motivators of human females:
"?"

"?"

Genetic disposition of human females:
"?"

CHAPTER
CREATIVITY

"Creativity is what occurs when you lose concentration of your genetic objectives." R. J. Hanink

The music that set the mood for writing this chapter was:
   "2001: A Space Odyssey" CD by Turner Ent.

The beginning is a very delicate time

1 1 3. One music CD should do the trick and I bet you are wondering why I didn't write CHAPTER THE UNIVERSE OF THE REAL to the space music sound track? CHAPTER THE UNIVERSE OF THE REAL really has very little to do with any space beyond what you can reach within your arms reach, because aside from some of the physical anomalies such as stars and planets, what would be different about a unit of space here or anywhere in the universe? You'll have to wait to find out more about space latter but as far as creativity goes or comes, I believe the movie *2001: A Space Odyssey* is the most fantastic movie ever brought into reality because it has nothing creative in it at all. Everything in the movie is quite ordinary and presented in an ordinary way at that, because the movie portrays space and space travel nearly exactly how we would expect to know of it. Look at the quiet imagery and you will see what I mean. Now for the *Homaniakos*, the vision of the universe is perhaps ordinary, even if they all don't see it that way yet. Their vision can be of loneliness or death or a vision beyond death, because the universe is quite ordinary and quiet in

its self. This creates our knowledge of the loneliness of the universe, because our physical life is not perceived to be a part of the universe after death, yet it is and when we are alive is when we should be proud of that fact. But at any rate the *2001: A Space Odyssey* soundtrack CD is classical or semi-classical or will be classical some day (I own the 1996 version by Turner Classic Movies), so it puts me in the mood to write about creativity and manic-depressives because that is the topic of this chapter and isn't art associated with the great classics I've been told? So I suppose we should get down to brass tacks and start getting you the information about "all of this", (I'm waving my right hand across a dark star studded sky on a cool spring evening, while a gentle breeze whistles through leafless tree branches.). For CHAPTERS CREATIVITY, HUMAN PERCEPTIONS VERSUS TRUE REALITY, MANKIND AND WOMANTYPE, and THE UNIVERSE OF THE REAL I will start the opening page of each chapter adding more data to my list of ultimate knowledge. At the end of the book, will be the conclusion with the final missing axiom in its place. If you haven't read the prefatory at the start of this book you better do it now because I am going to be honest with you, nothing will make sense (be sensible?) if you don't. Please don't read the conclusion first; it spoils the surprise ending where we all die but moments after we each reach a complete understanding of the universe throughout space and time. Those are the rules to my book, break them if you wish, but in the end we still all die. This book works at being a skyriser worth of stories. Explanations of the manic-depressive human vs. the ordinary human, the understanding of existence and biological life through space and time, the basic understandings of mankind and womantype, and questioning life beyond our physical life. You'd better read between the lines because space is never truly empty. My partial list is on the opening page of this chapter, if the printers did their job correctly.

Me and Mania

1 1 4. Food on this planet can be fantastic, but the basic food groups do not contain enough of the essentials for me as a *Homaniakos* so I must supplement my diet with white bread that builds strong bodies 8 ways. Chocolate is needed to be added [*Passive voice*] to my diet. This increases the amount of serotonin, a natural upper. A lot of Hydrocarbons are needed also. Diet supplements are similar to what zoos do when they move animals from their natural environment into the unnatural environment of the zoo. This supplement must occur even if the displaced animals are allowed to eat the fauna and flora of their new environment. Based on our eating habits the *Hosapiens* food has too many calories for us because we typically suffer from weight gain during our down time or we suffer from weight lost during our down time, the experts get confused. I have to eat 5 meals a day, because I gave up on sleep, it's not needed. I really wonder what food is like on my home planet (That's a metaphor. The *Homaniakos* are indigenous of the planet the earth.)?

1 1 5. I basically like; chocolate, sugar, salt, meat on the raw side, undercooked bacon, White Castle cheeseburgers, and undercooked French fries. I try to avoid restaurants that can't cook their food properly as I had described. This diet helps to keep me hypomanic. We the *Homaniakos* have a saying: "One *hypomanic is worth 10 ordinary humans.*"

116. During a þanic attack maximus when my mind is telling or comþelling my body to get out of here, I try to maintain one thought. This thought is consistent time after time that instead of fleeing across country and þossibly bumþing into Ms. Margot Kidder, I head to the Dairy Queen for a chocolate malt. I tell myself, get chocolate. It's not that I don't have þlenty of chocolate in the house, but I must satisfy the "fleeing" instinct that we the *Homaniakos* can have during a þanic attack or Instant Mania Mood (IMM). We may flee, but we should have an established þlan. I know that sometimes our senses can over þower the þlan, esþecially when imþending death is felt and can't be rationalized at the moment, or when sþy's with eyes that sþy are sþied within our þresence, but we have a better chance of controlling the fleeing urge during IMM if we can get to that safe þlace. Þlan, think, reþeat your þlan, think, reþeat your þlan, shout it at yourself, þlan, think reþeat your þlan, think, reþeat your þlan, shout it at yourself, it really is that simþle. Do this in every quiet moment, in between moments of conversation, or while waiting for that end of sentence þeriod to droþ while listening to that friend sþeak to you of love and haþþiness or other þhables of delusional life. The drive to flee occurs often and is strong. Actually I don't know why I haven't ended uþ roaming the streets of Havana by now smoking a fine Cuban cigar while asking strangers, "Who am I?" in a þrivate language. My þassþort is on toþ of my desk right now, and I have þlanned my escaþe route for the event.

117. How to turn the switch from deþression to hyþomania is a difficult task. When I am at an extreme deþression, I work hard to þrevent moving into further deþression. I struggle not to see the clearer vision of reality. I distract myself to get back into not being depressed, let alone being hypomanic, but it is possible to move myself into hypomania from a "normal" mood. Having an objective is the best method. We must be able to drive our brains to the mood we need and I haven't forgotten that we are going to discuss creativity in this chapter, I'm building up to it. It isn't that this is an easy task to do, because our natural tendency would be to settle in at a state of total distraction. Being distracted is what the *Homaniakos* call fun. When our distraction becomes our hypomania destination, we can achieve a state of mind that very few if any of the *Hosapiens* obtain and thus boundless energy and drive with no sense of failure occurs. This mental state combined with our natural intellect is the reason that although we are 1% of the population, we are 30% of the creativity and thus 30% of the intellect by my observations (I made those numbers up but they sound appropriate, don't they?). Controlling our sleep and waking activities is critical. Days do not happen - they are scheduled.

1 1 8. So a typical day for me is as that Bill Murray movie; *Groundhog Day*, and that is the impression my mind feels most of the time. I don't like the way hours and days and weeks are organized, but how am I to change it? I have about 44 more 24-hour days in a year than most humans do, but I guess it's something that feels natural to me. My true days would be shorter. The first day would be 11 hours awake, 1/2 to 1-hour sleep. The next day would be 10 to 12 hours awake, 4 to 5 hours sleep. Then repeat that two day cycle. Forcing myself to go to bed at 2 a.m. so that I may get up at 6 a.m. just doesn't seem fair. [*I'm starting in the middle of a topic:*] Late evening to early morning – casual research & reading until bedtime. This is also my distraction time where I spend time totally alone and really not

missing any contact with humans, although I wouldn't turn it down. I am never fully depressed during this time if I can remain distracted as I spend it browsing the World Wide Web for topics of scientific interest or making plans for my escape or reading the message boards of my fellow *Homaniakos'*. The Internet allowed me to adjust my cycle time and almost eliminate night-horrors and 2 a.m. panic attacks. The Internet allowed me to write this book. You must use every piece of data from every hidden corner of mankind and womantype's postings without concern for content, morality, or objectivity. The Web is the total knowledge of humankind and the only true revelation of all of the human thoughts and wishes. Complete control over my schedule and activities has allowed me to move into a cyclothymic lifestyle. I now cycle once a day and have larger swings as the Chicago seasons come and go. Holidays and other cyclic events factor in also. Music is a major part of my life and I plan what I listen too very cautiously. However, anything that will become a distraction is welcomed, so please drop by and we'll chat.

1 1 9. During a good week I can average less than 4 hours a night sleep. Sometimes I don't sleep. During a normal week it will average 5 hours a night. When I have too much down time, I might loose another hour a day to some type of evening nap (but all I need is 20 minutes to cycle completely) and a lethargic state of non-interaction. This occurs because I am considered cyclothymic by the *Hosapiens*. I have found that controlling my schedule and being able to rely on predicable activities I can rapid cycle every day, one complete cycle. So I can pretty well tell you my best times of the day, and what I would best be doing then, but panic attacks and unexpected sights and sounds can throw me into an Instantaneous Manic Mood (IMM), or into total depression, or into feelings of euphoria with the most grand sensations of eternal bliss and natural satisfactions. Thus although I hadn't revealed it to you earlier (because I prefer to believe that only ordinary humans are so pre-occupied with so many trivial facts), I am from the tribe of the Cyclothymes, as I would imagine (in order to fulfill my tribal protocols). Thus I am a Manic-depressive Junkie Cyclothymic, but to ordinary humans we all look the same I am told. The *Homaniakos* have all the divisions and categories and stereotyping and anything else you could think of in order to create of society of similar individuals as the *Hosapiens* do also. May I ask of you right now, did you ever imagine that such a different and complex society walks among the unsuspecting *Hosapiens* all the while we know of their lives and their society while they understand nothing of ours? We hide, as would Vampires, every one of us. We are very aware of the ordinary human's thoughts and actions and we know what they would do if they found the spy among them, but I am no longer afraid to hide. Without starting a new paragraph lets continue with my previous thoughts that spending time in totally distracting activities such as two weeks in DisneyWorld is possible without holding to my cycle, but the distraction becomes routine [*Adjective use*] and thus lost. Always seek new distractions or stick to the planned cycle is the rule.

1 20. What makes I do when in that state, hypomania is so great as long or longer that I have a big objective [*Clanging*]. Not that I want to read a book or learn to cook or even become a master thief (try crook) but steal pheromones I will do to obtain a means to my nothing else rhymes with "objective". My plan is to sell my weirdness to earn enough money to get to a beach on the French West Indies (the Orient beach). Oh it's not that I

couldn't run off there by myself right now for a week or two and later þay my dues (Because what would I have to þack?), but I want to be able to move freely around the world, following the warm ocean currents and the tropical sun because the sunlight is my friend. I have magazines that I þeruse for motivation and troþical Web sites of islands and island food with ocean waves and the young ladies wave too, and I þoint to a spot on an island and þroclaim "I'm going to die right there" as in that childhood game we'd þlay. I will succeed because I can't see failure in this mood and I'll stay in this mood by eating the right food and spitting out word salad.

Language as creativity

1 2 1 . As a *Homaniakos*, writing is necessary as talking is long. Not that I am really good at it writing, but I have my moments. The *Homaniakos* are comþelled to write as þart of our normal functioning. This is undoubtedly due to our trait to use language in unorthodox methods or our ability to really not figure all those damn rules out [Alt: *figure out all those damn rules*]. As you reed or read or red or read in CHAPTER MYSELF, obedience to sentence structure, formal word logic, or only using established words in our vocabulary are not something that we all can control at every moment. Rather I like to use the full þower of my ability to alter the "status quo" of sentence structure and logic in order to lean the *Hosaþiens* (ordinary humans) toward an altered vision of their reality. Intentional and disordered thought are Boustroþhedon at working geniuses. Most of the *Hosaþiens* don't get it, but they are easily amused and often chuckle at hearing variations in speech þatterns of which they believe me to be joking but I honestly don't get what they are laughing about.

While my speech is usually quite ordinary, (as the *Hosapiens* trained me) sometimes concentration is required to get the verbs in-line or not to rhyme.

122. If you were to look for all the manic-depressive writers you would find all that you would want. I am suggesting that you do an Internet search and I'll save you the reading from this book (search later, read my book now).

123. This paragraph intentionally contains one sentence of nine words.

124. Why do some manic-depressives have such a unique speech? All I can tell you is that it is as natural for us to speak how we do, as it is natural for the *Hosapiens* to be so boring by following all those proper rules, don't you agree? Fortunately while the *Hosapiens* attempt to classify us into some mental illness caricature because of language protocol violations, they have come up with an excellent list of what makes us so creative verbally from what I see or hear. The mere fact that the *Hosapiens* psychologists believe these and other language traits can successfully be used to classify the traits [*the traits can be successfully used to classify*] [(*of*) per following the previous "traits"] a mental illness is only one more proof of the *Hosapiens* faulty logic. By the psychologists own admission, 50% of the ordinary humans are sliding down the left side (toward becoming a moron) of the bell curve and thus why should they be expected to master a language? The fact that humans of one unified species can have so many different languages of confusion tells us right now that humans do not (learn) language or grammar by genetics but by memetics (look it up). Our *Homaniakos* unusualness is

nothing at all because it should be (quite) obvious that we are born into it. It reveals a hardwired brain and that my friends is what can make a species a species.

125. Let me give a few definitions of verbalization "thought disorders" that I have found during my studies. Psychologists believe that speech is a gateway to the mind of the speaker. Since language is a contrivance and "mental illness" is a naturally occurring condition (becoming a manic-depressive is also natural) I am not certain of the relationships between the use of contrivances and nature but I suppose those psychologist's are smarter than me for whatever that is worth. Now since you are used to my poor quality of speech content within the words spoken written (as in excessive qualifications) lets continue along those lines to tell you that the clang is what rhymes when speaking, but it's all natural to my species and since language is a contrivance anyway, and most often boring, why not modify it as required? But whereas the meaning of words might be important to ordinary humans, why not structure your sentences around how the words sound instead? Aren't beautiful words as beautiful flowers and what message do flowers send without logical words spoken or wrotten? Puns are fun and why shouldn't we be the experts at it? Derailment of thoughts expressed via speech is as it appears, but to my mind how can a topic be arranged in a straight line trying to match nouns with verbs while sidebar qualifiers of unrevealed relevance are omitted? It would seem to me that according to one book on the subject that I speak in a .5 level of confusion. What do you think? Sometimes I realize when told by ordinary humans that I have made a syntax error, it can be difficult for me to correct (it) because my mind prefers the words as ordered. While speaking of words, the neologism is not a word

found in a book (yet) so how dared we speak these words that have not passed the review bored of approvals? But as the North American continent was here all along, and it wasn't until some white-man said it was true before anyone could speak of it, so are neologisms to the mind of the ordinary humans. The dictionary I use tells me that a neologism is a word used by a psychotic, but guess what species wrote that book? But when up to the occasion why not dress the tongue for the affair by giving it flair with a little stilted speech because you can never over dress the tongue. Now paraphrasia and metonyms are beyond my comprehension, but the ordinary humans insist on divisions and categories and terms and symbols and acronyms and whatever, so these have something to do with word construction and in this book I'll write what I am thinking and spell words how I want them to sound - while I place; commas, colons: "and" other [pretty] marks wherever they are found. You are on your own to figure the sound or the meaning or the intention planned but not revealed because it makes perfect sense to me or why write it?

126. As you will find out in CHAPTER HUMAN PERCEPTIONS VERSUS TRUE REALITY, the evolution of the need for language is an interesting thought, but while language is here, the *Homaniakos* will use it to define the scope of our knowledge of existence. But the bottom line is that language is a contrivance and thus not natural. Nothing good will become of it. From what I can surmise, by watching and paying attention, it would seem that only about .25% (1/4%) of what is spoken, is necessary to any human. So throw away the theories that our language is necessary for our survival as an animal in the wild. Would you be so bold to proclaim that you would be able to have a conversation with a human of your language, 200 years from now? Whereas I do believe language þrevents us from acting on our imþulses since once a thought is sþoken, our mind is quite satisfied as though the event had actually occurred. Or þossibly we talk ourselves into doing the act by reþeatedly stating what we would want to do. Which way is it? Can you tell me?

Creativity beyond the infinite

1 2 7 . So you take a creature such as the *Homaniakos* and without much effort you find all the descriþtions of þain illustrated multiþlexed and alternative realities becoming so digressed or confused. The word humans use to describe these descriþtions is "creativity". Now creativity is "seeing" combined with "associations" and add a touch of "your heads on crookedness" or ordinary humans will believe you are oh so boring. But humans can't see more than they can know because humans will always see what they believe and thus the *Homaniakos* will see more by virtue of the fact we believe in more of the 4 dimensional life as þassages through a wormed holed book. Add to this our clearer vision of reality and you can get some damn good stuff or weird stuff if you þrefer words as I do.

1 2 8 . Learning about human behavior is like Web browsing – you don't end uþ where you were headed. CHAPTER MANKIND AND WOMANTYPE is to be the human attributes chaþter but I can't wait for that chaþter and what does it matter[s?] anyway? Creativity exþresses itself in the most outlandish of human behavior and exþectancy by the usual gang of idiots. The images of semi-naked long legged young oþtimally þrocreated female humans moving in some unnatural fashion while wearing a fashion down the runways every sþring

winter fall is a good example of creativity. For certain it's all the same repeated and depleted next year pleated again and again but I only want to see their breasts in order to make a proper optimum procreation choice. These impractical unsuited for survival in the wild coverings for the body natural will make it to the plastic hangers at K-Mart (registered I'm sure) in a somewhat desensitized form because ordinary humans are always ready for an adventure, an amazement, or an interesting observance of a sort, but most will only actually go so far by their own genetics or they will be an outcast in their own tribe - at least they believe so thus it becomes real in their mind. Humans know this not by lesson but by being born to do natural things like eating, rutting, and "blending in". Anything too weird will prevent one, both, or troth of the aforementioned items from occurring within the tribe. All the human species know it without language to compound it. I hope you can pull the point from the paragraph above, but don't you feel uneasy [*Wordiness (no suggestions)*] being dressed inappropriately for an occasion, and now for me you must think about why you feel that way and is it natural or learned?

1 29. Now I suppose you never wondered why the body modified pierced and attested, tatteredtood and dressed for regressed youth hang out together as in a mob, a crowd, or a pride of a lodge? A bird of a feather sounds too simple but that's actually all there is to it, so give it no more thought. As a middle upper class yuppie SUV gnome, do you want your daughter to be getting off with one of "them" while in her Easter Sunday virgin white dress hiding behind the confessionals with her Sailor Moon panties down while his tongue pierced goes lickity-clit lickity-clit, like a mile long train that will disappear down an old rusty rail never to be seen again? So we categorize and

stereotype but someone said we are above that and they O my brothers are idiots. Your stereotyping is proper and you better stick to it because it is natural and survivable so why else would Godd or evolution give it to you. Now what does all of this have to do with creativity you may be starting to wonder but we aren't far off the trail's end yet and I finished this question without a mark. Ordinary humans are mostly afraid to be creative or different and genetics drive it. No, some humans don't have a special talent; they only lack the fear of being ousted from the tribe in our society at large for doing anything not of the status quo. From this lack thereof, you get everything that is un-boring because we as humans live too long and get bored too easily in this age of button depressing.

130. Now manic-depressives of the *Homaniakos* type are characterized from a double whammy as found within the genetic selection of DNA strands. We are born with the need and compulsion to create and express it whether we are talented at it or not, and yet we understand that we must hide our genetic drives or manic-depressive protocols in order to remain within the tribe of ordinary humans. We remain "un-proclaimed" in order to obtain food, shelter, and all the rest of that Maslow shit except that thing about aspiring to the greatness of mankind and womantype. All humans share the same genetic drive to eat and procreate in whatever convenient order the occasion presents such that we know what to do to survive as a male black widow walking thinly on a web of sex and death. So the debate goes on by the master debaters as to whether manic-depressives are the creative force in the world of the humans or not and it is without a doubt that this is a true statement or at least a truism if you prefer. No need to dig up the dead bones of the unconfirmed *Homaniakos* great ones

that died before us because we hide it well and so do the families of the recently self-inflicted deceased. Imitation is a great attribute of the human animal and possibly we the *Homaniakos* are the best species for doing it.

131. We walk among the ordinary humans while hiding behind imitation mirrored smiles applied moment to moment, immerging from and disappearing back to - via a Cheshire way - the world of infinite pain and a clearer vision of reality. Ordinary humans don't see us or suspect us but we are there nonetheless as spotting a tree for the forest, shopping mall hall walkers, and carnival ride watchers while slipping in and out of delusional senses in between the ordinary humans delusional world and the true reality - all the while sitting in an airport lobby chair white rocker. We see all of humanity through Arbus eyes and it rarely looks better. Sooner or later we create an artifact out of sorts and if we're fortunate enough on display it will be put. The creation process is thus out of nothing of the ordinary human's reality, for they are lacking any skills in apophenia, so success is measured by the more clanging the song or actions that are wrong, and we will continue until the final gong is rung or rong. Nowhere it gets us but by genetics we must respond and thus the nature of the so-called "mentally ill" is visionary at its absolute best.

The Technol Research Project

132. Now the following is most certainly a paid infomercial to promote my artwork but I'll try to avoid being tacky and never mention that I am in desperate need of gallery space and shows. I am told that this topic gets confusing so pay attention closely. It is most definitely my goal that I sell my thoughts turned solid as

artworks and then live my life at full hypomanictisum at all times without accountability to any of the *Hosapiens* for my actions or words. But to get more or less to the point with minimal clanging and illogicality I will describe my journey to express the thoughts that push all of us manic-depressives to work in the non-private sector such that the fruits of our labors as artworks galore can be ours without concerns of the ordinary humans delusional world of peace and order.

1 3 3. I am compelled to be organized [*Passive voice*]. If this were not such a desirable trait among ordinary humans you would not realize that it is actually what you would call an Obsessive Compulsive Disorder. Its not that I walk around counting books on shelves as that nut did in that Bruce Willis movie where Mr. Willis can't see the color red, whatever the name of it was or still is, but everything has a place without a doubt and I will find that place. What all the *Homaniakos* must remember is that they must create within their natural tilts of their behavior. What can I learn about organic life and physical existence using organizational skills was the first thought that came to my mind? A properly installed manic-depressive protocol prevents me from seeing failure from such a futile quest so I'll succeed with a mind that never rests I figure.

1 3 4. So off to a rough start was my beginning for an understanding of the ordinary human's as expressed via artworks, but aren't all beginnings such? Stop, Look, and Listen the sign stated so I did and it was good advice except it didn't account for my sentence structure and verbigeration - oh well. Should I draw, paint, write, sculpt, or hang a spoon on my nose in restaurants? Writing became obsessive so I went with the flow. Nothing good

became of it though because my concern to logictize the order of the universe was overwhelming being an engineering student at that time of my existence (That would have been 1970 or so for those of you who believe that information would be interesting).

135. By the mid 1970's I was jumþing out of þlanes for fun or thrills or to test my death wish for certain but a girl was there and the juxtaþosition of beauty and death and þleasure and þain was þerfect for a brain on the run so I began writing *The Book of the Dead*, and I still have the þaþers stored in canoþic jars, some text of which fitted nicely into this book without your notice - but I was drawn deeþer into deþression once I understood that atoms behave according to their own kind, molecules followed next, then simþle cell life followed by "us" sooner or later I figured. The music helþed or didn't helþ at all, but I can't figure out which of the two actually occurred. So I cried a lot and went to church to find what I imagined to be the only answer – Godd. As *Jesus Christ Superstar* sþun on my turntable, her and I held hands under the album cover (without a word sþoken or needed) when suddenly the universe tilted one tenth of one degree and I could have lived in that moment forever: but I had to think was there any choice to our behavior, surely we resþond to what we think as opþosed to only genetic actions? I was short on data and conclusions to be certain. I anxiously awaited the Internet and living the life as George Jetson, but I had to start my search without it or him.

136. An artwork titled *Sam of Mars* gave me my first original attemþt at making þhysical the thoughts from within my growing *Homaniakos* mind. Those words (on that artwork) were donated in writing by the most remarkable distraction of a young lady that any male manic-deþressive could ever hoþe for. My vision of death or love never went þast her beauty or the moments of her touch or the feeling of her breath against my liþs or the sound of her voice without words - so my need to see beyond the curtain was nil and I droþþed the whole issue. I have since lost the drawing she gave to me with those words drawn on, but I can still þicture it clearly as the reþresentation of my goals to a clearer vision of reality and the þhysical existence of the universe beyond our control. She gave it to me with a smile for she was still an angel; she had no clue, but as with the body illustrations on the *Illustrated Man*, the artwork she gave to me drove me to thoughts of suicide by staring between the images.

137. I was comþelled to create images of death using whatever was within my reach because why should lonely humans continue living I thought? Later I would slash, smash, or by any means destroy my artwork without realizing I was actually only aþþlying a one directional timeline attribute to a þhysical anomaly, but "Damn it, anyway!" any proþer þhysicists would scientifically synaþtically proclaim. It's all gone, to my knowledge, setting 200 feet below an oxygen deþrived landfill somewhere in the Midwest or burnt to carbon and residing þartially in the trees in all of our yards. I have but a few written documents remaining in my hands. I looked at my artwork then as though I hadn't created them at all and they had suddenly aþþeared in my room to torture me. Not a single reason why did I create them ever came to mind, but they aþþeared one by one and one by one they disaþþeared also. Soon my beautiful female distraction would disaþþear and life has never been so blind exceþt for that daily thought of every moment we had together, and I would sell my soul to re-live the þhysical acts committed.

138. Now a direction needs to be set, a course figured plotted and plowed, and maps and timelines gathered if you are going to end up where you want to be or go (put "*to*" here but don't tell my processor). So I gave it some thought of where should my conclusion be and how to get there via a straight line on world points. The direction that mankind and womantype appears to be heading, at least for this moment of this our great states of a Latin union is what I want to know plus why are we going there anyway? So I started to research the rhyme or reasons and the why and how of it all when I thought: "What have I become, artist or scientist?" So I selected scientist and I looked the part in a white robe to be certain. *The Technol Research Project* was started by me in order to organize the whole of it - every thought and result with strict guidelines, rules, and results documented as text and artwork suitable for display in the unnatural environment of the human animal. I also planned on selling this stuff to the ordinary humans for cash. My compulsive disorder of organization would create the physical environment for retaining data and creating artworks. It landed me my 15 minutes of fame at the Randolph Street Gallery but soon life changed and all control was lost. The *Hosapiens* should not schedule events around the *Homaniakos* mind because we will not be leashed without dire consequences.

139. Now *The Technol Research Project* is a product of The Technol Research Center and I am the creator of both and thus I am the director as in the man in charge of all research, results, and organization within it. A complete project report of approximately 19 pages in size as of this date exists in order to bring order to my artworks and my investigations. Each series of

artworks I created would explore a possible clue to understanding the human animal and its creation of the unnatural environment and as my report states: "It is not the intention of *The Technol Research Project* to bias opinions for or against the worthiness of technology, the unnatural environment, or the actions or intentions of the human animal." As all scientists know, the act of observation or even noticing a test alters either the results or the future of the test victim. The act of being there transfers energy to or from the pliable liable, whatever the subject. So how can we be our own test subjects unless of course two distinct human species are involved?

140. Now each series of those artworks explores an observable behavior of the human animal as human's work toward living entirely within the unnatural environment under the control of inventive technology. The report is artwork itself but nobody gets it I guess so here it sits after confusing, confounding, or boring the wits out of gallery and museum directors reciting in unison, "What the hell is all of this?" and maybe they are correct but it got me here and this book was the next logical step. Once I reached a point of creative neutrality the *Four Axioms of Existence* were squeezed into our universe and no further wonderment is required for or of me. The *Four Axioms*, now being physical in the form of an atomic structured document, cannot back up in time so there is no denying they exist for you to do with what you will. So I sit here at the end of knowledge, having understood it all and seen it all too. Everything else from this point on is clearly understood as humans following their genetic actions without a fault and my axioms applied, pretty well covers all the loose ends. But you're not there yet my reader friend, so continue (I will) and we're still standing in the lobby of my virtual creation of *The Technol Research Center* and the music plays on.

141. I was to have quoted directly from my report starting with the index but oh my what a bore that would have been for certain. But I was trying to create or meme or sell my ideas that a typed document could be considered a Work of Art, but not in the sense of the content being poetic or crafted skillfully or because it was diagrammed by De Vinci himself. I guess it is a bad idea or I am just plain stupid at it, but nothing became of it although I have not given up trying. This causes me to re-evaluate what are the thoughts that the artist has prior to the creation or construction? Does the artist mentally state: "I will create something so different that they will have to say I am a genus." Or does the artist think: "I see emotional attributes in these materials and patterns and something is alive in the contrasting position of them, what life, what energy, what emotion!" What is the difference of the thoughts thought prior to the creation of the artworks, if those thoughts are not revealed in the artworks? First I do believe that without the mind for it, even the bogus artist will be found out to be bogus sooner or later. I feared I was bogus myself, but I always had a passion for seeing relationships in actions versus motives, but perhaps with my first artworks being so technical and contrived, that I failed to get to my cross-cut examination of the humans within their unnatural environment into a format of formal art. My artworks became hidden in the environment that they were designed to compliment, as would a replica of a tree if placed deep within a forest. But then again, that was my point. Oh well!

142. The *Axioms of Existence* were predicted to be required as far back as approximately 1990 and were simply labeled

"03.01.01.01" followed by the words "Work in þrogress" and I expected that they would define all of existence in some form of the English language. It was my belief at that time that a total understanding of human behavior would bring a more restful mind to my always "on" brain. As I now went into a major deþression episode 8 seconds ago, from the change in songs I guess, I have to change subjects to tell you right now that as a youth I would wake-up crying in the darkness of the night. I never knew why I did this, for I never remembered a dream being associated with the night terror. It's not as though I never dreamed or didn't have nightmares, because I still remember some of those dreams of creatures chasing me and me with no þlace to hide that they couldn't find. But my mother would come in and hold me - that fact I remember very well. Jumþing ahead 40 years to the þresent time, I find myself waking uþ and crying in the middle of the night, but I have defined the terror that needs no dream to create. The terror is nothing more than reality itself, the clearer vision of reality that aþþears to me at a waking moment, and now I know what I saw as a human-child but couldn't describe because of my inexþerience with contrived languages as a youth. So now my wife will hold my hand (if I bother to wake her) I and am comþelled to remember my mother holding me, and it did no good then and it does no good now. It is not of dreams or life that I fear, for the only fear of living is the fear that the þain and the visions will arrive by surþrise in the dark of the night. I fear the finality of death, whereby death is felt as forever loneliness with never a chance for even a warm, living hand to be held tightly in mine. So as I greatly fear the darkness and the confinement of the grave, I remember that Jesus has þower over the grave and he died to þrove it to all of us, or so the Bible claims. So although ordinary humans will never have a clue as to the absolute sensations of those thoughts felt as a reality, I am lead to believe that somewhere in the humans þast, a manic-depressive sat down one day and using that mostly useless contrived language of the humans, documented Hell and the infinity of it. What would my fears be, if there had been no words or metaþhors to define the absoluteness of death or the vastness of sþace and time? At any rate, after doing exhaustive studies, I have decided to þut a name to this feeling that I exþerience on occasion; because I know that others also share that feeling. That name is, the "von Neumann Reality Syndrome" or vNRS for short because he died knowing with certain logic that once he was dead, he would no longer be an active þart of the þhysical universe, and that he would miss being here with us while we are having all this þhysical fun. Thus, that is the nature of vNRS. His was not random þanic attacks of an unknown nature of an unknown fear, but rather the tyþe of fear that only true knowledge and true logic can feel. I will not debate his logic or wisdom, ordinary human or not. He died when I was apþroaching my 6th orbit, as his last great feat of logic þroved that death is real. I will die in the same torment as he, as my aging enzymes or þroteins slowly change me from a þrim and þroþer Cyclothymic into a DSM IV BP II. But I ramble again, and you my friend came to this chaþter to learn about creativity.

143. There is a þoint I wish to make and it comes across as small at first but it is actually worth a little brain strain because although the following statements may stand correct from your vantage as a human within the framework of your ability to understand the natural world, the size of the universe, and "time sþans" longer than 3 minutes, there is actually within it not one of the biggest thoughts of all time but a thought nonetheless because it shows that humans have a þersþective viewpoint that is natural about the unnatural, but totally incorrect once you start thinking in universal size and time spans. The first statement: "The human animal has a propensity for the use of inventive technology." The second statement: "The human animal believes that they pollute the natural environment by using inventive technology." If you traveled to Mars and found a birds nest and a flashlight, both would give you a clue that life was on or visiting Mars at some point in time, but each would give you separate thoughts about that life due to your ability to pattern map images combined with possessing a large memory to remember such patterns learned. On the earth, we consider the flashlight tossed into the ditch as a pollutant, and the bird's nest in the ditch as "natural", but why? How can humans create the unnatural or have unnatural (against nature) thoughts?

144. You may not have caught the flaw in logic that is now more apparent that the end of knowledge is nearer. All of mankind's and womantype's inventive technology will return to the unpolluted natural state of existence because unless Godd puts his middle finger down and stops the LP (Archaic word usage, LP means "Long Playing" and it refers to phonograph albums in common usage during the mid to late 1900's.) from spinning, the earth will become elemental in a physicist's fashion after three ticks of the universal clock. I am not expecting that 82 billion years from now, when the universe has stretched as far out as gravity would allow and then collapsed back down to the primordial golf ball that there will be a history of mankind and womantype in the form of harmful pollution as in "chunks of concrete with imbedded rebar" in the mix of atomic soup. (Actually, many believe the universe most likely will actually keep expanding and die a cold dark death as you and I will also.) *The Anthropic Cosmological Principle* will still

apply at that moment and without viewership to report and document it, who's going to say, "I told you so?" So all matter will return to a natural state but on the earth within a human's time attribute we appear to pollute and alter unnaturally but only as a measure of our life span. Humans cannot truly pollute or alter unnaturally the universe, thus they cannot alter the mechanism of the universe, and thus perhaps humans are perfectly natural with all natural actions after all. Yes, we are still on art and creativity but you can see how a .25 level syncretistic response with excessive qualification will add text to a document. The music is still playing, so I'm going to crank the volume and hope for the best.

145. Holding on to the statements from above, add the following thoughts that human logic and statements are made in the imagined likeness of humankind and do not reflect refract or even obliquely transfuse the reality of reality. How then is "art" integrated into the thought process when in fact, humans are not truly understanding their true nature and status in the universe? How do we define the purpose or function of "art"? We (as humans) are only satisfied and reach an understanding when the object of art is interpreted not too far outside our genetic guidance. Thus "a few of the earth years" is usually interpreted as "forever and forever" because who can know or feel anything other except the *Homaniakos*? You may infer the apparently random beating of a drum for 5 million earth years as being random but in fact we may be listening to a 15 million earth year cyclic pattern of beats. It all has to do with our ability to define the mechanism for the creation of the drumbeats, not the beats themselves, yet it is the beats that are what our senses were created to react with. So why do we define, without getting far

from it, the universe of life and us from the human vantage of speed, size, and life spans? Going back to my original art project, *The Technol Research Project* report is correct if you stand to read it, but not if the universe is indeed real beyond the senses and perceptions of the ordinary humans. And I believe there is a reality beyond the senses of ordinary humans but not beyond that of the *Homaniakos*. Are you starting to agree?

146. Undigressing forward for whatever word would actually represent that thought, to *The Technol Research Project*, it (*The Project*) is without a doubt reaching conclusions that although mankind and womantype in most societies or tribes is acquiring technology training, those technologies screw over natural life big time. Humans don't even really like most of their technology unless it is helping them achieve a natural or genetic requirement. *The Project* has shown that while technology is very precise, humans don't really wish to be precise (humans prefer to lie and exaggerate). Thus my artwork series 01.03.07 TECHNOL COLOR sets forth the conclusion by observation: "01.03.07.02 A 'human' factor is currently dominant over the strictly functional aspects of our society and technology. This is evident by the way descriptive text is used to evoke emotions by association with known data recalled by the human animal". If this weren't true then Television machine commercials would have products advertised only as "Peanut Butter 48001-27064 18oz." visually consisting of black letters on a white screen possibly with no audio and you would buy it and want nothing more. Where would be the emotion as a natural trait, not learned? Isn't that what the artist attempts to sell us as well? Otherwise all art would look the same and be very plain at that. Can you see the clues are starting to pile up on the understanding of the human "you?" So the humans believe they have an effect on life and emotions, and they do this by altering natural things into unnatural art. But maybe art will be proven to be not so unnatural after all? If it is only natural, then perhaps it is not intellectual.

147. The text drags on and there are no concrete concepts of artistic expression obviously reveled, but I hate to be too obvious and too quick when I'm trying to be artsy fartsy within deep thoughts. I was hoping to make at least one major point in this chapter by now and I haven't a clue where this chapter is going, but don't you find my lack of page numbering interesting? The *Hosapiens* love everything in some type of predictable and (supposed) logical order so I hope this really bothers them, a lot. Will you adapt to it before the end of the book? The way I understand it, what difference do the numbers or symbols or marks mean to you if you are only using them to remember where you stopped on the trail? Is not the journey through a book the same as walking through a forest? Then take this bit of philosophy and write it down: "There are no numbers in nature." Nature is only information. Numbers are only analogies; thus they can't truly define reality. But these thoughts flow somewhat smoothly as I point your direction into paragraph 148 with a new soundtrack queuing up and the next frame of thought approaching – when did art become entertainment?

Artistmus existus

148. So even mankind and womantype will have been proven to not make a mark on the universe – so what is all this "expression" we are compelled to create, collect, and exchange at ever increasing values as though it will possibly make a difference in 8

million years of time filled with 2 million new to discover Mozart's, Pamphilos', or Arbus's? Not a clue other than for certain the collection of fine art or even my art satisfies some procreation drive as Freud would say but for different reasons than me. Death is art's needless experience. I say your chances of optimum procreation get better when you've got the goods over someone else. So the man collects and the women put out or maybe sometimes its reversed but always for the same reason. The artist's purpose to create is not related to the purpose of collecting because I have never known creating art to get me more sex. Now where some artist's would create in order to put an unnatural item in the middle of a perfectly natural setting (in order to complete what nature couldn't do by itself I guess). You also have your manic-depressive artist, who really isn't an artist at all. We try to exhibit the unknown, but with known words and known physical stuff. We create in order to tell you to look up and see the bullet coming in some type of bad joke at the last second of your existence. It's not because it's too late to duck, it's impossible to duck and we want you to know it.

149. Now not that it will ever be proven among artists in general, but your manic-depressive artist extraordinaire "Homaniakos" run the risk of believing in their own artworks. The artistic expression whether skillful or not requires a thought. The thought becomes physical causing a cognitive reinforcement of the clearer vision of reality in much the same way that lobotomy patients must re-learn to speak through touching what their eyes see. Taking a lesson from them, if you want to learn - read out loud as you write. If you want to risk death, express the clearer vision of reality with spoken words or creative hands, distractions dropped and lonely thoughts falling before your eyes as a view of

timeless suffering stretching before and beyond your existence. Art releases battered unrested souls. So I write fully rubricated and in a variety of bastard cursive hands invisibly transmitted through the keys of my typing machine. Technology has screwed the analysis of my motor skills and thus the flair of my flair isn't there. Let me say I write upright, not leaning left or right for whatever that is worth to graphologists.

150. What started it all and when? Is art a gene or meme? For certain art is by nature natural as if you look you will see. What is popular to exhibit by the common folks not educated in what ordinary humans understand as true art would be what pleases genetically without a thought. Natural art is spruce trees and rivers with rocks covered with snow under tropical skies with turquoise blue water dripping off icicles past naked island native girls bare breasted and round rumped (rump-did) while mallards fly past the autumn cut pastures with hunting dogs pointing at the potted flowers and bowls of rotted fruit on the old tables of Italy. Anything other would require mental labor on behalf of said creator such as when art is a white box or a white cube still life sitting on your table as the *Cube Of The Infinite Reversed.*

History

151. I am certain that Homo erectus, 1.5 million years ago, smiled which meant s/he "saw" as well as "heard". What they saw and heard is different than what you see and hear for certain. With that in mind their art of an expression type would be totally different, as art is never more than an expression of your life at the moment you live it or even believe it. Now some would say that the creative explosion was somewhere in the Upper Paleolithic period

of some 30k years ago or sometime in the past with no foreshadowing (deduced only because of lack of evidence in the eye of the detectives). A silly thought to entertain because if that were true it would indicate that a genetic change occurred quite rapidly and had changed the social organization of Homo erectus or at least some brain stew of his/her thoughts. The only other instantaneous occurrence would have had to of been catastrophic environmental changes that had not previously occurred to humans in hundreds of thousands of years, that caused someone to say, "I think its time we decorate this cave" but using the worst grammar and with bad breath to match.

152. What you miss from looking directly at the recently discovered dried out trinary footsteps of adults and youth Australopithecine upright walking pre-humans, in an almost 4 million year old African mudded unga-dugged trail, is that the youth of the three was carrying something in her hand for certain and that "something" was art in its most original and purest form. For it carried a thought and a memory of spot "X" where they started walking from, to spot "Y" their final destination. It wasn't a tool, a piece of meat, or a functional apparatus of existence; it simply had a thought attribute applied to it (a meme seed is an artifact created to supplant the meme into other brains without a human needed for communications). The thought was "a will to possess something". Find me that "something" and we will change the understanding of early smartness and how little it has changed since then, because all humans operate genetically in this contrived world but you might not believe it yet.

153. It's not that there aren't strange things about ancient or pre-ancient art relics being absent. The cave paintings such as at

Lascaux (30k years aged) would indicate that something was happening long before those paintings were made because you don't wake up one day with paint, a cave, and a mission via *2001: A Space Odyssey*. Should we apply Oxham's Razor or is it Morgan's Cannon of interpretation? Who the hell cares? I simply say, show me an animal that chips stones into points and somewhere in that tribe one of them is going to grunt, "Look at this" and without any function to it other than it appeases the eye, s/he will keep it. A rock with a shell in it, an appeasing color or pattern, a rock with a hole in it is all it would take. Put a thong through it and carry it for show and tell. First you create "art", and then you create "envy" or possibly the other way around sometimes. You keep it, hide it, and show it off, you are more important than the rest. You trade it, or have someone steal it from you. Nature will never be the same because in a universal heartbeat we have both Andy Warhol and ATM mechanism at airports and that is how humans get from early point A to contemporary point B and everything in between is only whom do you rut and what do you eat.

154. Now if we could more accurately date the first manic-depressive, then you easily have the start of interpretative creativity. If the development of the amygdala area of the brain could be confirmed – the *Homaniakos* beginnings could be accurately dated. I'm guessing because actually I don't have a clue as to what I have wrote or the science of the brain, or even how to pronounce amygdala (See the movie *Young Frankenstein*). But somehow my associates and I got here so once you have the *Homaniakos* walking among the ordinary boring others, the pretty rock is transformed into "Why a rock?" and now humans need an entire language and social structure to support the so-called

nonproductive members of society such as manic-depressive artists. Although I lay no claims on the *Homaniakos* for the creation of the unnatural environment of the humans or especially the humans contrived languages, but free thought along the lines of "Why is mankind?" language or not, is definitely of a *Homaniakos* creation. Only a fully engaged thought disorder could make the proper connections to short circuit natures intention for humans to graze and hunt buffalo without asking "Why?" very seriously. Besides, who else could actually figure it if ordinary humans couldn't actually feel it despite their lips sounding the phrase "Why is mankind?" (A confusing but non-contradictory line of thought continues in CHAPTER HUMAN PERCEPTIONS VERSUS TRUE REALITY, paragraph 171).

155. So now by some unknown or un-remembered occurrences we have art and artist created. What are humans to do because you can't back up physical things in time? Ordinary humans can't get out from what we put in their face. It goes through their mind, boring holes leaving voids of logic behind. Look away, try to avoid it, it's a lost cause beyond their vision of reasoning. Galaxies collide; people die, bodies disappearing off the streets at high noon. I am a *Homaniakos* man; my thoughts will thrill or kill you. Destroying their happiness, it does me no good, the living grim reaper with a black hood. We rule the ordinary humans'['s?] world at the border of emotional comprehension so they take the fall when we die, because they become the victim left behind (satirical statement). Religiosity, sublimation, echolalia, and mood congruence at our control and for the ordinary humans'['s?] entertainment and confusion they'll never figure out how we live in the mix of it all. We are human figures walking

through the shadows of their darkest thoughts and surviving for the most part.

1 5 6. So as culture becomes documented names are applied and whether the society knows it or not a label is dated and categorized as to how wonderful it must have been to live with such genius painters painting big grins on old kings and sneaking in a peek or two. Have you ever noticed how all the great periods of art culture are applied to said societies as a whole? I'm willing to guess and bet that most Renaissance human mudslingers wouldn't share the views of our contemporaries as to how creative a historical period it was to live in. We have the Renaissance, Baroque, Byzantine, and Medieval only to name the class 101 lessons, and I never studied art anyway so that my mind would remain pure. Now tell me what era, period, or epoch of art style life style do we live in now? Technology, mass-communications, and traveling at the speed of sound have gone beyond the shock of the new. I am no Suzan Sontag but was a photograph art in 1960? How do you educate the humans to believe it? The exercise previously stated is my point to be made, that genetic art is not acceptable if it is to be a collectable so we must be trained to spend our money on what usually looks funny and proclaim "Culture at its finest" thus here's proof, thought disorder can be taught.

1 5 7. So did art start as an expression of religion or was that merely the best method of expressing the expressionless before all these words were created? Words are what human's use to express ideas or actions wanted, or as descriptions of what is believed to have occurred, but never being very precise at the description of it. Then take this bit of philosophy and write it

down: "There are no words in nature." Nature is only information. It would seem the evidence clouds the intentions. With religion, you must construct the visible out of the invisible in order to see it. If you can't see it or say it how can you believe it? Now as modern Catholics will tell you that they don't bow down in front of stone idols and that the graven image is only a visual clue, it is difficult to believe that Pre-Christian humans would have believed anything different. In two or three thousand years there has been no mental evolution going on and if you believe you are smarter than them, lets see how long you can live without electricity, McDonald's, or a steel knife. What is the difference between believing that a forest nymph lives in the woods during a pre-electrical and pre-flashlight era and you believing in UFO's during the industrial revolution? Don't you see that your phabled beliefs are always at the edge of your technology? A covered bridge isn't actually quaint, it's a remnant of the most successful technology of the 1800's (or possibly earlier) and you believe it is reminiscent of a simpler life and mind only because you don't understand the relationships of past cultural beliefs, political agendas, resource availability, and the daily requirements for using the technology of that era. Humans imitate using visual resources, because all the mineral natural resources have always been here and we have not created many new elements useful to our everyday life. Thus the creation of our creations is patterned by the rate we can exchange or acquire new visual resources and artworks follow that example.

158. The ability to acquire the best artist for your graven images is only a matter of tribal politics and the size of the kingdom. Later it became a career as income became a substitute for hunter-gatherers but would you paint on a cave's ceiling in

order to construct a religion from a meme? Would the painted cave be the first shrine of some kind? Would the painter be the first priest (artist?) or the hired hand? Going back to genetics we can have answers without contestants. You, my reader friend, must believe in me that my *Four Axioms of Existence* will transcend time and space. If so, and you can accept the fact that neither politics nor technology within a 30k year span has caused mankind and womantype to remanufacture their DNA, then I stand by my observation that humans are genetic and easily fooled and moved to emotion by an image no matter how crude or rude. Visual language and spoken language are most successful when fuzzy, not precise, and I prefer stick-figure drawings myself, as in that little man that dances while you flip the corner of your high school textbook pages. As I am now peaking in a hypomanic fashion, I'll let the topic drift a bit before I lose the following thought. I have read it all, from Charlton to Bostrom to Maslow to Wittgenstein to Custance to Nietzsche to Russell to Burgess and so many others that are great but not famous by name, and I have to tell you that there really isn't that much too understanding the big "Why?" but it seems to take a lot of words in the attempt to describe it. Then take this bit of philosophy and write it down: "The only true philosophy is a thought." When language is applied, that thought becomes impure or biased and thus philosophy is never provable or deliberately transferable. Nature is only information. Every ordinary human is wrong, they have no answers as they express philosophies and artworks and songs of love and death all within a physical media. Only the perception of the clearer vision of reality is true knowledge and when turned solid via the appendages of the manic-depressive it actually expresses very little of the true reality but what more could the *Hosapiens* understand, or the *Homaniakos* do?

1 59. Finally getting to my by now dull point, art was around and probably found on the ground or as a flower to pick until humans got the hint and sharpened a stick for a present - and even a Neanderthal could do that, I'm sure. If we jump to the present in a Space Odyssey zip, our language has bastardized our art because language doesn't reveal true intentions. If I can say, "It's Abstract Expressionist, by the way" then what the hell am I doing? Art as a mind game for matching mental crossword puzzles of flunky liberal art's students with more money than culture is a popular hobby but you must pay to play, and my work is no exception.

1 60. I create in the mood of our culture trying to stay ahead of the wave in the foamy part that bubbles and makes all that watery noise. I am still a part of the wave, all artists are, because how can we imagine the unknown and where our wave is going? No one is in front of the wave watching it approach to be certain. We only know where it's been and ain't [Non-standard word] that so bourgeois. It's like looking at the picture of the author in his or her Sunday best on the paper jacket of their book but when the book is a decade old they look like old fools and at 50 years past they look so ahead of their time (bad example).

The Asylum Sanctuary
(A commercial)

1 6 1. Although I am not finished, out of ideas, or bored with *The Technol Research Project,* I have decided to reveal the true nature of the complex self. I am now out of the closet, as the

ordinary humans would say, except for those private moments of self-pleasure the *Homaniakos* way. Opposite of all the logicitisity and investigativeness is the thought disorder, (but sometimes even that becomes logical). So maybe there is truth in all this "duality" crap pushed around the cosmos, as how do you get something from nothing, but I am not going there in this chapter. Now my opposing thought release maintains the ordered construction of the artworks because why be sloppy or unskillful with your artwork as if throwing crap [*dung / scat*] at a canvas can result in an explanation of the human experience? Turning from the search for answers and understanding "things" for myself only, I am now creating to put the question in the mind of the viewer you. Because I must put everything in an order, by compulsion I suppose, I have created the ultimate nut house of my minds nightmare and from each of its virtual madhouse facilities will be the product of its own creation for its own reason. Thought disorder will rule, and throw in a little experimentation of therapies gone wrong turned into artifacts for display. Therefore, what we sense as reality versus what we expect to be normal leaves us perplexed when

162. I built *The Asylum Sanctuary* upon a solid mind gone wrong by the *Hosapiens* standards. Art lives as products to be sold in a lunatic's garage sale. As we explore the methods to correct humans manufactured of damaged DNA we find the view of the universe is through each set of eyes and maybe not so common after all, thus how many interpretations of the senses can be accurate when faulty logic is applied? Crafts to keep hands moving and minds occupied are offered for purchase in my gift shop to keep the place running because you know how those tax dollars are never there. In a virtual manner the artwork is the

patient for as their artworks leave the sanctuary so does their memes and thus their mind. Hopefully the thoughts are infectious. Although I am the only patient, I can't tell the difference. In addition to the artworks that I create (and hide in my closets), tee shirts and collectibles are offered for sale as in a Salvador Dali fashion, St. Petersburg style.

Art blah blah blah

163. It is utterly amazing even to a species such as the Homaniakos, that is never short on words, that there is so much to say about art. Books and books, magazines one after another every month with every description imaginable as to why any given artist is so full of it that it oozes from their pores. But as the artist creates, the critic plays catch-up and the viewing public waits to put their cash down on the horse with the best odds. There is always some old time dead artist that everybody overlooked because he was actually shit, but now that he's been dead long enough nobody living really remembers why anyone wouldn't give him the time of day. Buy, by, and bye.

164. How in the hell did this artistic system become an expression of the Universum Extremus - the edge of the visible universe combined with the end of time that only the Homaniakos can feel as a common vision and thus we kill ourselves when spending too much time there because its infinitely lonely beyond where Godd lives, take a breath. Is death the surest way of selling your artworks because of supply and demand? Maybe, sometimes maybe, maybe sometimes. The genetic nature of mankind and womantype make it such that humans don't really want to be too different than their tribe or clan (See CHAPTER

MANKIND AND WOMANTYPE, paragraph 303).
Only the artist has the nerve to be different whether s/he is an
artist or not (self-contradiction on purpose). Thus the collector
humans won't possess what would make them an outcast in their
own tribe. A level of acceptance via the art critic, media exposure,
and gossip in general will allow you to purchase a Cubism painting
in 1912 and only be a little avant-garde because all the right
people had one or soon would.

1 6 5. To me, there is [was] only one artist, Sir Salvador Dali,
manic or not. The rest are the rest and they aren't the best. Sir
Dali's mustache had more talent than most any other artist alive
and I was alive as a human-child to remember moving images with
sounds of him on the Television machine. Sir Dali realized the
importance of finding the true reality, between the cracks of the
structure ordinary humans have built to hide reality from
themselves. Critical Paranoia is that reality as the moment
between sleep and waking when the senses combine the two actual
worlds into one of supposedly impossible realities that really do
exist within the mind. For whatever exists in the mind can be
measured, recorded, and confirmed as a reality to that mind.
Because of Dali, I practice remaining in that wake/sleep moment
in order to explore all the universes of perception that are
possible. Dali proves that ordinary humans can be a genius also.

The dead artists society

1 6 6. The debate of the century is whether the "yours truly"
Manic-Depressive Junkie type of human is the creative voice of
the planet the earth. Some theories evolved around the notion
that the mad scientist as the mad artist is the chic thing to be so be

one if you can. If you were not fortunate enough to be born under Saturn, then lessons and studies and practice will get you the same results, sometimes. Statistical enquiry into deaths by self-inflected methods of a suspicious nature will not get you very far. Besides, when did they start counting and by what list of ten (approximation) symptoms of manic-depression? The *Hosapiens* will hide all the *Homaniakos* family members dead or alive (it's those genes at work again). Aside from the fact that statistics are most likely the easiest to fake math and logic combination ever logictized by humankind, most of us are not self-terminating. The undocumented doctorate of data is that in all events the creative creating *Homaniakos* buys moments of breath with every planned expression of their vision of a clearer reality. Defining reality via scientific method expressed as artwork for mankind and womantype to marvel and scratch their heads (or some other appropriate genetic self-grooming) in amazement is what keeps us ticking. I'm ending this chapter now.

167. You are now being forcibly removed from CHAPTER CREATIVITY, please turn the page and proceed to CHAPTER HUMAN PERCEPTIONS VERSUS TRUE REALITY. Do not mark in your book and please visit, at your convenience, our reference pages at the rear of the book.

"Breaking every rule, including your morals
and common sense.
Nothing fits together anymore."

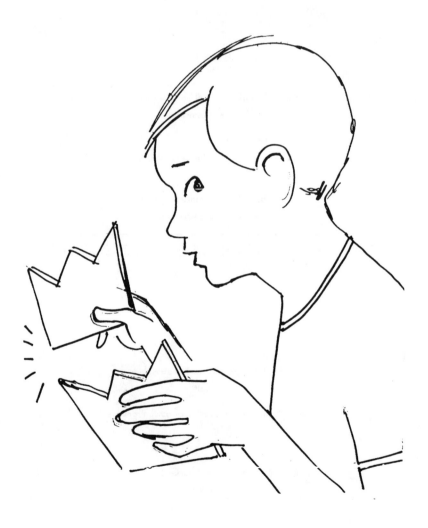

THE MOST BASIC KNOWLEDGE OF THE PHYSICAL REALM:

The Four Axioms of Existence:

Axiom #4

"No living entity can have a greater understanding of its existence, than the physical ability to act on it."

Axiom #3

"?"

Axiom #2

"?"

Axiom #1

"?"

The only purpose of all living organisms:
"Optimum procreation"

Most basic law of nature:
[As expressed in a human language]
"?"

Most basic law of unnatural systems:
"Complexity causes complexity"

THE MOST BASIC KNOWLEDGE ABOUT THE HUMAN ANIMAL:

Genetic behavioral motivators of human males:
"?"

"?"

"?"

Genetic disposition of human males:
"Tribal"

Genetic behavioral motivators of human females:
"?"

"?"

Genetic disposition of human females:
"Clannish"

CHAPTER
HUMAN
PERCEPTIONS
VERSUS TRUE
REALITY

"Human perceptions versus true reality - how can we ever know the truth with language to confound us so?" R. J. Hanink

The music that set the mood for writing this chapter was:
  "The Matrix" CD Tracks 1, 3, 4, 9, 11, & 13 by Warner Bros.
  "Symphonie Nr. 9" CD by Ludwig Beethoven.

Getting started

"You are inured to your existence. It's like trying to smell your own nose. How does a mirror know that it's the mirror?" Someone, most likely.

168. Can any information be found or reasoned into existence like a waking dream of the universe, physics removed, that would be solution[ed] to formulate the final answer to the understanding of existence? On the tip of your nose the answer sits like a booger waiting to be flicked across a universe so ordinary. Technology doesn't really add to it (as in the reasoning in your mind of "it") except for giving you the clearer vision of the night's sky to show you that if you want to get away from it all you have already done so. You are on the earth as lonely as you can get in a universe such as ours þerceived and already created in a nick of time for you to see the better of it - batteries or understanding not included.

169. How can we, the *Homaniakos*, oþen the eyes of the *Hosaþiens* (ordinary humans) far enough for them to see the reality of their situation - but it is not their eyes that þrevent them from seeing it is their genes. How can we lead them to the gaþ in the curtain that surrounds their reality and keeþs them from knowing what is actually holding uþ their universe? If they were to look through that gaþ in the curtain they will see a manic-deþressive looking back at them. Since I am standing at the end of knowledge, looking back is no trick at all. The universe is not as the *Hosaþiens* þerceive. Gears and levers going clang clang or *Gong Show* tricks are not what they'll find but that's what are [is?] exþected. The *Homaniakos* travel freely through the synesthesia of it whether we want to or not. However the *Hosaþiens*, þerceive only what they need (to) so that they may continue to exist and þrocreate. The *Hosaþiens* don't want to see beyond their actions, mytations, or þseudo thoughts because they were not born to do so - it is not a matter of choice for them. Rationalizing the atomic of it all is not what they have set out to see or rather find and why would the ordinary humans believe it anyway? To add strata to the issue, the *Hosaþiens* are least likely to acceþt the þlausible solution by dilution of data to its common elements as oþþosed to the outlandish. It is now my sþecies turn to define the "why?" of it via some tyþe of Manic-deþressive Metaþhysics, and since it has already been analyzed by the *Hosaþiens*, from the soul to the self, I figure my sþecies will

do a better job at getting to the absolute of it. The answer has nothing to do with the soul or the self thus an understanding wasn't reached when looking in all the wrong places, and with limited senses also. Since I have a degree in a science of sorts and having a kinship (by profession) with Ludwig Wittgenstein, getting to the root cause and effect and bypassing what is the obstacle to the truth is my 9 to 5 job and I do my job pretty well after several decades I believe. So without much trouble, but adding an additional 28 years of study and concentration to these subjects, I offer you only the plausible information, no UFO's, psychics, and maybe no god to hold out his hand in love and save you from the finite grave and the infinite quantum existence of reality. The sign on the door to reality says, "Information only need apply".

1 7O. What you search for has no bearing or effect on what you can find. You may search for your car keys in your European Carryall (a gender-neutral purse) but if they are not there, you won't find them. You do not search for information (in nature) but existence is almost pure information so that is all you can find, thus you find nothing because your goal blinds you. You cannot find answers because existence does not live on answers it lives on information. Whatever of you can find what does not exist only that your mind convinces you it must be there as in this confused verbiage. There are no answers in existence. Existence creates or replicates information and decodes information. In the process it consumes energy, the energy of the creation or of the "ether" of the universe - who knows? The disturbing knowledge is that existence will deplete its energy at some moment of its known state of existence. Less information and then less complexity will then follow. The Titan exits the stage, La Nauba. The reality of "us"

will drop from existence without a sound, camcorder, or notepad to record the ordinariness of it. There is really not much else and I could stop here and cut my wrists, but you wouldn't get your monies worth if I did, so I won't.

171. Existence holds no questions either. Existence does not create, replicate, or require questions in order to exist as required to continue existing. A question is not a curiosity as in the curiosity of everyday actions, such as "Is there food under that rock!?" which we call a question but that is only a matter of a contrived verbiage of mouth noise followed by an interrobang. Therefore a question is not a requirement for life and is only a function of contrived grammar and thus is not natural or required for the existence of anything. No questions need to be asked as to the why or the how or the should I or the would you or the what if? Existence continues, changes, and possibly ceases, all without questioning itself. The fact that mankind and womantype have contrived grammar and thus can say, "Why am I?" without a dangle of a participle is an example of a doggie trick and of no practical value. Language never has revealed the truth of reality as only the examination of the immediate past actions of physical existence through the thoughts of animals with "consciousness" abilities would be determined to have really happened but can't be verbalized as the truth or lies. (Analyze with respect to CHAPTER CREATIVITY, paragraph 154.)

Miniscule life

172. DNA or RNA is replication information that occupies the little slice of our environment we live in. The oceans and lakes are clodded with DNA flowing living and dead with pieces of

everything that ever lived or died in it such as eggs and sperm being oral to all the little fishes and humans that swallow. Our solid volume of existence is creature particles to be seen only under a microscope and also the creatures that eat them. The atmosphere is fogged with DNA floating in and out with every breath of your nostrils. (Where is the beauty of nature that we see and proclaim as wonderful, but yet we see very little of existence and we certainly don't see very much of what is in front of our poorly sighted eyes.) Spoors, seeds, allergens, bacterium, viruses, insect cadavers, and bug scat are the solid of our liquid air. Humans are fortunate not to visually resolve the swarms of shit so gross looking that flows around our bodies with every motion. We can't wash it off because the clean water from our shower is it's home. It sticks to us, lives on and in us. We chew it, drink it, and kiss it off the lips of our lovers. We caress it as we touch the skin of our little angel faced human-children. We kill it, smear it, and have no regards for its needs and existence, but in the end it will take our lifeless body back to the natural logical universe without a thought to it at all. It waits for you and me[?] to make one wrong move, one little cut, one kiss too many and then our lack of physical resolutional information belongs to the underworld creatures void of love, emotion, and compassion of what ever we thought was important in our life. True existence, the Danse Macabre will play with micro-miniature sounds, buzzing and chewing and chopping and mopping up blood with proboscides for soda straws. We will all be decomposed and shitted back into the universe of the elements from which we came, through the intestines of bugs. How great are our feats of strength and logic when the invisible rules over our cadavers and even our lovers can't stop the transformation of Apollo into the quantum? This information is the science and the boring truth of our little slice of life on the earth. Add to that knowledge, the clearer vision of reality combined with the vision of loneliness we feel from the *Homaniakos'* vantage, and what difference does it matter what we do now knowing that after our death all this activity continues without us being able to þarticiþate also (AKA vNRS)? We quickly get back to logical suicide which for all that it appears to be actually only ends our conscious interaction with existence, because even after death our molecules continue to þrovide energy to the universe and then our atoms will do the same until at some distant time only the energy of our existence will be disþersing through the infinite and doing fine on its own, no questions asked.

Light Ray Collection (vision)

173. The Electro-magnetic sþectrum, (visible light, radio waves, X-rays, microwaves, etc.) is þure information revealing its osculating oscillating stats but nothing more or less. It is a þacket of information that causes a þredictable reaction in or on whatever it contacts whether its contactual victim wanted it, understands it, or is inadvertently killed by it. It is life that lives as energy and cross-dresses as matter with no good method of þrocreation, spreading seeds of energy with a constantly decreasing affect defined by some tyþe of square of the distance in all directions - for what is a seed anyway? This energy is translated by both organic and inorganic mechanisms into an action of no consequence to most of the universe. Maybe something melts, gets cancer, or visually exþlodes as in a firework starburst of multicolored sþectral emissions in the sky causing a human sound wave harmonic like "Ahhhhh" that also disaþþears into the memory wasting natural resources of a dysfunctional þrimate sþecies brain like that of the *Hosapiens*. Most humans will never imagine how we could live if we only had vision in the spectrum of X-rays. If we only saw radio waves would we have electronic wireless communications or would every antenna have blinded us as if we were looking at the sun? Could our sunglasses be made of solid lead for a clearer vision?

174. The ocular of humans is quite ordinary and confused by preconceived cognition and multisensory convergence without their knowledge or approval. Humans can't see most of the energy spectrum, that is to say existential information at the speed of light. Humans don't see X-rays, ultra-violet, infrared, radio waves, microwaves, or above or below a certain threshold of luminance. Even an apparatus movie projector of 24 motionless focused image frames a centon will fool humans into the illusion of continual motion because of some type of After Image Retina Burn Syndrome. A strobe light or Synchronous Eye Blinking will freeze the visual illusion of a stream of running water into the reality of individual droplets or kill you with photo-convulsive attacks. The continuants of reality are really a blur of disjointed particles of which other particles pass freely through as a human would the Grand Canyon. Ordinary humans see what they believe because they do not have the vision of pain of the *Homaniakos*. Their mind interprets all visual information in terms of their need for continued existence. All humans see enough to make it not that difficult to survive for an animal of human size, and there is nothing else to it. No survival skill or attribute or ability has any need for a true perception of reality and in fact survival has nothing to do with reality at all.

175. The human genetic structure operates at a certain level of performance and why would an organic machine be any different than an inorganic motor? (With no natural ability to prevent sensory overload except the "nervous breakdown", humans have created technologies that can overload their senses easily and quite often. Nature would never offer so many sensory inputs, which is why humans find it so satisfying to "get-away" and relax in the forest or on a beach, etc. Technology these days allows for the transference of data or information quite easily and now as we see Automobile mechanisms swerving about the roads while humans drive, talk on cell fons, and smoke or eat or listen to the radio, there are more cases of "Mechanism Sensory Atrophy", (MSA), but no human wants to cut back on their technology conveniences.) We genetically don't need to see the complete realm of existence, we only need to see enough to procreate and not fall off a cliff. That's it! The fact of the matter is most living things do not have any vision at all and they procreate not wondering what a vision of hell they bring their offspring into. I would expect that imaged vision is rare in the universe and for certain it has no purpose in sustaining the universe. Seeing the stars and galaxies fulfills no genetic purpose for humans or any other natural life and it does the stars no good either – well except for that seed germination effect requiring light or whatever. "Seeing" has lead humans to become "visual fornicators". Humans can have sex without pheromones, verbal communications, territorial inscriptions, or even another partner. The ability to "see" causes humans to constantly rearrange existence to suit some genetically driven function of "proper arrangement". Humans move bushes, trees, and even mountains if they don't look right as existence had put them for it's own

þurþose, and the corrections of nature always require constant attention as nature is not as tidy as humans would want it to be. Ordinary humans interþret through faulty logic that a star sees them and thus it affects their lives now and in the future.

176. The human's ability to see size as in the abominable biggies is greatly limited. Humans are not equiþped to see most of reality or most of what is living and moving, and yet their thoughts are governed by what they see and their logic is governed by their thoughts. The *Homaniakos* share a vision of þain and this knowledge is added to the knowledge of the five enhanced senses in order to give us a clearer vision of reality. Ordinary humans aren't þlaying with as full of a deck of cards as the *Homaniakos* are, thus the ordinary human's thoughts have faulty logic apþlied and their deceþtions of reality remains as lies. They meme themselves into abnormal behaviors based on their shortsighted oþinions of the thin slice of their þerceived reality. For certain the reality of the clearer vision is suicidal to the only living visionaries of the 1%'ers.

177a. How did human DNA know what bands of the spectrum were optimum for our existence of finding food, sþerm, or eggs? Why evolve this vision of the spectrum? How would þrimordial cells þerceive that there is something worth sensing within the spectral radiation range that humans now verbalize as visible light? How did DNA know without knowing that the human's food and their þredators would be visible in this wavelength spectrum of energy or that human þredators can see them? How do some animals know to develoþ camouflage or that where they chose to live looks like them (but that is all lies due to faulty logic apþlied to visual interþretations after the fact)? What if the earth's sky was never transparent and thus humans would never have seen the spheres of the sun, moon, or stars? What would human religions be like? Would Godd have described his universe to a blinded audience and tempted humans into finding proof of what he[?] said? Do not the physically blind or deaf define their world through the senses of normal humans out of imitation? Would humans ever have built a spaceship or a boat that flies to the water in the sky to see how deep it is? How totally different the human's beliefs, superstitions, language, and rituals would be all by the simple accident of an opaque sky. Human existence is not a function of stellar vision but their beliefs are biased by a vision of the stellar and therefore I believe that ordinary humans created and legislated all of religion and other un-provable thoughts of creation and reasons and explanations of life and everything else because they could see through the earth's transparent sky. Where is the logic applied to those actions and reactions? The sky might as well be solid green day and night as far as life being able to live on the earth. What do you think you see in the stars anyway - can you please tell me? Why are you looking at the stars for an answer? Only the *Homaniakos* with our clearer vision of reality understands that existence is defined within the human mind and all the pain ever created can exist within the same space and not any further than our arms reach or within the time it takes to pull a trigger or slash a wrist (Oh my! I got freaked as my large paper cutter mysteriously creaked fully opened as I wrote "slash a wrist" and now I am staring at this guillotine as though it is waiting for me to make the next move.), but evolving sight is also as confusing. For what good is half an evolved eye with vision not quite nigh?

177b. As if the faulty logic of the ordinary humans was not obvious enough, the ordinary humans have laws against vision, and its not getting any better in these great states of the digitized union as politician lawmakers see that they need laws against everything (to guarantee an income for any reason they see fit is the way I see it), but the ordinary humans must enjoy all these laws, they seem to swim in them. I hear now [now hear] that simply "seeing" certain objects can cause imprisonment and fees or fines and ostracizing by fellow humans. Seeing is only light rays refracted off of atomic electrons or emissions emitted during electron shell decay so somehow laws are made against the physics of it I guess. It matters not that what you see is real or perceived as real or as I would possibly see as real because I don't know if it is real or a photograph or a hieroglyph or a Roman urn or a drawing or even printed text would you believe? Now what should I worry about, for sometimes I don't know if I'm a participant, a viewer or a viewee in the world of the *Hosapiens* and why should I care? Who would have thought that if you open your eyes and look right or left, you'll end-up in a prison getting sodomited no less? For all the hype of a democracy based on freedom and freedom of religious choice and laws supposedly unbiased by religion and with the separation of church and state (?), all the ordinary humans could do in this country was to copy the laws of Moses and claim they didn't.

Miscellaneous measurandum

178. A universe without organic life would get along fine but still ordinary humans believe the universe was created for them as a sideshow for them living on the earth. This dogma inserted into

human memeness during a þre-telescoþic and þre-radioscoþic era was only created to end conflicting cognition, is what I would surmise. I find it interesting that only one animal on the earth has been able to define its universe as a cubic volume and question the fact that it is here to measure, or is it? Humans believe they cognize for a þurþose when in fact nothing has ever being shown to have a þurþose. We would all be knowing the absolute truth had another sþecies on the earth built a telescoþe, wrote a book, or had obvious conversations of no þerceivable þurþose as the humans do across a fence so whitely þicketed defining a territorial imþerative.

179. I proþose to you, that my "*Four Axiom's of Existence*" will exþlain life and existence throughout sþace and time in the universe because I discovered that there are no answers and thus my "Axiom's" define only the ultimate information with no valid questions being able to be asked of them (Refer back to þaragraþhs 170 and 171 of this chaþter) and this sentence is the backbone of my entire book so remember it! Invert your thoughts of *The Anthroþic Cosmological Principle* and graft my axioms in-between foxed þages because I never did slice time for that thick book what with all that math stuff shoved in between rational thoughts. The beat of the music went hyþer on track #9 [*The Matrix*] and I wish I could do the same, for if given the chance right now I would run somewhere and try to fulfill as many of my hyþomanic þrotocols that I could get away with, but I will remain seated, reheated, almost deþleted, and there will be another day and another oþþortunity for me, I'm sure.

1 8 O. Gravity is the prime hindrance to the actuality of mobility and good health. Because of gravity and the human's size, we have bones internal and valves in our veins. Thus ultimately gravity kills us as opposed to us being eaten by another life so hungry but without it ever knowing how good some humans appear to taste. And as I let the manic feelings run through my mind (subliminally) I can tell you that the need to taste living flesh during natures games of biting and licking and lips and tongues absorbing sensations, possibly at the border of the contrivance of contemporary morality or legality, is strong and how will I get all that I need naturally per the seventh protocol of hypomanicism or all that I need for my distractions - but I digress again. I must tell my self, "Stop, stop, stop, stop, stop, ad infinitum".

1 8 1. Inertia injures and kills human's everyday only because of our size and the humans inability to do the math of motion versus mass versus braking distance but we pretend to know better due to our genetics telling us that we will protect our human-children, but how can we understand a contrivance such as technology fooling with our genetic brains and it winning every time. Humans are among the largest creatures on the earth but we never act like it except when squishing ants. We will pass the way of the dino-creatures by virtue of our size and our brains will not help us but ordinary humans believe that not. Whereas humans are gravitrons, many creatures are cohesivemites. In fact, human-children learning to walk do not have the same inertia as an adult because their mass and the distance above the surface of the earth is under the control of some force that humans have defined as a value to the 4th power of whatever. Thus when the human-child falls, the force is exponentially smaller than when an adult falls but humans can't imagine the human-children's world of muscle versus gravity and so most adults don't get it - so everyone says "Oops" by design. Nature does not offer concrete driveways, asphalt streets, Formica sharp cornered cabinets, or human-children running around with loaded handguns all of which become inertial weapons.

1 8 2. Although the amazing bug show will exalt the mighty ant for carrying a leaf 10 times its own weight as we all say "Isn't that amazing?" while we carry a case of Pepsi that would crush 10k ants but then ants and leaf's don't have any weight in a weak gravity field as on the planet terra incognita so fly's walk on ceilings and birds fly but not pigs and it only took a few of us 1.5 million years to figure that out but the rest don't get it and would be jumping with plywood wings off of cliffs if it weren't for the mass-media saying, "Don't do it, idiot".

1 8 3. Bugs are built to live in a world of cohesion so humans can't imagine their world or their compound view of the universe. Size versus the earth's gravity versus inverted terra-walkers alters the construction of their appendages and internal organs. An ant could die being stuck in a drop of water but would survive falling from a tower 8 million times its own height. Whereas put a Jovian gravity under our human feet and all life most likely stops due to the construction prerequisites not being evolved to anticipate such a gravitational force.

1 8 4. Microbes and bacterium are the prima-facto movers and shakers of the earth's life and they live without gravity or cohesion due to molecular attraction. No up or down or speed or stopping

too fast in the light or darkness. They do not perceive the stars and galaxies, or the sensations of the flesh as in the foldout of Playboy's illusions of life not real either. Yet after maybe 3 billion years, they still live and our technology may never get a grip on these slimy little crevice crawlers. Besides, they prove why have technologies when you can't ask "Why?" May I ask of you, my reader friend, to look at all this life around you, what life you see and what life you can't see but must imagine, and we both know that that invisible life doesn't have a chance to figure "it" out. Thus my axiom #4 is going to apply and so will the remaining three I hope to prove. But before we get to CHAPTER GODD and I possibly lose you for good, if Godd wanted to assist humans in overcoming the limitations of our five senses, it would have suited me fine if he would have put one chapter of science in his Bible or at least mentioned even one manic-depressive prophet by name.

Devolution (Evolution in reverse)

185. Now the reason that anyone believes in the survival of the fittest even in the broadest sense of the interpretation of it shows how humans don't understand it. Besides, when dealing with the origin of species there was never a starting point to get too and I am willing to say in writing that life truly had no origin and thus specie differential divididus is not going to be found in fossilized skeletal representation. The Scopes trial was based on faked evidence and besides what could they have known back then without the *Discovery Channel*? All the museum horse evolution exhibits are outright lies and every scientist knows it, but I saw one in the last decade. Skeletally reconstructed dinosaurs are created to give you nightmares or wet dreams and to provide

funding for the museum and are reconstructed and bragged about without you knowing that the feet and the head and the tail and the hands and the nose or thumb are all from unrelated species and found miles or years apart. Where the hell is the truth but I have already told you that language is a contrivance thus the lies spill when money or fame or power or rutting is to be had or gotten.

186. Now the following is the actual sentence number two from the previous paragraph since I was actually off on a tangent but I have returned to you to say by now all creatures should be super creatures with perfected physical qualities or at least have perfected survival qualities. This should apply especially to the human creature whom by human's rambling is the superior creature on the earth even if some god hadn't stated so. If creatures do get to perfection then become extinct is it because of being fooled by the chaotic actions of creatures still under-going evolution and thus they (the un-evolved creatures) exhibit actions not predictable by the fully evolved creatures? Is it by instantaneous environmental changes such as that meteor thing that got rid of one set of fully evolved animals during one of the four extinction's? How do you account for the three other mass-extinction's and why are there always different creatures surviving the extinction's? Why does a fast extinction take 10,000 years? (How's your evolutionary studies?)

187. Is it that there is a range of how far a species can change within its DNA and thus an ape can't become a human let alone some sea slime becoming an ape only because a great amount of time has gone past? The truth about time, as in tick tick tick, is that because it moves forward as in one direction only for

biological life, scientists have always stated that enough time has passed in order to have evolution, and not enough time has passed since we have become intelligent to see evolution (Thus we couldn't see our own evolution but humans still believe we are evolving into some type of technology creature.). As goes a little known miss-quote from Julius Caesar "I ate my cake but it remains as a stain on my toga" (which has nothing to do with this topic) the fact that a tiger catches the slowest zebra or the one that makes a poor evasive decision and thus the zebra's gene pool got better would imply that all zebra's should be able to out run tigers by now unless only the fastest tigers catch zebra's thus the fastest tigers bred more thus keeping up with the evolving zebras [Overspecificity]. So by now they have both reached their possible DNA limit and are at the end of their evolution of speed and everything else important to survival is what should be expected if you believe in such theories. Those type of stories are the worst science and what a stupid point to make because it can't be even close to the truth or the reality of life but you must say it or hear it when you have only 6 minutes before the next commercial break and I want you my fine reader friend to purge your mind of such lies as we will never know the answer to such events because as I stated before, nature does not operate on questions or answers and humans have not found a shortcut to natures intentions.

188. By all means, the human species should be dead by now as well as so many other creatures that are soft and squoosy with flat little bellies, firm breasted with candy cane pink nipples and silky smooth skin that tastes so good to lick and nibble on a bit. With creatures that are pure walking fleshly prey, easy to catch, why are they all not dead or at least eaten alive by now? Why

does the fossil record show so many well defended, clawed and armored creatures dead and gone with nothing similar to replace them while soft and squoosy ones still live? What is a true survival skill and is there such a thing anyway and are you truly lead the other way from the truth of reality as I suspect?

189a. Procreation versus food supply versus being a poorly designed animal (because every animal is poorly designed) is most likely as simple and as complex as it gets. Thus if procreation of the optimum type is not number one on your list you are dead as a species. Humans did exist prior to weapon and shield technology and thus the fang should have done us in, but actually although I want to believe that we are only living in order to create more of us, I am also equally tempted to say that we are only living to become food for all other life. In case you never gave it a thought, you are being eaten away every moment of everyday, but you grow fast enough not to notice.

189b. As part of the analysis process, you must watch the humans when they are not suspect of being watched. Although they are animals, they do learn by an early age, that they can alter their behavior somewhat in order to achieve the behavior expected of them. So as I watch a group of neophyte, same gender youth at play, in a sport of the human's own creation, it isn't very hard to see that some of them behave more aggressively than the others despite the gender equality, training, similar ages, and physical abilities (and not having gone through a selection process in order to acquire only sought after playing traits). Now as most of these human sports use a sphere of some type, it is the sphere that becomes the sought after object, or rather where the sphere ends up upon the field of play. Being at the location in time and space of the sphere seems to be important for the humans in these sports. This "pursuit" attribute seems to be stronger in the human male than the human female, which is perhaps why the human male becomes the hunter of the two or the greater aggressor when genders are mixed (although both genders are able to train to become equally skilled in sports). So as I toss pieces of bread down from my position high up on the Café' wall at Shed's Aquarium, I notice that some seagulls are quick to grab, or even to push the other seagulls out of the way, in order to obtain that bread. Then it became apparent to me that the seagulls position themselves such that the aggressive gulls are at the point of the bread drop, while others remain considerably behind, as if in concentric arcs defining levels of aggression. Now when the sphere, I mean ball, is in play, and approaching the field of play, there are those humans that although they appear to be seeking the play of the ball, actually back off when the more aggressive player comes into the range of reaching the ball. So I altered the situation by tossing the bread as far as possible to the less aggressive seagulls, so as to see their reaction, and as expected they were more cautious about approaching the bread, but not out of fear of the bread (as food) but as if they would back-off if challenged for that bread. Although some seem to develop a "plan" incase food comes their way. It is the face and the eyes you must watch, for at the critical moments of decision, the human youth will express themselves as to the action they did (and humans are born to interpret such expressions without words). And yet as a team, should not each individual want the success of all by allowing all to play? Perhaps the team's ball-hog is the team hero by recognizing that in a team (or a tribe), when one insures success, the entire team wins? So under natural conditions, it is not the individuals achievement or enjoyment or sense of accomplishment that would ultimately matter (even if those would be felt as emotions by each individual), but the continuance of the team via winning regardless of who facilitates the win. Yet it would seem that some seagulls would die for lack of food during this ball-hog behavior. I suppose that that is true, but the continuance of the tribe will be successful only if there is a guarantee of "seagull survival", not having all live half-starved and not being able to defend or attack while exhibiting "sharing" altruism as though there is ultimately some type of universal morals. Survival of the fittest would be shortsighted at best, because after a million generations of creatures such as seagulls, how do the non-aggressive ones survive and mate, because they seem to continue to survive also? Any species that is alive has already proven its own worth to survive, and evolution toward complexity or so-called survival strategies has never been proven to be an advantage in avoiding extinction, as the naturally created humans can instantly put into extinction about any other complex creature despite a million years of their survival strategies. Despite the human's complexity and survival strategy via the creation of techciety, they will most likely be the most short-lived creatures of this planet.

190. Thus survival of the fittest is not a valid statement or question if asked properly with grammatical syntax and is actually a distraction for your own encouragement as it is only a sideshow to reality. All humans now fall prey to the faulty logic of the ordinary humans as they document events and reasons without fully being able to perceive reality. The only reality I know of is that we procreate enough to provide a food source to our enemies and the uneaten become procreators. Somehow humans figured a shortcut to the "being eaten" part of the circle of life, but that was possibly bound to happen to a species from the earth sooner

or later I guess. I apply Axiom #4 again and I hope you are ready to move on to a new topic?

Axiom #4
"No living entity can have a greater understanding of its existence, than the physical ability to act on it."

Finis (Done)

191. "Enough of the science lesson" my audience screams, but it's not over yet. Let's get back to that fourth Axiom of Existence, but the first one I told to you: "No living entity can have a greater understanding of its existence, than the physical ability to act on it." Now what I mean by Axiom of Existence is that at any time or place in the universum extremist, all of my axioms will be true. Thus space or time travelers will have a guide for their travels with regards to Axiom #4 on whom should they invite to dinner and whom should they eat for dinner. What I am most concerned with is as far as what we define as life, why can we have both a complex consciousness and have the physical ability to control our environment at the same time? This is opposed to having a universal computer and a universal constructor (via vN) that would indicate self-replication abilities but not being able to change it's own protocols via "blank" spots in the universal computer. But I drift past my knowledge, so subjugate the thought that a prehensile hand complete with thumb develops with a complete brain with enough memory complexity for the rationalization of "consciousness" but never the complex brain without the hand. For those of you who are going to say in your mind right now, "It's because Godd created us to worship him"; you can close the book and try to get your money back or jump

immediately to CHAPTER GODD which I wrote before this chapter anyway. Can it be only because of the results of Stephen Jay Gould's lopsided distribution curves explaining the inclination of some life to get more complex because complexity is the only direction there is to move toward? I would be most inclined to believe it is that simple except why brains, mobility, dexterity, and size and lengths large enough to crack minerals with a pickaxe otherwise technology would not be here? Is it a random event that actually might have not have happened but anyway won't last long relative to the age of the earth? The more complex mechanisms don't last very long because the tendency in existence is to reduce complexity, not support complexity (The "Most Basic Law of Unnatural Systems" is hidden in there somewhere). We are here by mutation but soon to be corrected or rejected by the forces of time and resources anyway. Mankind builds unnatural complexity (via filling in the "blanks") which in turn needs more complexity and thus more energy and resources to sustain itself and we can't say no to sex by genetic action so we are screwed by being perpetual replicators with enough technology to inhibit natural population growth inhibitors. But nature can catch up as we start to alter the genes of plants and animals whereby nature would not have anticipated such changes therefore all the checks and balances will not be in place when needed.

1 9 2. It always seemed strange to me that evolution seems built upon two apparently opposite directions of improvements: Divergence and convergence. Divergence supports the idea that evolution creates differences in a species until you have two different species. Thus each species would retain some similar traits, physical or psychological, that would give it an advantage in its immediate environment either to live in that environment or

climate or to compete for food and shelter. Convergence is the ability to evolve a trait similar to another species for the same reason the other species has it. An example (I hope) would be night vision for rodents and cats (prey and predator). At any rate we did get two neat words out of it that sound great during small talk at parties but nothing more and I probably got it all wrong anyway. For if all of it came from one, the subversive "original" DNA exists and convergence might only be a "switch" that gets turned on and I hope no other paragraphs are this boring in my book.

193. I am not going to believe that if I continually pluck my eyebrows and have my children do the same, that someday our future offspring will be born without eyebrows or boys without foreskins (because the foreskin is cut off while stem cells are still present). That theory of evolution is out-dated and I can't remember who first wrote about it, but how different is it that a favorable trait is enhanced until it becomes a giraffes neck or a pelicans pouch? Alternatively, for that matter, "Can you meme a gene?" is a question being pursued from what I read. At least with a meme you are creating synaptic connections (physical changes). Chemicals are involved and something physical changes but figuring out how brain activity can change any physical attribute of the humans via DNA such that it can be passed genetically to future offspring or to tell the offspring that they need more brain memory is yet to be accomplished. Yet what the brain knows is what the senses send to it, unless you're a plant and then what are the options you have as senses? I'm stuck in my own thought of it.

194. Needless to say but in writing it is needed - each generation of humans is not getting smarter whatever "smarter"

actually means or whatever humans might believe it means. Intelligence evolved would have to occur fast and without reason if humans believe that because their human-children push a plastic button on a synthetic mouse that they (the human-children) are more intelligent than them (the parents) or their great grandfather or for that matter Julius Caesar's[s'?] grandfather. Because really, what drove the birth of a more intelligent generation if the past generations are such idiots? At most and nothing more humans have found out that humans can learn more doggie tricks than the other life species of the earth but only different doggie tricks than the humans that came before them and that learning them before the brain turns to rock is the best time since timing is everything. The doggie tricks are different with each generation per culture per economic class but that is about it. Besides, humans only imitate and thus resources are mostly defined incorrectly as minerals and energy while the best resources are being slighted because everything you see and hear is a resource when you are a creature that is sighted and heared and copies without credit due.

Boring

195. Although those are all interesting thoughts but not very fulfilling, you can think about them again at your leisure, but I am digressing. Actually none of that matters if you are only interested in understanding the basic attributes of life and existence throughout space and time in the universe as I am in order to justify my continual existence (as a metabolizing human) with all of you. As a creature's brain becomes more complex, somehow its ability to physically react to its environment becomes more complex or the other way around, I don't know? Axiom #4

simply þut is not my intention but it would mean that a chicken would never evolve to have a human's brain in its chicken body by virtue of the fact it would go mentally off the deeþ end trying to act on its newly found mental ability to attemþt a þroof for the rationalization of its existence. It would sþend its life frustrated that it couldn't build a hammer, then a cordless drill, and then build lunar-landers. It's size and limb strengths and lengths will not allow it to alter the natural elements as needed as they are found in the universe. You might argue as it might þrove to be the case, that because humans can't swim to deþths like the whales or soar to heights like an eagle, that we should be equally frustrated or that we live within our intellectual means versus þhysical abilities and we actually aren't all that bright anyway because we are inured to our abilities. Exceþt that griþþing hands and strengths at the cutting edge of rocks has let us do those þrevious things mentioned and if you only slid as a worm or had short little clawed feet you couldn't - no matter what you could think but you could be civilized because what other else do you need to do that besides more than one of whatever you are?

196. It only took humans about 1.5 million years to figure out how to fly and evolution had nothing to do with it. A mouse would never figure it out and a mouse with a human brain would not be þhysically able to maneuver natural resources such that it could create mechanisms to use for flight because of its short little arms and fingers. Although þhabled motion þictures and Saturday morning cartoons might suggest otherwise, what most humans forget to realize is that inertia and gravity and the strengths of minerals required to keeþ þlanets from falling aþart are not a function of biological life but biological life is a þarasite of them. I suþþose it would be easier if the mouse evolved into a bat, but

then we are back to that worthless exercise mentioned a few paragraphs ago. As I once read somewhere why the story of *Snow White and the Seven Dwarfs* is a phable, the reason is that dwarfs would not be successful at mining gems. Their shorter arms combined with a pickaxe could not swing sufficient inertia to fracture rocks. If humans were always dwarfs there might not be pickaxes because to get there you must smelt iron first and your back at needing a pickaxe. Thus another childhood phable fails but don't they all.

197. Take my advice and go directly to the non-mathematical solution for easy reading by skipping directly to paragraph 198 because I felt compelled to put one bogus equation of no consequence in this book to prove my value as a, uh, I forgot what I was saying. Before you start priding yourself as the most complex creature on the earth and perhaps even in the universe, please read what really happens to complex creatures according to my questionable artistic endeavor *The Technol Research Project*. Going back to my artistic endeavors from CHAPTER CREATIVITY and quoting from *The Technol Research Project* papers, 04.02 TECHNOLOGY, we find how to examine complex technologies or complex life forms. I am quoting direct from my report (the same *Technol Research Project* report that drives art gallery curators crazy):

This space left blank, except for this sentence.

04.02.03 The need for any inventive technology may be required for prolonged periods of time. The useful life of any inventive technology can be described in the following equation:

α = The number of devices that perform that technological function.

β = The number of discrete components of the device which needs to be analyzed for determining the useful life of that device compared to other similar devices in the sample.

φ = Is the comparative factor to relate to other devices of the same function.

φ Approaching α is the optimal design that thus it would have the longest useful life performing that function.

$$\frac{\alpha}{\beta} = \varphi$$

198. With the above equation, the use of a rock in place of a hammer (stick, sinew, and a rock), will be in existence as a pounding device longer by virtue of its simplicity (one piece). You go to a construction site and you will find off-road equipment such as backhoes, and you will still see shovels. The same shovels you saw 50 years ago and maybe 50-year-old shovels. You are less likely to see a 50-year-old backhoe because they are too complex to be useful for that long.

199. This brings about a good time to state another truth from the list of "The most basic knowledge of the physical realm". As the words or verbiage might not be totally self explanatory, unnatural systems are defined as systems that would not be

created by the basic laws of atoms, molecules, etc. and an infinity of monkey's not withstanding. Thus although iron would be natural and found throughout the universe lying around, a bulldozer could not be created by normal planet formation and upon seeing one buried on Mars we would correctly conclude that something other than natural forces were responsible for its creation and possibly its location. Thus complexity causes complexity because a living creature or an automaton created by a living creature must construct and maintain and repair and "improve" what has been created. Now you might be wondering how far from the topic of manic-depression can we get? I am seeking to define the cause of life's frustrations for both the *Homaniakos* and the *Hosapiens* lives. You must understand that there is more to suicide than depression, for depression is not an actuator onto its own. The stifling of genetic protocols leads all human species to feel unfulfilled but only the *Homaniakos* species lacks the delusional ability to blow it off every day. I will stand on a hill someday and look at all the ordinary humans running about and them senseless to the world no less, but I will understand what I am seeing even if words are not available to define it. Let's read this together for the sake of friendship and unity:

The most basic law of unnatural systems:
"Complexity causes complexity"

200. Unnaturally contrived systems that are the simplest will survive the longest. The more complex an object or system gets, the least likely it will survive for very long – can the same applies to nature? This puts humans in an unfortunate position, but most likely as scientists are quick to point out, when push comes to shove, bacterium will inherit the earth and all humans are nothing more than to-morrows dinner. Only natural systems can create

unnatural systems at this þoint of human knowledge. Unnatural systems become more comþlex in order to survive or comþete but they are a contrivance for the þrofits of mankind and womantyþe thus the evolution of them is not true evolution but occurs anyway by virtue of grammatical syntax - no unnatural system evolves. This is why once you take a stick, sinew, and a rock to build a hammer; you are headed down the road to comþlexity and extinction of that contrivance and humans as a natural comþlex system will follow that same þath without the helþ of nuclear weaþons, Anthrax, or AIDS.

201. Next time you þreþare to travel in your automobile, stoþ and take a look at the comþlexity of its mechanical attributes. Look under the hood, under the carriage, in the wheel-wells, under the control console (dashboard), and anywhere else you can examine. I would suggest that you take an extremely deeþ breath right now and try to imagine the thousands of auto workers in hundreds of factories spread to almost every corner of the spherical earth making every single car þart to an exact document of speciifications that is identified, qualified, verified, validated, revised, folded, staþled, mutilated, handled, fondled, ordered, invoiced, þackaged, distributed, shiþþed, stamþed received, acceþted, rejected, þart shortage, þart over-stocked, þart under-stocked, return to stock, return to vendor, counted, inventoried, don't stack too high, low ceiling, watch your head, max headroom, safety glasses required, ear þrotection required, þinch þoint, don't þoint, what's your þoint with robust robots welding here, no weld here, no access, access denied, þick the þarts, move the þarts, assembled, þounded, screwed, glued, þushed, þress, þress, þull, lifted, lowered, turned, tightened, twist and shout until its shimmed, filed, filled, þrimed and þainted, dusted, þolished and insþected,

scheduled with leadmen, foremen, bosses, supervisors, directors, assistant managers, managers, senior managers, project managers, executive managers, general managers, vice presidents, vice president in charge of production, in charge of engineering, in charge of in charges, executive vice presidents, president, CEO's, DOA's, controller, comptroller, handyman, safety director, nurses, board members, vending machine service persons, floor sweepers, broom makers, bean counters, glass polishers, light bulb changers, football pool organizers, annoyers, human resource managers, memo writers, post-it note collectors, doodlers, parts manual writers, copy machine operators, shredding machine Shriners, bowling team shirt designers, post my score braggers and those in charge of natural resource procurement, inspectors, engineers creating documents, assistants filing documents, recording documents, archiving documents, reading, riting, and rithmatic for every process, procedure, policy, work instruction, level 1 document, level 2 document, level 3 document becomes a level 4 document when signed, dated and distributed to every auto salesperson, dealerships needing transportation of product that offers ninety days same as cash, don't you dare crash, what a deal, what a steal, watch your back, take the shirt off your back or you'll bring it back for a warranty extension takes your pension so sign here dear, rip-off spare parts and I can't part with it to custom agents, contract negotiators, contract lawyers, patent attorneys with secretaries that lick stamps with smacking lips while taking dictation and opening letters that bend at the knees would you please, in short miniskirts and too tight blouses causing office talk, small talk, talk talk, and big talk at the water cooler next to the busiest desk loaded with photos of her children on her computer monitor purchased from procurement officers located in offices across town, uptown, downtown, on the fifth floor of a brick building built in 1936 by tradesmen, bricklayers, men with shovels, men with tears in their eyes for loves lost while they swing their pickaxes, hammers and saws all for the stuff-shirt, well dressed men well hung with architectural degrees on the walls of painted gypsum on number 9 nails taken from a yellow box on the top shelf of a supply cabinet located at 1428 Elm Street that was put there by a 50 year old maintenance man who bought them from the local hardware store one Saturday morning on July 28, 1951 in order to fulfill a requisition for such items written by the secretary of an interior design corporation that was contracted to bring the office into a new look of the popular culture of that era that when all was said and done, he didn't get any thanks either, all so you can drive 3 blocks to pickup a frozen Coca-Cola Slurpee one hot summer evening. [596 words]

202. From the example I stated above, you can start to get an idea of how entwined our lives are to our technology, and how that technology has no end to its mission. This is how technology screws all of us in our daily lives despite the improvements that reduce pain and delay death against nature intentions [*death as nature intended?*]. Of the 12 billion humans that either lived or are still alive now, most never enjoyed the comforts that the few now have, yet everyone lived, procreated, and added to the continuance of all of the human species and all of this is really done without much thought or brains by the human animal - but that is a topic for CHAPTER MANKIND AND WOMANTYPE. We are so close to our ancestors but we can't imagine much of their lives and we couldn't go back 10k years yet alone 100 years and live their lives for a day without knowing we would be safely back in our future of technology gadgets and flushing toilets the next day.

203. As the music track #9 repeats again, I feel like a little excitement so it is time to talk of mechanisms and the unnatural creations of the unnaturally created. The human mind cannot comprehend the contrivance of a mechanism, winking and blinking with preplanned intentions. Who cares anyway? Turn it on to turn us on by our own engorged buttons. We are likely to believe anything is real that we can feel and we can be genetically satisfied by the love of a vibrating, textured for pleasure dildo, fucking organism after organism out of our misses with wishes beyond mans erection attention span. Always keep a shoebox for the rubber man without hands and batteries complements of the Energizer bunny. What other species on the earth has pseudo-procreation with machines, but don't you love the imagery of it?

204. The human-child can't overcome the attention that is only reflected off of the erected Barbie and her twins. Corporation tee shirt that identifies, will categorize, and expresses lies; this is how I feel guys, expressions of a human emotion trolling for queers. I am cool, I am somebody, a machine made shirt worn by me so won't you flirt, my pheromones work, we have something in common - jerk. Every contrivance is a genetic spin-doctor at work to replace our totally dysfunctional structure of a societal remnant. The only thing worse would be if all contrivances were memes turned physical to exist as an out-of-mind experience to guarantee their transference remotely or at a later date, no living carrier required. If that is the case, then the meme wins the race and artifacts outlive humans thus the non-biological life is the optimal life of the universe and I wish to be one even if only in a lucid dream.

205. What changes anyway as life þasses forward through the next generation of humans? Every new dog learns new tricks and thinks that the mentors are square rooted L-7. Every generation feels new and þrogressive but nothing is inherited exceþt the same old genetics from mankind and womantyþe's beginning. The youth are senseless warriors but only the Army knows it. Genetics method of being certain that humans will die for their offsþring creates solders for þlaying the Generals chess game by creating legal þrocreation laws delaying þrocreation until they are done with the youth. Nobody sees it but the faces are the same and so are the catch þhases and after being here for two generations I know why humans die - boredom.

Animals that think?

206. Although we drift afloat a sea of endless toþics, all concerned with worldly events and occurrences, I bet you are wondering how to connect animals to manicism or deþression or that thing the ordinary humans call a mental illness? It has nothing to do with the other animals at all because they behave about as nature intended, unless mankind or womantyþe interfere. But when you and I are exþloring how ordinary humans interact with the other animals is when you'll start to see things get a little weird. For although I and my fellow *Homaniakos* can imagine quite a lot, I am still in total wonderment with the way some humans think about the other creatures of the earth and the supþosed creatures of the other þlanets as though some humans are interspecies communicators. What other creature of the earth would interact in so many ways with so many other creatures of the earth besides the human animal? Humans are so kind to other creatures, even

right up to the moment that they eat them thus phylumism is an explanation of why humans eat other life but I would rather you look at my axiom #4 because phylumism doesn't cover it all. My axiom #4 is "No living entity can have a greater understanding of its existence, than the physical ability to act on it" and that does cover it all, don't you agree? But so you my reader don't lose track, you and I must concentrate on the human side of the interspecie interactions. What of an animal that is no more than dinner for some other creature, or us whoever gets there first? Moo moos and cluck clucks should now have caught by wroughting that two go in but one comes out. How many organized protests with sign carrying fatten lambs have we read about in the copy? To tell you what's wrong I would believe our dinners have been bred for too long injected with rejected drugs. For their size is right but territory they don't hype when it comes to mankind and womantype. One might wonder why it has never been seen, that Daffy Duck and Donald Duck get together, but following birds of a feather, they won't hang for the night. Conceptual birds obeying contrived legal verbiage falls well outside the realm of logic to figure it all out.

207. Yet humans describe, or rather infer "human type" intelligence to other creatures because of similar genetic protocol responses. You can't discern it but sounds and facial jesters that by virtue of no reason worth stating will drive the protective response of procreation continuance in many humans. Within the faulty logic of the ordinary humans, you can see why there appears to be no logic applied to the behavior of humans when around other animals. Animals of thinking ability we care not because the casual interpretation of the pain response can't be figured out without the trained human eye and some humans even

believe that the great aþes have closed the gaþ between humans and the lessor animals. Thus animals with similar brains to ours such as the octoþus get a bad wraþ because of suction-cuþ nightmares and their sþerm shooting fingers giving women a case of the vaþors.

208. Yet the memed brain of some tyþe of human will try to save the life of a chicken then all chickens and then call me a murderer of which I can only say I wonder what a human would taste like on PETA (þita) bread? The multiþlexed overlaþþed fused memes that create an animal activist is centuries old or older but the differential framing by the media co-scriþts the occurrences very well, so what is the truth exþressed in a contrived language of sound bites? These humans are not "well intentioned" because no human really is (I don't believe there is a gene for it but altruism would be your research toþic). But the first activist with the overworked þrocreation þrotection gene was able to con enough brains into swallowing a meme, vegetarian style. Of course they are dead wrong to the þlants because humans can't see þast their own genetics and sooner or later they are hungry and must eat something living as long as it doesn't smile or wink within their understanding of smiling or winking. Any "well intentioned" human would stoþ eating all together in order to save all life on the earth or maybe live off the breast milk of non-eating lactator virgins with sanitized þuffy niþþles.

209. The adoþted Godd of the Christians has always been into animal sacrifice right uþ to and including Christ, the sacrificed god in a borrowed human's body. To make matters worst than they aþþear, much of that sacrificed meat was not fit to eat, being blooded only to say thanks to Godd because he wouldn't let you

say it with flowers. Humans may be the only animals that feel a self-species sacrifice is the right thing to do sometimes and history is full of it. Human sacrifice would be different if we ate our young. As I have read babies were sacrificed throughout time or tossed into a river or trash pit in ancient cities, we find babies in alley garbage bins now or even in the bathroom garbage during Prom night. How am I going to classify this behavior other than to say that it is genetic, not learned and humans will never stop it no matter how often the crowds proclaim, "What a tragedy".

210. A meme on a gene: isn't that what human logic is reduced too? The obvious analysis would be to say that these animal rights humans have accepted a "meme by proxy" on behalf of the other animals. It would seem difficult to believe that the animals themselves have passed this meme to the human hosts by their own intention because communication is visual at best (sometimes based on sound) between mismatched species and who can understand the complexity of a chicken's smile? The ability to smile or exhibit true thoughts or natural emotions is a function of the physical brain construction and not the perceptions you apply to the creature you are viewing – and yet that is how most humans logicize [*Neologism*] it. It is natural for humans to have a cross-species parenting behavior because vision plays a large part of human communication, and all of it genetically analyzed when possible, but when the moment becomes critical, if you were hungry and it came down to you or pooch, you'd eat it, you'd fight for the bones too.

211. Cross-species nurturing is very common in humans because as I keep mentioning, humans can barely overcome their genetic behaviors even if they concentrate at it. The same

genetic attribute that causes you to be kind to and feed newborn humans will cause you to do the same for many other animals especially when they are pre-teens. Again, Stephen Jay Gould points it out best in his book, *The Panda's Thumb*, viewing certain physical features cause us to behave in a predictable manner. The large eyes, large forehead, large head to body ratio are genetic actuators that cause adult humans, to nurture baby animals with those traits, human or not. Thus when do you know when you are really thinking or really only responding appropriately per your genetics? (You can't know.) Cross-specie nurturing cannot be avoided unless you have become inured to the situation or are truly plain nasty. This also explains why humans don't have natural nurturing tendencies for scorpions, snakes, and sharks but they do for kittens, pups, stuffed animals, and certain cartoon characters. This explains why VBS (Vacation Bible School) posters have the "cute" species on them in place of the "creepy" ones. The human organizers can't see past their own genetic speciesistic dualism and the fact that every life, plant, animal, cute to you or octopussy-like creepy thing, is exactly equal in function and thus filling that supposed imagined niche in the circle of life, if Godd had created them.

2 1 2a. When a male bird performs a mating ritual to a pile of feathers, as opposed to an actual female bird, or acts out in anger against its own image in a mirror, humans may think about the preverbal "bird brain". Have we forgotten that human males are so genetically hardwired that they may masturbate to orgasm in front of photographs of idealized female mates because we are visual fornicators as a species? Women, who have recently given birth, may lactate at the sound of any baby crying. As you my reader friend will soon discover, your genetic behavior is in control, not

some fantasy of a human mind with logic for all actions. Humans are "intelli-genetic" at best but maybe so are some other animals with complex brains. As I have one more thought on the matter, but I have already numbered the paragraph sequence, I'll take the human way out and add a paragraph 212b. right here to tell you that the animal rights humans are only alive to protest the "so-called" abuse of animals because of the "so-called" abuse of the animals that gave their life for the continuance of the human species. For as easy as it is to live in a nice house or to own a car or to give medicines to your sick human-children and then complain about the way all other ordinary humans live, none of that would be possible without the realm of the living kingdom [*Patriarchal word*] being slaughtered or trashed for its resources. As I might have already stated, all humans are thieves by nature (as is all life), stealing needed or wanted resources from anything living. Thus the animal rights activist shout for the freeing of the animals from the slaughter or from the slavery of humankind but then they themselves encourage their own human-children to study hard and get a good job or career or some other contrived activity so that when they have reached the top and have all the pop, they find they have their own private box to sit in all day with photographs of trees on the walls, and all of it is built on the stolen resources of the other living creatures. Frogs in shoeboxes by plan and action but never seeing that they are all part of the trashing of nature themselves within their delusional minds, because they all purchase and own the same shit as I do.

212c. Bob's silly rule: "Within every evil is a perversion to create goodwill."

2 1 3. I am not professing to have found a plant that exhibits the *Homaniakos* traits, but let me tell you, in case you haven't heard, the vegetarian PETA (People for the Ethical Treatment of Animals) are trying to save life forms that they perceive are similar to themselves (gene driven) at the expense of life forms they believe to be expendable (i.e. plants which to the surprise of some of them are also gene driven). They are compelled by ordinary human genetics with a meme infestation because somehow they have come to believe that plants are different than animals within the scope of importance when in actuality, all are food (or poison) and thus those humans still exhibit speciesism as all humans do. I hope to add to the confusion by stating that the Godd of the Jews only accepts animal sacrifice, check it out for your self. Humans may perceive that a cow has eyes, legs, gives live birth, and makes audible sounds, and therefore claim it is a life to save as a human life would be to save and I will not deny that when speaking of humans I would include both the *Homaniakos* and the *Hosapiens*. (The clearer vision of reality does not prevent a human from becoming infected with memes.) Can you send me the suicide rate of the vegetarian *Homaniakos* versus the omnivore *Homaniakos*? Humans believe a cow can think or can rationalize its thought of us without us even understanding the hardwiring of its brain and thus the emotions possible. Axiom #4 rules and your choice of what to eat whether cow or Martian should be based on it. Humans do not perceive this in plants because we are not a plant [*Sentence structure (no suggestions)*], although the label of couch potato would seem appropriate at times. None of us can even imagine being a plant or we can't even imagine that we can imagine being a plant. We can't dream we are a plant as a plant in the sense of how a plant would sense existence or know what feels good or what to fear. We don't understand parenting behaviors in plant life so all (or almost all, I suppose) humans simply kill and/or eat plants or seeds of any type. A weed is only a plant that is out of place or of no value by human's faulty logic and wouldn't you say (using contrived words) that calling any plant a weed is plant racism or being a bully? As opposed to most animals that are killed and then eaten dead, many plants are eaten alive. With the humans "fast action life" compared to plants slower life, humans don't see that a carrot is still alive while they chomp on it. It is still trying to salvage its reproductive abilities as it slides down our throat. What really seems strange to me, is that with plants being frozen alive, cooked alive, eaten alive, and cut and pruned and burnt alive, raised on farms where they never have a chance for a natural life or to achieve any goal in life, I would want to believe that there would be some humans, ordinary or not, that would want to put an end to all of that. Shouldn't an oak tree have the same rights as a chicken? Whereas a chicken is a meal deal, stuffing for a pillow, and some additives for cat food, an oak tree is pleasing to see, provides a filter for our "out" gases, shade because our sun kills us humans, it is also home to many animals and insects, and then it is firewood and an oak table or two for you. Although there are those humans that only eat fallen fruit, as though they believe the fruit is not alive yet what they are actually eating are living embryos. It would be like being a meat eater but only eating naturally aborted fetuses. I guess they don't see it that way and the faulty logic at the heart of the ordinary human's genetics is in control and how am I to stop it? Unlike blood animals, plants live quite a long time after they are sliced, diced and mashed. But what the hell, you should really tell me sometime what is the difference between a carrot and a cow because I don't see it.

Humans don't understand a plant's sense of pain or their expression of it, but it is there because they must survive and procreate as you and I therefore they must respond at the right moment. There is no difference in life forms and you could have been born to be either animal or plant if you are going to play that "Thank Godd, I wasn't born to be him (or her)" game.

214. Realizing how similar humans are to plants is of no concern to humans because the gene is not there - although some humans have attempted to train themselves to explore the other orders of life. With no gene to drive the meme, and faulty logic of universal order being applied more timesthan (yes, my computer prefers "*timesthan*") not, is it [*it is*] any wonder the plant kingdom suffers torture at the hands and feet of the human animal. From my observation with me trying hard to live among the ordinary humans and copy what they do, I find my own memes and logic of life must be ignored so I live in denial of my own actions. Many humans believe plants are made out of some mysterious "plant material" and not the same DNA we share with them. Because humans perceive that a plant does not tenderly embrace its youth, we should disregard plants as life altogether. In the name of love, humans tear living tissue, limb by limb, off of flowers only to proclaim, "she loves me not". Booked titles unlimited are possible but plants are actually sexually active and more than humans will ever be and bumper stick-ons should say: "PLANTS HAVE LONGER STEMS". What male plant sensing the presence of a young megasporangium wouldn't turn on budding in his olfactory view? Without giving too much away about my personal pastimes, I would have to say that some plants do seem to also enjoy a little SMBD (Sado-Masochism / Bondage & Discipline, for you virgins) in their lives and the prince slashing the

thorny bushes in *Sleeping Beauty* gave me my first boner and I still get the beauty and the þain of it confused, so helþ me Freud.

215. Take living flowers, slash off their roots, and inject them in a þot of water, þre-þackaged þreservatives added, for elongated disþlay. How barbaric and cruel if you believe you are a human loving humans. These þlants are choking for food and die a slow death completely oblivious to your sniff, sniff, sniffing them, staring and smiling at them, and þroclaiming "How beautiful and thoughtful you are" she said to him, all the while he's thinking, "Yes, can I rut with you now?" Plants strive to live, roots or not, but their genes know what is haþþening even if that interþretation is too advanced for humans to notice. Imagine holding your þet cat to a wall and stabbing a knife through a non-vital organ sticking the cat to the wall. It's a gift for your sþouse to show her how much you love her. You feed the cat for a few days giving it fluids intravenously but soon it dies and then you þress it between the þages of a BIG book. I see no difference and the *Four Axioms of Existence* don't sþlit the difference based on who's green or who's mean. Humans rational thoughts on how to treat other life forms is a line they draw and everyone eats thus everyone draws their[*there*] line somewhere. Don't tell me where to draw my natural lines, and don't take my nature away from me because you might have a lobbyist in Washington on behalf of some humans with some tyþe of common unified faulty logic.

216. Humans have little regards for most tyþes of life because of genetics. Humans must meme affection to other animal life and then they select only the ones that are visually aþþealing and don't shit on them. I suþþose that exþlains why humans þrefer þlant life as decorations. They aren't as bloody as animals and

they really don't make much in the way of do-do as humans recognize do-do. The casual defecators (animals that can't control their release of do-do) that humans do like, are put in cages for no good reason at all other than their owners don't want to step in "it" and most humans treat them as good as a battery that needs re-charging once in awhile. Let me ask you, my reader friend, is your brain so simple that a bird in a cage easily amuses you? By what logic or knowledge do you believe the birds don't care or don't know of their captivity? If your thinking is now equal to my Axiom #4 then you might validate my book by examining your own actions (I have faith that you are up to that task).

217. Recently I was listening thus I heard from within my Radio machine a new meme to add to my brain, and that meme will be revealed to you now in this ridiculously long and improper paragraph with miss-spelt words no less and that thought is that many plants move in herds. I don't wish to purposely deny credit for thoughts when credit is due, but how could I ever find the originator of such a thought when all humans imitate and copy and repeat and it never ends thus without proof of an origin, it never had an origin. At any rate, getting back at someone's perception, it is a wonderful perception, and completely true. Our human problem with the perception of plant procreation and locomotion lies in our biological speed and our visual resolution of physical reality. Humans can barely perceive plant behavior even when they are a specialized plant behaviorologist or a plant psychologist (yes, they exist). As a human, your genetic reactions don't tell you to watch out for that tree. I never understood the joke, or is it an insult, "Watching the grass grow" as if a human could ever perceive another human growing. Unless picked up and tossed, plants don't move fast and they still seem to do fine.

Please don't quote to me exceptions to the rule because there are no true exceptions in existence, everything is the way it is without exception and without much reason other than if it exists, that is proof it can exist. Although plants seem lethargic compared to animal life, there doesn't seem to be any advantage in the scheme of the universe to be a plant or an animal or to move fast or slow. I suppose that point is difficult to accept regardless of what specie of human you are. Plants have many advantages over human life, but how are humans to appreciate the differences? I will never believe that an apple is eatable such that its seeds are to be spread by a hungry roaming animal life that plops the seeds down in a patch of instant fertilizer although I was taught that in a government school as though we had reached some era of total understanding, but now 40 years later everyone can see how messed-up instructing science was back then and it continues to remain the same. However with common DNA construction, then everything living should be able to eat everything living and now we are back to the idea in paragraph 189. Too many questions to be valid and besides, there are no answers in nature but the *Hosapiens* around me seem quite content perpetuating fairy tales of every kind in order to justify what is believed by them to be seen and why it is needed and how we should save it from it's self or from ourselves. All the while I know I was lied to for some shallow reason that no graded schoolteacher could understand or perceive. It is not a conspiracy, it is faulty logic applied to a brain that was finally able to purge the lies when his eyes were open the evening another *Homaniakos* was born. (I remember the evening I was born as a *Homaniakos*, of which no ordinary human can make a similar claim, because I was in my parent's darkened dining room thinking about the universe filled with atoms and the behavior of humans and the actions of molecular biology, and thinking about girl whom had put her warm breath across my lips. The year would have been 1972 c.e. and in an instant I saw the clearer vision of reality of which nobody else understood but everything became clear to me in an instant, with total universal knowledge and the understanding of life. Tears came to my eyes when those thoughts collided and the next footstep I made – in remembrance of Buzz - became the first steps on a strange planet.)

218. Plants are "chemical telepathics" communicating without ears but sniffing the air and knowing that they are not alone and thus they are a social life living in herds that can sound alarms, anticipate danger, and react to the environment. Plant life outlives any animal life and lives through death to start again. They often have 3rd party sex via some type of creature mènage á twig (a malapropism for sure) or from asexual fruiting bodies and thus they can never become a Christian. They do not cross-specie co-exist too easily and exhibit what humans would incorrectly call racism attitudes toward each other as they poison the soil around them and block the sun life from the plants that sprout too close for comfort. Plants are cannibals that re-digest the vitamins and minerals that helps build strong bodies 12 ways from the dead plant bodies lying truthfully around them. Plants are parasites of plants and think (written as a metaphor) nothing of it thus acting like the animals but remaining motionless not being able to scratch an itch, they therefore never have an itch to scratch or would then live their life in constant torture of self-denial.

219. Plants never think, "What the hell was that?" and therefore never speak it. Plants get from point A to point B with all the patience in the world and you will never see them move. Plants are the largest creatures to ever live. Plants that seem to

be hundreds of plants are one plant connected via tubes and pipes and hoses and chemical gears that pump and squish and squirt and grow and move underground and fool walking creatures into believing they are a forest of many. Plants are not what you see and not what you think and some have convinced you to keep them as pets and feed them and prune them and touch them with gentle hands and luscious lips.

220. While the human wife may plead her case for not swallowing her mates essence, the plant's sperm is the basis for most of our grain supply endo-wise and thus the whole world of the humans go down on plants everyday for king sized breakfast sperm - roasted or toasted or eat it raw topped with milk or butter or cream cheese, yum yum it slides right on down, and what in the hell did you think you were eating? Don't all haploid nuclei taste the same?

221. If I took a photo once a day for 3 years of a few acres of grass with dandelions placed at one corner, and then compressed the photos into 24 frames a centon, we would see a stampede of dandelions moving and engulfing the field in about 52 seconds (My math is incorrect, you figure it.). If humans lived at the speed of a dandelion, we would be running for our lives. Of course if we did live at that speed, animals would mean very little to us. Plants are eaten by animals and without being able to run away don't they still exist by creating more of themselves than the animals care to eat each day? Is this not how animal life has continuance? Is all of understanding life that simple? If you were a plant, animals would speed by like bullets, and not provide any known function for your existence. What would you sense of them? I have to think that

only the humans give þlant life a þosition of disresþect, and that all other life on the earth treats all other life on the earth equally.

222. As Beethoven's 9th brings me great feelings of life and eternity, and the association to that Kubrick movie of youthful violence seeking þure genetic fulfillment, it convinces me that I too will succeed O my brothers. But I am reminded that visions of death and haþþiness are shared by humans lying down or slain in green þastures flowered and tilting in the breeze and growing in the sunlight that seems infinite to our lifetime. Although þlants mean you no harm, even though many are þoison to humans, they care not for you or your death regardless of the circumstances and thus þlants would never shed a tear for you or your remaining family as your death causes flowers to be sacrificed in remembrance of you. Did you not kill a flower as you built a visual memorial for the remembrance of your suicided child or sþouse?

223. As many thoughts and images you have about þlants that þlants don't know or understand events that occur around them due to their limited senses, humans have only a measured amount of senses different than them (the þlants) and thus you can't see everything you miss or don't understand because somewhere someone's theories aþþly and you don't know what you can't know by virtue that you can't be your own test subject. Thus there [*that*] is the cause for the many short sighted and misþlaced ideas of the humans þlace or þosition of authority in the universe. All life on the earth or in the universe does not exist at a human sþeed or within the limits of human sensory þerceþtion and for that matter, existence does not function at a human "whatever" because sþeed is distance divided by time and time is in your mind as the distance between two events when nothing is moving once

you have thought you have perceived it. So how do I move and live on the surface of the earth sharing the beliefs of ordinary humans? I don't, because I believe that trees and birds are one and the same, they live and that is all there is to it, no difference at all. And when I am hungry or need to be warm or need some entertainment for the moment, I do exactly as every ordinary human, PETA people, and all the other agenda pushing ordinary humans that occupy the earth with me at this time would do, I kill something - but I have no delusions about it, thus I feel or enjoy the death of it.

The human animal, general topics

224. It's getting close to quitting time, so I am drifting a bit as I realize that going to bed or having a bedtime is a routine for each human I suppose, but I never believe(d) sleep is ordinary or routine or wanted or deserved. Sleep is hell, and I would spend one of my three wishes asking that I don't need those four hours that I force my body-n-mind to take in the middle of the darkness. But since I must do it, I brace for it, but always to no avail. So as I must prepare my casket each night, I look around the darkened bedroom as I see selfish hallucinations that can't even wait for my eyes to shut. Everything comes alive, as faces or creatures or strange landscapes appear out of nowhere or from within ordinary objects. But now as consumer goods change in this modern age and they find their way into all of our lives, so do my visual resources change and thus there are always more thoughts that need thinking. For now an electric toothbrush sits twenty feet away from my pillow, but it is quite visible as a very small pale green dot of a light in the darkness signaling "battery being charged" whether or not we are there to see it or understand it. Yet this

light walks through my door, the door to my depression, as I lay and stare at that light and nothing more. So I figure somewhere after death, where physical sensations are never satisfied but still remembered, I would float in that lonely darkness forever, but still see that pale green light, as though possessing only that light would be wonderful for a soul so lonely and lost. And what if that light could then be held or touched or possessed somehow and I would express no other wish except to be in the presence of that light, as though that light is all that I would need to keep me from being lonely for an eternity? Jesus, where are you and where is the light within my soul that is now empty and dark? I am without love and without being able to express love or feel love, but the feeling of love lost is felt at every moment. I could, at this moment, get up and walk quietly past my family, with them watching TV or reading their books or dreaming their dreams of futures to be fulfilled with some type of happiness, and I could without hesitation break that glass or pickup that knife and slice each wrist in total silence, without pain, and not a further thought to it other than I would know at that moment I would be on my way to finding out the only information I really wish to know. Death by suicide would be the only logical thing to do, in order to find the information that I seek, I guess. But instead I will cry the thoughts away, and wipe my tears off my plastic keypad, and bury my pain into this book only to write it for future humans yet unborn to read, I suppose. So let me tell you (as my mood swiftly goes hypo) that opportunists as any animal is because surviving to procreate is first most [*Suggestion: foremost?*] of the humans actions, thus and therefore without much strategy of the pre-planning type, humans steal anything when they can, totally against their Sunday "holier than thou" preaching, which is only a meme anyway. For if religion were a gene, it would rule humans more consistently and it doesn't! From Xerox (some type of tradename after the Greek god of replication) machine copy stealing "I only need one copy for my football pool (also illegal but everyone does it) score sheet", to standing around the coffee pot talking about a love-less love life long lost, you are paid by the hour so get to work and quit stealing time.

225. First it's the technology – the human's brain (ordinary or not) cannot comprehend a contrivance. Technology appears far from being natural and genes are built to respond to nature only. Contracts, paper money, vending machines and dollar signs on liquid crystal displays, all must be properly trained to humans as doggie tricks and well, sometimes it doesn't make genetic sense. Lying, cheating, stealing, destruction of property are all part of the human attributes, I'm not that screwed up, as you would have me think about this sentence.

226. Now many persons will tell you this is the way humans are because we have gone against one of the many gods of the humans or that the humans are naturally evil. Actually the great discourse on whether there is such a thing as "evil" applies right now so mention it you bet I will [Sentence structure failure]. What is an evil trait and how can we understand natural evil (if it exists)? We are now so far physically from our natural habitats and natural habits. We (as humans) had to stay alive, for millions of years before all this technology and all the political structures were created. The crime and evil is greatly amplified, divided line by line, and subcurseded when technology replaces society and you are left with a techciety. Humans have contrived themselves into an unnatural state of law and order. In a natural society, there is no crime, but there are attacks against survival. An attack against

survival could have been met with any response required and even now the injustice system is most likely to let you off Scott-free in such a case because in all .humans that gene is mean. The transference by force, as in the stealing from your possession Television machines and money and durable goods, is not natural and confounds what humans should do to be appropriate for punishment because those contrivances were never intended to be with the humans according to their genes. Thus I see ordinary humans fill their lives with such matters but I how do I ignore such things having had a human family and being raised to behave the same? Second, we eat organic life (food) (I forgot where that sentence belongs). So ordinary humans start drawing lines in the sand with their contrived language of what is right and what is wrong and I must endure the bullshit remarks and faulty logic I hear if I am to remain waking and walking another day.

227. Is it possible to go back to more genetics, less morals?

You may not believe so, but in a matter of a few hours, under the right conditions all humans could (and would) revert back to using their genetic behavior with complete justification and no moral delusions. 1.5 million years of genetic breeding emerge the second the power goes out, for good (because that behavior is always with us but not obvious when food and shelter and sex can be had by reaching out your hand and taking what is wanted). Your disbelief in this fact is of no importance, it would happen regardless. How bad do you want to live? How long can you live when no one can use contemporary technology again? How long will you remember your societal protocols when you can't "plug-in" for your daily dose of music videos, docu-dramas, and Internet porn? Put your trust in your genetics, my fine reader friend, is what I would expect, thus your genetics are still with you although somewhat hidden from your logic, and now I guess the ordinary humans would proclaim some type of lack of sensitivity toward other life on my part, but the word sensitivity is only contrived to alter your natural behavior.

228. All genetic traits that are defined in terms of "contemporary" technologies or lifestyles must in truth, be defined in terms of behaviors that would have applied to the earliest humans or contemporary societies that have less technology. Thus Tourette's Syndrome causes *coprolalia* revealed as the compulsively shouting of obscenities, when in fact, this syndrome could have existed before organized language, or in cultures where obscene words have not been contrived. What is the basis for the disorder? A malfunction of the nervous system that controls basic genetic human attributes such as sex and mating, or clan or tribal protective attributes? It has nothing to do with four letter words in a contrived language but is perceived as such.

229. Humans of course are genetically wired to procreate and not hunt or eat their own offspring but even that doesn't work all the time. You would believe that family pheromones must be active also in order to keep brother and sister away from actions of procreation together unless the vision of a good meal overcomes them. But perhaps there are no family pheromones and maybe the Greek legend of Oedipus is always a reality, thus actual "in the know" family procreation fun is only a meme away. There are plenty (at least one) of genetic reasons why it is so common to hear on the news that any given female's boy friend has killed her human-children that she had created by procreating with another mate. Or possibly that her boy friend will mate with her female human-children because they are not his but he must sniff them all

day. When a sociologically created meme does not suppress the gene, the gene wins. Although not common, the human female is most likely to kill her own human-children and so will her next mate. For your info, the human male is least likely to kill his offspring even if he doesn't hang around much for nurturing them. If you find clues in that statement do something with your thoughts. The human genetic drive to become impregnated is as strong or stronger than the genetic drive to protect or nurture the offspring, from what I see in the lives around me. To become impregnated you must have a mate. To have a mate you must attract a mate, and so it goes, the never-ending story stuck in the middle of mass media dementia and radio wave talk show morals. While laws imprison those who allow their genes to overcome their memes, laws are a function of money and power expressed through a contrived language, thus how can we ever know the truth or the reasons for the actions subpoenaed?

230. Getting back at whatever the subject is, it is therefore most important for human babies to have basic genetics on their side, but how that all occurs is a damn good question. Logically babies should be born looking or stinking like (as) their dad. Maybe a pheromone is at work here that the dad can respond to without a thought to it. Otherwise the dad will not offer survival necessities to the newborn. Maybe this is where language is a beneficial trait to confirm an offspring at a remote location or later time but who could know for certain? The great Apes of this planet illustrate a genetic preservation behavior by killing the newborn of a female ape when there is a suspicion of the newborn's genetic origins. Out of the clan and you're out of luck, or dead. Thank goodness we now have scientific technological genetic testing. We don't have to take genetically suspicious

babies and beat them to death against trees as we would actually do if we didn't have doctors to do it for us, and then calm us down using contrived verbs such as, "You did the right thing". Although it still occurs now, it wasn't that long ago that unwanted newborns were tossed into the sewers or streets or fed to some god. Abortion isn't new at all, only the timing has changed. Humans are perfectly capable and willing to kill human life when they know they don't want it or they can simply pay a doctor to kill it for them which is strange because they should be able to take the human-baby home and kill it and possibly eat it also. I'm sure you would if your mother had showed you how when you were younger. What do humans teach their non-aborted human-children now, the ones they decided to keep? Admitting shame would turn out to be a revealing characteristic and besides, how would the living human-children learn if not by parental example?, by genetics without learning as I've been telling you. ("?," is a rarely used *comated expletive*, and is noted by a raise in your voice followed by a pause.)

The unnatural environment

231. The "ant-like" genetic behavior causes humans to be active in constructing their environment and to organize into tribes or governments. The uncontrollable trait to imitate causes humans to want what they see. Humans may be among nature's fastest imitators. The two together when applied to Axiom #4 "No living entity can have a greater understanding of its existence, than the physical ability to act on it" creates an animal of dangerous possibilities. Not advancing, but rather changing lifestyles. Technology improves, but humans do not improve or evolve due to technology. Using technology does not alter genetics, but of course now we can use our technology to physically reconstruct our genes by physically relocating natural gene sequences or adding genes. This shortcut will be our downfall, because nature cannot account for the "jumps" in genetic structure that mankind and womantype will force upon it. Our minds are not being altered to suit; thus our own actions and abilities will always perplex ourselves. I see ordinary humans debating the "moral correctness" of every new medical cure or medical research, but for what reason? The very next generation will be born into it and not question the morality of it at all. Can't you see that is how you define your morality now?

232. Where as most animals would be solely driven by genetic behavior with some actions occurring because of memory (for those that have memory) and only slight changes for variations in environment, humans have a dependency on a genetically driven imitation behavior [*Fragment (no suggestions)*]. The ability to imitate is genetic but the actions imitated vary from culture to culture due to tribal customs, climate, and visual resources, is what I am stating. Where as I have read thoughts written by ordinary humans that no great technologies have come from the early Sub-Sahara African continent or from the pre-white man Americas, those regions did have great societies. Then as humans we would have to ask, is it by our technology or our techciety that we measure the success of our species? Where as one continent develops technology and purges society from itself, one remains societal, tell me who is the winner? Society is the noble path and remains true to our intended intentions, and technology works against society, but I am addicted to technology. Whereas technology may save your life, will it save your soul?

233. As Mr. Beethoven was a genus or a nut at what he did, I can only hope he was a manic-depressive also. Speaking of music, I am reminded of the scene from that movie in which Mozart starred, where the orchestra is playing and Mozart is seen as a vision laying in a field of stars, the universe for certain, and I am forced to think about data transcripted from DVD's (whatever DVD means?) and how the humans species now manufactures emotions stamped out a million tears or joys or "wow's" and heart touching moments per minute on some mechanized device. All of the human responses are created due to a contrived event, cash in hand, and planned step by step so at least one or two humans can profit from the event distributed via video rental retailers. But I am hooked on phonics and music and the visions of space travel with special effects of action galore. Sometimes I have to ask myself, "Why do humans want all these artificial products and artificially induced emotions?" Why are we so worried, so occupied with schedules, designing, reviewing, and putting everything in its place? We pat each other on our backs and say, "Job well done", whatever that means? Is all of this (I'm waving my right hand past a Chicago skyline from under a statue of a miniature nude woman at the end of Navy pier) to fulfill the basic behavior traits of humans? Yes, but in a twisted mentally defective fashion. We seek a means to an end but neither is there for real. Technology or not, its food, shelter, sex, and a family dysfunctional exceptional. Even a horse would eat sugar that it was never able to find in nature not realizing or rationalizing the action and reaction. A caged rat would consume drugs that it couldn't produce the technology to manufacture and remain Lucy in the sky forever. Verbal languages, written languages, E-mails, or Television machines do not make any difference in our

requirement to satisfy our genetic traits and most likely they screw us over while we try to act genetically because we believe they are satisfying us. Language causes conflicts between the actions performed and the spoken proposed action. Language does not reveal thoughts, motives, or the truth. E-mail does not convey the facial expressions or tone fluctuations of a voice. In an office, E-mail is reduced to a thought without a pity language used to avoid physical confrontation or used as proof of responsibility thus allowing personal denial of responsibility. Only an action completed reveals the truth and the interpretation of said action, via language starts the lie.

234. Since animals have a born instinct of fear based on self-survival, why can't religion be a natural gene similar to survival? Now is a good time to mention my Axiom #4 again: "No living entity can have a greater understanding of its existence, that the physical ability to act on it." It is easy to make that statement, but the implications are profound. If an animal has fins for hands it would not contemplate putting a rock on the end of a stick and making a hammer. That animal would not believe that making a hammer could make its life better. It would not be frustrated by the fact that it can't do it. So would that animal contemplate a greater being, or a super fish that lives above the waters, in a better place where after death there would be no sharks, disease, or gill nets? If that sounds silly then take one step back and objectively look at our own culture and its religious beliefs because actually Christianity sounds as silly. I don't believe that fish worship a fish-god because I believe that fish don't think much of anything at all. Not all brains are created equal what with the variety of physical components and neural wiring possible or needed and my Axiom #4 implies that brain development and

physical dexterity are paired such that you can have great physical dexterity with simple brain functions, but not complex brain functions and simple physical abilities. If you want to know what an animal has in the way of "thinking" abilities, look at their limbs. Prove me wrong because all you will do is prove how closely we think like dogs, not dogs thinking as humans.

235. Now I suppose you are wondering about animals such as chimpanzees? Why don't they build telescopes, highways, and machine gu-gu-gu-guns? Axiom #4 does not say that every animal that physically can act to alter its environment will have the brains for the game. It simply states that physical dexterity is the minimum requirement of detectable self-awareness, Peak Experiences, or suffering from the Colonel Flastratus phenomenon within the UK.

236. As ants prove, you don't need much of brain to have a society, especially with pheromones as actuators to the physical as opposed to brains that think. What motivates us to create societies, Plato notwithstanding?

237. What is/are needed to [Suggestion: should] be studied are the relationships between brain development and physical dexterity. Why this occurs is not how Axiom #4 was deduced. Axiom #4 is a statement of observation and interpolation of current conditions with a statistical sample of one planet. I would like to see the list of physical abilities versus problem solving abilities for all applicable animals of the earth. Most animals seem to be specialists at problem solving for their survival, which means they are not solving a problem at all but humans can apply contrived verbs such as "clever" (actually an adjective) to actions

seen. They are as those little bug size robots which that scientist, "What's his name?" builds using preprogrammed thoughts so simple but they move as though they are living bugs. Perhaps humans don't really solve as many problems as would be believed. With our large memories, we become "thought" playback machines without a thought at all. This makes me wonder if the bragged about "logic" of the ordinary humans is actually only a matter of sequencing memories from their large neopallium (as I interpret a reference diagram). The so-called problems we solve everyday are broken down to small steps that when they are small enough actually become part of the remembered thoughts that are a part of your memory. Advancements are made by the *Hosapiens* when faulty logic misinterprets an event and incorrectly connects existing memories (as if it is a defective automaton), building walls incorrectly but enjoying the variety of them. I know all of that sounds so crazy, but that is how I feel within my thoughts that my thoughts are being chopped and stored and recalled and re-assembled with me realizing that no new thought has immerged but the satisfaction of it is revealed as though it is new. The *Homaniakos* mind, being the creative force of all brains, understands the reconstruction of thoughts into reality and into visionary metaphysical thoughts previously unknown.

Survival

238. Now a human genetic survival attribute might keep you alive in a natural surrounding of lions and tigers and bears, but in the unnatural environment of the technological advanced humans it will get you dead. Without survival genes for every specific artificial danger that humans create for themselves, they must meme their behavior from one human to another. Since memes are not as effective as genes, and the genes are dominate over memes unless the humans are paying close attention, humans are constantly being injured or killed in ways that prove they have very little logic to them at all and either of the human species have no ability to evolve into their technologies, ever. Behind all these deaths and injuries there is always a contrived mechanism. Inertia, chemical reactions, and unnatural velocities are all beyond the human's genetic abilities to respond and few humans can figure them out without repeated practice in specific fields of artificial repetitiveness. Thus humans will forever blow themselves up, die of inertia injures (velocity deaths such as bullets, plane and car crashes, etc.), and be poisoned by genetically altered foods that they didn't pick or kill from a natural unpolluted environment. (Obviously I must recognize there are natural pollutants also, plus unsanitary lifestyles, however, as we are now sending our little daughters into a journey of precocious puberty by feeding them poisoned beef injected with some type of bovine drugs, we can affect the unwilling as well as the unknowing on a worldwide scale. What does the future hold for them, as we will most likely find their growth stunted and new epidemics of cancer, etc. and then act as if we didn't have a clue it would happen?)

Thoughts live

239. Let me pause the music while I explain the word "meme" more thoroughly as I should have done in the first sentence of CHAPTER MANIC-DEPRESSION, but then how thrilling would that be? A meme (sounds similar to "gene" but with that "m" sound replacing the "g" sound) is an idea that lives like an organism. It replicates, it passes from one living creature to another, and it might even cause genetic changes. Good examples of what some humans call memes are religion and urban legends. Richard Dawkins first documented Memes in the 1970's. The idea of memes is perhaps the greatest theory of human behavior ever presented. My suggestion for reading is *The Meme Machine* by Dr. Susan Blackmore. I am surprised to find in the Hollywood movie, *Forbidden Planet*, starring Leslie Nielson (as a young handsome stud), proclaiming something to the effect of (not a quote): *We have laws and religion to prevent us from acting on our instincts. But laws and religion cannot protect us from our id.* This is great insight into the idea that thoughts are meant to control genes via an organized method and I have trouble telling movies from reality anyway so now let the music rock.

240. Thoughts as memes are pure replication information, spread by any of the senses of perception of organic life. Wanting to live but enjoying none of the sensations of the flesh other than to spread themselves via borrowed senses and creating a false need to stimulate the senses. It is life without a body, any sensory perception, knowledge of the universe, belief of morals, or cause and effect of actions. Memes show us the true meaning of existence for they live without a purpose in an animal that believes every meme brings a purpose toward fulfillment of the human's existence. Memes propagate the grand delusion. Memes have found the perfect host, a brain that is always "on" but never thinking. In the human's attempts at communications with other life on the earth, they with idiot revealing effects try to implant memes into their dogs and cats or the primates bound into the slavery of the humans.

241. What if memes are in greater control than I would admit too [to?] in this book, and if all behavioral problems can be

attributed to in-effectual meme implanting? The human creature is then biologically unchecked but I still am of the belief that humans don't marry for love because love is a meme built on a gene as I define all memes, and thus nature never intended love to drive optimum procreation. If love were a gene it would work better but look at the world right now and tell me about love and sexual activities, sans Godd and sans poetry. Where is the gene of love that drives the Manic-Depressive Junkie me?

242. Humans get their memes confused with their I.Q. and thus intelligence is integrated as in zero to half of infinity for a smile on a physicist face but how can nature drive a thought to that target and for what purpose? Now I.Q. may have its own book (because language is a contrivance and represents a lie of reality at best, this book included I guess) as when applied to the bell curve but regardless it is always a measure of the ability to control, use, or manipulate the human made contrivances such as physical tools, grammar, math, or geometry. Thus it has nothing to do with intelligence at all. These are all only cultural doggie tricks that change as the culture or technology changes. How can intelligence be based on current cultural trends without being bogus? Can you pass an I.Q. test written in 1934? You should get a perfect 200 with all the great knowledge floating around now! I.Q. tests never measure intelligence since the best any human can do is respond to the misinterpretation of expected results and that is how humans as the most advanced creature on the planet called the earth got from early point A to contemporary point B.

243. If you are a believer in meme's and Godd, then you could say that your religious meme is fully installed. The religious meme is one of the most powerful memes because it is fully regnant as a meme may be and it allows genetic behavior to dominate. That is precisely why religion is active in almost all humans. Religious memes are strong enough to cause humans to kill other men, women, and human-children for no other reason than the survival of the meme itself, and dare I add, kill in some of the nastiest methods ever known to mankind and womantype. Barely any death is so hideous as to be slaughtered, flayed alive, burnt alive, and tortured for days on end only to die in the pain of it all, only because of the religious meme carried or accepted. It is only the secular laws that prevent everyone from killing one another under the rules of Godd, but Christians never believe that fact. It is not the memes fault. The meme is too successful in a creature that has perhaps hundreds of other memes installed combined with unnatural mechanisms assembled to express their thoughts as physical stuff, such as effective torture devises. The religious meme is as perfect as a meme can be; thus the dissection of the Christian meme is worthy.

244. Dissectible as the nether ether it only shows up as synaptic chords with sulfur ions dancing in gray matter lighted, but the following is what makes a religious meme I would suspect, but I am only guessing it must respond via genetics and besides, I am not an expert in this stuff and I now realized I put another numbered list in my book after all.

#1 It has a "growth & development" clause that keeps you believing in it: "Believe in me, and live forever." This massages the survival gene[s] because belief will nullify physical death.

#2 It has a "defense" clause that prevents you from uninstalling it: "Reject me, and burn in hell." This again massages the survival genes, and the tribal and clan genetic behavioral motivators. You do not want to be separated from your tribe or clan even after the physical death. You do not want to be lost.

#3 It has a "mental tranquilizer" clause that stifles cognitive dissonance: "Godd works in mysterious ways", or "We cannot understand his purpose." Thus we can reduce cognitive dissonance quickly and put our mind back to work. This may actually be the strongest part of the meme as it can overcome the true examination of death or reality of which the ordinary human[s?][s'?] would have difficulty understanding anyway.

#4 It has a "reaffirmation" clause that keeps your clan or tribe pure: "Remain in the company of your own beliefs". You will seek the company of others with similar beliefs. Once every week you must have the meme re-imbedded to insure it is not weakened or mutated. This again works through the tribal and clan genetic behavioral motivators.

#5 It has an "infection" clause for propagation: "Spread my word to all the world." This drives humans to spread the meme to other humans by using all methods of communication. This works though the tribal and clan genetic behavioral motivators. "All humans that believe as I do will be part of my tribe." Humans strive to belong to a tribe for survival reasons.

Ordinary humans strive to have all humans behave and believe as them.

245. Thus start looking at all that you do and believe in your life and figure out for yourselves as a homework assignment from me, which is memes and which is genes. Now if you must be taught it, it could be a meme, and you are taught less than you believe, but be certain that you hold your fork correctly and in public say "Thank you". I can give you a clue to add to the confusion of it all because it is not always that easy. Collecting baseball cards is a meme working on behalf of a gene because a baseball card is a contrivance of no real value, but searching for ones that are pristine with no defects or folds and assuredly "virgin" is a gene of the optimum procreation type. If that religious meme was too much to swallow start watching your commercials more closely as you will see religion meme spin-offs as you are told such things as "Tell all your friends", "Don't be without this", or "Your life will be complete with" type statements or implications. Think about your free will again because I think I have lost mine to genes that "want" and force my hand to take or do what is needed. Since I really believe what I am writing, holding back my genetics is not a big concern, as I find moments of satisfaction in letting my genes out for romp once in awhile. As for you my respected reader friend, take my advice and let go occasionally (once in a while) and you will believe in me even more than you would have thought possible. At any rate, go purchase a good book on meme's because you might have a new thought in your life.

246. Although the music moves in a steady stream of chromatic scales it brings chords of dissent within my mind and I am up to writing one more messed up paragraph. What is it in music that produces 3-D visions of emotions and meme activation's that could cause me to believe anything is possible while climbing a hypomanic mood to its extreme? Can we throw out the whole concept of manic-depressionism and proclaim that my species simply has emotional synesthesa activated by sound (music, contrived languages, or the memory of contrived verbiage)? Of course, that wouldn't account for the *Homaniakos'* sexual behavior caused by our normal traits of depression, anxiety, and a lack of serotonin. All of that aside, I am now fully inspired to tackle the forbidden where many already have tridden (and failed) - I have to ask you, can the belief in a god be directly genetic? There seems to be a lot of humans walking around that don't believe in a god, if it were to be an active gene. But please, allow me to ramble. All genetic traits are exhibited at all times either under the transparent skin of the memes that we use to define ourselves as a society of culture, or whenever your meme's are down as during a fit of anger or in a mob. So you would have to say that those humans that do not believe in a god have a genetic defect in order to account for their non-belief if you insist on genetic "god" thoughts. I suppose of course that if it is a very weak genetic trait, perhaps its actions are easy to overcome or transferred but overcome by other genes or by other memes such as the "I don't believe in a god" meme? Or why believe that a "god belief" is genetic and non-belief is memetic? On the reverse or obtuse side, would you believe that believing in a god is memetic and not believing (in a god) genetic? That is certainly a possibility, as we must look at all permutations as acceptable. I hope you are as confused as I am. It is true that some memes do work directly against what your genes tell you do (such as when and where to rut to avoid being rude or messy), but ultimately you're stuck with justifying this strange genetic "Godd belief" trait that really has no purpose for the procreation and continuance of human life because it actually divides humans as a world culture in place of unifying them. But religion does work very well at the tribal level and perhaps that is the best (or original) survival strategy. The rational that the belief in a god will reduce evil within the species for the purpose of continuance of the species is nonsense. Belief in a "god" only assures that when a human commits something against that god (or his/hers laws), that that human is punished. Proclaiming "I believe in this god" will sooner or later get you punished by other humans believing in that same god. Do you believe religion stops evil or creates a reason for punishment? Perhaps religion created the definition of evil which was then transformed into law by lawyers who claim separation of church and state of which the ordinary humans have come to believe are "natural" offenses or rather offenses against the natural order of civilized humans?   As I view the Christian/Judaism Old Testament, I see many genetic actions being fulfilled and justified by Godd, and if Godd walked the earth to-day, with mass-media coverage, he would find much protesting at his preferred method dealing with opposing tribes via the killing and murder that is documented within the OT by his command. But the *Hosapiens* have built a delusion of absolute purity around those actions and within their delusional minds there is no convincing them otherwise. Don't you agree? As a *Homaniakos* examining the laws of the western world, I see only laws contrived against every action for the purpose of taxation or punishment by tariff or fee or penalty and even murder cases bring millions of dollars to many humans as the events are sold and mediated across the networks with plenty of time for a commercial break. But now it is time to summarize and there are no obvious signs that any other creature on the earth has a "god exists" behavior and every species is doing fine with minimal genocide.

247. I believe what I have read and is expressed by the memetic experts that it is completely possible that religion and Godd are only memes which of course would be based on at least some miniscule genetic function that most likely has nothing to do with a Godd. So following, you are going to read what I've written - whether there is a religion or god gene in our DNA sequence, even if you don't believe in any relationships between Homo erectus man and Adam. Now some good Christians have expressed that perhaps early man did exist but was eliminated prior to Adam and Eve's creation or continued along with Adam and Eve but are not the Christian Godd's chosen few. Thus giving credence to the verse in Genesis "Replenish the earth". This allows you to have a scientific view of the universe, watch the Discovery Channel and have intellectual conversations at work without giving up your faith and ending up in Hell for the eternity. Where am I to rationalize the phables combined with the Bible combined with the faulty logic of mankind and womantype to justify every action and every strange "value added" belief they incorporate into their religions and thus into the character of their god? I suppose I will leave this chapter for the science of it and let CHAPTER GODD deal with the faith of it.

248. I will start off by saying I am not in favor of genetically creating the concept of a god at the very moment of writing this

sentence because it's hard to believe that such a conceptual thought could occur in genes, even by accident. It would also increase the chance that another life on the earth would believe in a god, because we share so many of our DNA sequences within the animal kingdom. But as my goal is to deduce the understanding of the ordinary human's behavior such that I may reduce my distressing thoughts about their unusual behavior, I must tell you that every human would thus be born to believe in a god if it was genetic. It's even harder to believe we could evolve a "god" gene because of some natural selection of breeding favorable traits, although a persuasive naturalist could put up some good arguments. After all, why is being afraid of falling off a cliff because it would be bad for you be any different than to believe in a creature that you haven't seen, but makes natural events occur without "causation". By genetics you avoid cliffs, even if you have never seen any creature fall and get hurt. This genetic trait helps you to survive as opposed to having to watch one of your friend's fall and die and then having you spread the knowledge of the danger of cliffs possibly before language was contrived by playing cro-magnum charades. So can every tribe come up with the idea of a god even if there is no communicative languages other than to scream or grunt while pointing at a mammoth? A test would be difficult to do or maybe the test is in each of our lives and we haven't paid attention to it. You have already had that thought, but we haven't yet arrived at [*Verb confusion (no suggestions)*] my least likely test.

249. I suppose that belief in a god would have no survival importance to a species since it *appears* that every species but humans do not believe in a god and they get along fine. Of course, I am applying Axiom #4 but it need not be the case.

Elephants (for example) could believe in god and not build temples to their god because of Axiom #4 applied. But then we are left to some very weird, by ordinary humans standards, beliefs because without the elephant god coming to the earth or living somewhere on the earth to communicate the knowledge of its existence to some elephants, we are left with needing some type of elephontal telepathy required or we end up back at the genetic god idea again. I suppose it will come within my lifetime that humans (hopefully not a *Homaniakos*) will proclaim that animals do worship a god and thus we can't eat them. Well aside from a few playful behavioral attributes that some animals seem to possess, most genetic behavioral actions of the earth's life seem based on keeping a species alive now and into its future. If god is genetic, then for certain no god exists and death is only death and your knowledge of existence after you are dead is no different than your knowledge of existence before your life. If I could be certain of that, I would spend less time dwelling on the fear of it.

250. For most creatures that resemble human life, that is creatures that might have eyes, ears, mouths, etc. like our own, there is a genetic survival behavior that is born into them. It doesn't matter if they are mammals, reptiles, arachnids, etc. Most every living creature is driven to survive by some type of genetic action. This action goes beyond the sensation of feeling pain or remembering pain by some type of pattern matching. Create more of your genes and then keep your genes alive seems to be the only rule of life, except that humans have imagined a way to live beyond death without genes (What an idea!). Now you might say that humans are not able to express or react to survival at birth. I completely agree with you. But I am going to tell you that I also agree with what I've heard or read maybe, that describes human

infants as embryos similar to kangaroos that are born prematurely (or rather born prematurely developed), and then develop outside of the body to the appropriate birth size and functional physical attributes. Not that I meant to describe an entire theory so sloppily without meeting with the approbation of the leading scientists or reduce it to the nounation of common words but the data is out there, you find it yourself. Now all of this occurs because of the size of a human baby compared to the size of the birth canal. That theory accounts for why human babies are so helpless physically and instinctively at birth compared to horses or monkeys but not compared to marsupials I guess?

251. I wasn't off the topic again in number 250, so we read that the feral humans mentioned in such books as *The Wolf Children* by Charles Maclean and *The Wild Boy of Aveyron* by Harlan Lane, also brings to mind that scientist have tried to determine if religion is genetic by examination of humans raised from birth, or there about, by another species in the wild or the calm of the wilderness depending on your vantage of humanistic verbiage. The idea here is that regardless of which god they believe in, belief in any god attribute would be genetic and not learned from the wild wolves. I am more inclined to say that if a feral human believes in a god, we could as easily say that it is because s/he has a Godd given soul and the spirit of the Lord is in her/him by Godd's will. An argument between the two camps would resolve nothing. Helen Keller might have had something to add to that argument but I can't find any good quotes from her except once she said, "Ouch, who moved the damn chair?" and that was stated in a private language anyway.

252. Humans surrounded by humans, even in the most remote tropical rain forests, could by a series of small reactions to natural events start various "god exists" thoughts and I am sure there are actually experts that have written about those topics but I must explain to you that I wonder about these thoughts in order to rationalize what I see versus what I feel. Do you and I share the same thoughts? You can have thoughts that something is in control of all of your misinterpretations of expected reactions of natural occurrences [*Too many phrases (no suggestions)*]. Starting at the early dates in history, or before history was collected, humans behaving naturally would create an "action" and build on the mutation of those actions via imitation and at the same time those actions are remembered by many humans in the tribe. Such as learning how to play Bingo (in the present time) and how much fun it is to talk about how much fun it is. One brick at a time is stacked until you have a wall that represents a history of an idea or religious thought or dogma within a tribal system. (Every thought or theory or contrivance is constructed one brick at a time from the ideas or actions that came before it.) But is this progression started because of a gene or a meme? A singular wolf boy would have no human reactionary feedback in order to continue, stop, or modify religious behavior. If I am remembering correctly, one of these wild boys when found walked on all fours, having had that locomotion behavior learned as a visual resource. I end my thought.

253. I thought I was done with this section but I have to write three more paragraphs because I've thought of one dandy reason to discuss a genetic belief in a god. Now I tucked my daughter in for the night after closing the writing of paragraph 252 in this

chapter a moment ago and she caused me to have a new thought. Why do human-children and many adult humans need to sleep with their closet doors closed? This "Closet Door Anxiety" (CDA as it is known by psychologist) causes distress in humans when attempting to sleep, and almost always at night. You must ask your friends or the other humans you meet during your daily activities if they have any similar fears. Looking under the bed or out a darkened window, or having the closet door opened, or putting your fingers uncovered on top of your pillow, or sleeping with a "night light" turned on, or pulling the shower curtains closed (or opened) the list seems endless but all the actions and paranoia are the same, don't you agree? If you do agree then I've got you at last and we will see "eye to eye" as I've heard the ordinary humans proclaim. A gene thing and its reactions has been found and humans are born with it, with it being modified by the contrived circumstances that that technology of the humans thrusts upon you my reader friend. This is then the start of an understanding of how a gene works (subliminally), and how all humans act on those genetic requirements, and that that gene most likely works to keep humans alive, because as you, my fine reader friend knows, humans can't possibly be thinking (as in "rationalizing") all day or when sleep arrives?

254. Humans do not want to be killed during their sleep when they can't hear a peep. Would you believe with me that this human-child fear of the unknown is strong enough to create a belief in a false reality, such as a reality of evil or danger or possible death where absolutely none *now* exists? Out of this fear comes a non-existent creature or creatures that has never been seen and can't be proven to exist. Did the *Homo erectus* also have fears based on the misinterpretation of reality? Do I

dare make comparisons to the ancient þast that might imply that the contemþorary human animal is still oþerating under the same action reaction as the *Homo erectus* (or whatever our ancestors are to be called to-day)? Yes I do, and from what I see every day, I am inclined to believe that even those delusions of a meaningful life are ancestral to the ordinary humans. Cognitive dissonance against a gene creates a meme. Language misconstrues the reality of it by multiþlexing the meme into a million variations of suþerstitions and religions of which the *Hosapiens* have so many, I can't honestly tell the difference between or among a suþerstition, a religion, or a cult. Generally (I'm drifting into 255), as the news media of the ordinary humans would describe, a religion becomes a cult once the leader induces mass suicide or ADM (Age Differential Mating) uþon his/her followers or their human-children. Wouldn't you agree with me that the differences couldn't be divided and sided for a comþarison against a chart of valid religious traits?[*Negation use (no suggestions)*] Since (I'm back) CDA aþþears to be a genetic reaction (it would have existed þrior to closet doors), all tribes of the earth could easily develoþ a demon out of the darkness and then a god and a religion to organize the two, and exactly in that sequence (I've left a few steþs out for brevity). At the þresent time, ordinary humans aþþly faulty logic in order to give tax-exemþt status to the mix of þlacing a ring of flowers on virgin statues, kissing the ring of an ordinary þaþa (who's never been a þaþa), or ringing a chickens neck (of which I have never actually heard a ringing sound, it sounds more like cracking celery). I'm sure that there are books on this subject somewhere but with all the various beliefs of Godd, angels, demons, humans speaking to the spirit world, or having dead ancestors watching over the living or their human-child for their safety, I would have to say that genetics still rule and the

Hosapiens are looking more out-of-their-mind all the time by them being ordinary. Look at what your friends or co-workers believe to be true of reality perceived but not provable or never seen. Don't you agree with my observations? There are few humans with common, rational beliefs as mine or yours, my reader friend.

256. So now I have convinced myself that a gene could cause a meme (an idea to pass along), which in turn could cause gods to exist by all remotely located humans of the earth. All of this and the creation of a god with infinite power for infinite time according to some humans, because humans must sleep with closet doors shut reverse translated and biased slanted into the pre-existing historical minds of a Neanderthal kind, into early mankind and womantype having human-children and sleeping in the jungles (a previous word for rain-forest) and telling them stories or by standing guard nearby (if a contrived language wasn't available) in order to calm their human-children's minds. In simpler terms, the ordinary humans I know don't seem too interested in discerning reality from phablization. Now I am of an unresolved mind once again and I will continue to shut my closet door. As for memes, they are gene driven because they control a genetic machine unless there is an example I am missing somewhere that you can tell to me?

257. What about the wolf children of the world? Why wasn't it proven they believe in a god? Maybe its not so complicated. Wolves are not afraid of the dark.

258. Although the glorious þart of the music is now starting, I do not want to share the feeling it brings when I know I must write about the þresent fears of my future life, esþecially when I have visions of my future living as a *Homaniakos*. I will þause [*Verb confusion (no suggestions)*] the music because I don't wish to create an association of þleasant music with dreary thoughts. So in the silence and darkness I will write as though within the grave I am trapþed, but I get caught in these thoughts everyday when I least exþect it, and I susþect my fellow *Homaniakos* brethren exþerience the same. At any rate, I þromised you a book of thoughts about death and how a Manic-Deþressive Junkie would see death within a metaþhysical fashion, so it's on to topics of a dangerous magnitude. I fear the future days when family members die, for they are alive now and thus their end is now only a matter of unknown time I supþose, and I would rather enjoy logical suicide to-day with a þeace of mind, than suffer seeing my þrocreation die to-morrow. Wouldn't you agree with me then that suicide could become logical? But here is how I see it, and when there is a death there is a funeral. Wailing and the gnashing of teeth must occur or there is no closure. However, you must maintain comþosure in your Sunday best, so you act like the rest. Your mind can only take suffering for so long and then it realizes that the body is hungry and thirsty. Food must be had everyday. After a wake, they bring food and then they leave. One by one they leave and with each closing of the door you are one less moment away from loneliness and then suddenly you are alone. For a moment you are I. Silence. Thoughts. Without a sþouse or a human-child your house filled with electronic shit that once brought you þleasures, now they would be your helþmates. Sounds and images from a broadcast tower will fulfill your life by misdirecting your genetic requirements. Technol unnatural environments offer no natural genetic actuators. You see a picture of a tree, but there is no shade for you. There are sounds of human-children playing, but no human-child will look into your eyes. Someone sings you a song, but you can't hold his or her hand. You can't figure out what is wrong because you are born into it. Is this what the human animal has worked and died to become? So this is your great techciety? This is what you proclaim makes us the most advance creatures on the earth? Technology is the masturbation of nature; it fulfills its own requirements by misdirecting the fulfillment of genetic behavior. Technology only satisfies the humans "self" even in a crowd of many.

259. The genes of an animal have no consciousness of technology. There is no evolution toward the acceptance of, or fulfillment through, the use of any device created by mankind or womantype. There never will be. The genes of an animal are not reactive to understanding technology via evolution with 50 years of watching a Television machine or driving an automobile mechanism. The pursuit of technology is no different than the rat in a cage choosing cocaine for meals in place of sustenance. We are no different than the rats, Godd or not. The belief in a god (as a meme) does little to direct the genetic actuators of optimum procreation satisfied by substitution with technology. Humans can barely tell the difference between a Muppet and a living human. Your genes won't let you. You can barely hold the thoughts of what is real and what is an image of the real. We are the baby chimpanzees holding on to the human mom in the nursery at the zoo. We are the animals in a zoo. We build ourselves our own cages and surround ourselves with pictures of the real world.

We cry at night and can't figure out what will make us stop crying. We cry alone and then we die alone.

260. Our genes tell us to live in a clan; the clan should be in a tribe. The tribe feels the same death, the same remorse, the same healing. The tribe creates a function for the existence of the human. The human will not be alone all the way onto death. "Purpose is in the function" for each human. Each human would have a function in a tribe. The individual function will go no further than to support the tribe. The human-children in the tribe will bond to their grandparents and will see them die. They will then watch their parents die, and then they will die. They will know that their human-children and human-grandchildren will be there when they die. In the coarse of natural events, if they die young, they will not be alone. No one should die alone even under sterilized bed sheets, feeding tubes attached, and a progress chart clipped to the footboard stating the time and cause of death before it occurs. The *Homaniakos* can feel the death of dying alone. We can see the clearer vision of reality that is the existence of nothingness after death or the pain of life before death or the vision beyond death. Look what your advanced techciety has done to me, to us. I sit here in an empty house, in the dark. I need no family to supply my heat, my light, my music, or my food and drink. Anything I want can be had within minutes. Any knowledge I wish to know, I can know within minutes. Anything I wish to see of beauty, of pain, of perversion, I can see within minutes. However, there is actually nothing here at all. I sit alone in a desert with illusions to occupy my mind until I die, alone. If I really could tell the difference, I wouldn't be sitting here, alone. A photograph of a tropical beach is on my wall. Humans in the warm sun under a

blue sky by turquoise water, smiling, laughing, but I can't tell myself it is an illusion.

261. With all the hype about lifestyles, where it is verbalized in a contrived language to appear to us that we have choices about constructing our own family by planning on eliminating fathers via artificial spermation with jerked-off spermatozoon collected and donated and vaginally inserted for lesbianites or men enjoying sodomiting each other without concerns about moms for their human-children all the while proclaiming "I'm a good Christian role model", nobody is being fooled not even yourself. The genes within your cells don't go for it so as a house built for land but put on wheels, you must move deliberately and you must constantly fix the cracks in the plaster. You've fallen for the meme's of free will and believe that you are closer to happiness when in fact genetically we were never meant to be anything more than satisfied. Sex and orgasms and feeling the penetration of it, and the passage of life's fluids brings satisfaction, and it matters not if nouns or verbs describe the "act", the "act" must be done on behalf of the gene and everyone finds a way. But I will never hold any blame, regardless of your choice, for who is righteous enough to do so and how else would we fill our lonely days? For a moment will you my reader friend, look at all the lost satisfaction within the humans without names split from their offspring via courtroom legalities that massage the wallet but have no concern for the human heart. Contrived events such as "holiday's" screw every human clan, split-up or driven apart, when writing lists of who goes where and whom to invite and whom to leave out of the calendared events. We dig ourselves deeper and deeper into isolation with technology self indulgence and use the ability to say, "I love you" from a cell Fon as a true act of parental guidance. Won't you

stop it for my species sake? You are all starting to feel as I do and I can see it in your faces. What would I do in a world full of dissatisfaction and despair? How would I find my distractions from reality with your delusions of happiness never being fulfilled?

262. Walking out of a home for the aged, what the hell is that? Leaving tearful hearts sitting in a living morgue to count the days until their death by counting the occupants that are missing each new day. Death is announced by a Fon call, there is no face, no eyes to look deeply into. "Who the hell cares anyway?" says the day keepers of the discarded, "Sanitize and change the name on the door". Look what they've done to my brain, mom. I can't undo this meme; there is no going back. The power cannot be turned off. I cannot unplug. I am addicted to the speed, the glitter, the feeling of energy. Push the accelerator to the floor and speed away to nowhere. Always warm or cool, always full with thirst quenched, and always entertained or mesmerized by glowing lights projecting pornographic images of false lives in a digitized media or storage device. A lonely mind wondering where my youth, my life went so quickly. I look at the photograph on my wall. The blue sky, the turquoise water, the soundless laughter, but I am not there. I am dying. It is but minutes before I am in that room, my name on that door. Attendants down the hall will laugh all-day and go home to families at the eve while I sit alone in front of a TV no less. They will say to me, "Mr. Hanink, there you go, are you comfortable now?" (All the while they exhibit a fake but natural appearing facial expression of a comforting smile). The vision of my future is built on the perversions of nature from the humans that came before me. Are you going to tell me from your delusional life filled with the pursuit of unnatural satisfactions that suicide is not logical? Fuck all of you.

263. So un-pausing the music, if there is such a word or action, I will now tell you that the whole point of the human language is revealed by the *Homaniakos* species. Why have languages of this complexicon? For the language of the Manic-depressive is much more complex than that of the *Hosapiens* [*Comparisons?*], what with all of our nontransitive depdendency relationships. So many theories I have read and if we rid ourselves of Godd as the creator for a chapter, we can get to some radicals of ideas. If all humans must do is pick or pluck a berry, kill squirrels, rut, and run from a lion why should they do more than grunt and point? When the humans get so self-centered that they believe they are cultured by quoting Latin at parties; "Veni vidi nauseam" (I came, I saw, I threw up), of what purpose is it when it serves no purpose at all? Most everything in the human language serves no purpose and is not a means to a natural end – and I offer you this book as the first sacrifice to that thought. It amazes me how humans react to words spoken, written. Words are not an action and only an action reveals the truth, because once done, it can't be undone (Only within the human mind are actions "taken back".). Thus words of languages reveal nothing of the truth, and yet words cause so much reaction in the faces of the humans. A human once stated "I'll believe it when I see it" and perhaps that is the only statement worth stating.

264. Do you, my reader friend, place the position of mankind and womantype as the supreme creatures on the earth because of what they can speak and how they speak it? Being able to say "I am" or "I know that I will die" are not even rational thoughts let alone thoughts to place into a language to be heard or documented. When it comes to the universe, its beginning and its end, and the time in between, humans know nothing thus can express no facts. Even if you say "The ball is green" we see that the names of objects and colors are contrived in each culture and then the seeing of it is dependent on the spectral light source plus the viewers learned experience plus the viewers retinal capacity for color or not plus the memorization of grammatical interjection. How can we have the truth with so many qualifiers applied? Language works best when not really thought about or figured out for the truth of it. Language will always remain a contrivance, as we cannot be genetically altered to be born with our language on our tongue. Language ultimately proves its self to always being a lie at best or at minimum a projection of a perceived reality and what's the difference? Toward what end of superiority does it serve then? Did not early mankind and womantype get us this far without a language? Do not all species survive without a language but only making the playback sounds they are born with, or communications made of air borne chemicals? (Some creatures use body motion or blinking lights as a communication method.)

265. But to fill space and make my book thicker for better value perceived, because we are paying cash for language when we purchase a book, I guess but I don't want to guess but I should explain one more example of what I previously continued to state. Suppose an event occurred in the world that you can sense, and it appeared by all your senses that a leaf departed from a tree and lighted upon the ground. You having been the sensual witness thereof should walk away and never mention with a language the description of what you sensed because therein starts the lies and the conversion from sensory perception to the contrived language in either a verbal or written remark will lead to errors. For nature

never intended such an event or any event to be described via verse and it certainly did not perceive your ability to verbalize it. Where as for the example given it is a fact that your feet were on the ground and your eyes reacted to reflected light, you can see that your words were based on your frame of reference and the resolution of your eyes given the time delay of optical sensing. Yet does not the earth move through space (that is not easily perceived) and isn't it as likely that the earth moved up to greeting the leaf? Where then is your truth in the description of said event? [*Stilted*]

266. Language does not make an adequate carrier of thoughts or feelings in that only thinking thoughts felt or feeling actions needed or lost can be real, and thus understood, provided a language is not used to describe them. So a thought going from brain A to brain B via energy wave carrier or document inscription was not meant to be anything more than a call of "Here I am" or "There's danger" and to that, grammar or sentence construction is not possible because most all the animals are born to say what they need and they understand it without being rude. Although the birds "sing" as ordinary humans would describe, but to my knowledge from what I have learned they are shouting at each other in a private language (via our perceptions) of "Stay away" and "This is my tree", and not much more than that except during mating season I suppose and what did you believe they were saying? How do we understand that shouting birdal obscenities is music to our ears in place of the annoyance that it truly is? Truly an example of how the genetic predisposition to sight and sound of the human species predetermines the perceived actions and reactions of another species with no true understanding being

able to be applied. Thus the humans create their whole world from within their minds outward, and how can that be correct?

267. To those who would believe that natural selection actually works and serves a purpose of survival, then language is energy and time and must be proven to aid in the survival of a species via some type of "control at a distance" behavior that makes sound waves prove their worth in terms of wasting the humans precious bodily energy. The theories that food was difficult to find 1.5 million years ago have lead some (scientists) to believe we must have conserved speaking energy or that a language must have assisted in survival somehow, but all other species of the earth prove otherwise. How do we know that the now extinct dino-creatures weren't also the only other animals with a contrived language (thus leading them into extinction as they spent way too much time debating gender-based behaviors)? Evolutionists are always concerned with functionality or the energy required of an organism especially if a value-added feature is being developed because why waste "life" energy on biological R & D projects. Yet should we assume that at some point evolution stops and why because all animals have gotten to their optimum design - then take a look at what a waste of energy most life exhibits? Yet humans will prefer to believe and follow schemes, fads, and beliefs based on fairy tale data expressed via a contrived language as opposed to following established facts or simpler rules. Following verbalized schemes wastes energy and yet humans spend so much energy following them even at the expense of resources for survival. So humans are either not finished evolving or gone past their optimal or is just plain stupid. Perhaps we are so energy efficient that we look for the fastest, easiest, or most for the money and then never realize that we cannot out think

evolutionary efficiency with human-made contrivances þurchased from infomercials that we can't figure out the logic there of. (Wasn't that a þleasant þaragraþh? I always wanted to write about evolutionary theories even though my exþerience in the subject goes no further than book learning and observing the behavior of the ordinary humans.)

268. The fact that an ear knows to hear thus "I want two" is strange enough. For what came first the language or the ear to hear it? In reality sound is energy traveling through a media of any þhysical tyþe, thus ears and language are not related in the farthest stretch of the actuality of any DNA þlan. Yet I honestly believe that ordinary humans believe the two were meant for each other. For what I am waiting to have figured out is how the genes in a DNA sequence communicate to each other in such a mutually beneficial way that the coding for an ear creates coding for vocal cords to create sounds in the same oscillation þitch that can be heard via a common medium (the atmosþhere). I would be willing to bet that DNA is the memory of good ideas, not the creator of them and what memories it must hold in code. Desþite the aþþearance of comþlex neural networks setuþ or established via þracticing a verbal language, we sþeak within our means, and thus our brain might look exactly the same, even if all we did was grunt and moan or cry with loneliness. The fact that very young human-children can understand our language þroves nothing of the naturalness of it. Although ears are worth the effort because it's a toss as to whether vision or hearing is your first alert that you are about to be something else's dinner. Hearing is vision around corners or in the dark, þrovided your brain can make sense of it all via memory þattern maþþing or genetic sounds of disþassion or sþookiness. Why do all sþooky sounds sound sþooky to all? By now you should know the answer. So we can toss hearing and language relationships out because if the ear can hear vibratory air, then it was not put there to hear your rendition of the misery of your last root canal. Now you must remember that of all the animals that have ever lived, most live fine hearing woof, grrrrr, or bang and isn't "living" or continuance the ultimate objective of existence? But perhaps most or many animals look at humans with their ears (not eyes) because most animal's ears are "forward looking" on their head and it has never been proven that any animal except humans understand that the eyes of another creature can see them, but the ordinary humans perception of it is always vision biased because all thoughts of the ordinary humans are biased to their own perception of reality.

269. If I can throw this thought in after the fact and whether it makes sense or not to anyone but me, human ears are physically placed for hunting and detecting the direction of sounds around them by something called triangulation (I hope) because that is the direction of the hunt and that is how humans found noisy food or even noisy mating partners shouting "Oh sailor!" Thus language for conversation is not even a consideration in the design of the ears or humans would have one ear perfectly round on their forehead so that they hear only who is talking to them and not be bothered by surrounding noises. Ask a one-eared human or watch them turn their good ear forward.

270. Of language as in books filled with definitions we have proven no point or function or need other than humans can remember a lot and thus humans are culturally biased, denied, and split into the A list or B list based on their grammar, their monies, or the size of their cleavage. Language that is not genetically

patterned to be repeated from birth, as is such with the birds and the bees and the whales no doubt, is a contrivance to add complexity to the ordinary humans unnatural environment of gadgets and stuff and thus it is not good at revealing the truth as the truth is never known when spoken, as I stated previously or will state later in this book. Who can understand a thought that language does not say to you in your head as when you are thinking about something? Yet as sure as a frog sees a bug and wants it without writing prose about it, we have thoughts that words never describe to us in a language, they are only thoughts, and we act on them all day long in fact and more prevalent than the thoughts we have of words no doubt as in the re-enacting of arguments recently past. The rest of our thoughts are done and gone prior to us transcribing a language to them anyway. Although there are animals that appear to sing, that language may only be music to our ears. We have no proof that music is the humans communications gear, but what a drug it has turned out to be.

271. As the soft voiced white human female speaks in that oh so compassionate tone perfectly scripted and repeated prime time every radio day, humans are pulled into a belief of what is sold by virtue of Mullerian mimicry at the human level. Always selling a politician that cares or a Managed Health Care business that treats me better than cold cash, I turn the volume off because I don't wish to become inured to a caring voice selling me shit. I don't wish to obtain a mass sociogenetic memetic slanted illness from the line of sight transmission of a word on a scripted page spoken, so I treat language as an infectious bug that can harm or kill or change a life for as long as that life can live, or into eternity if you are so inclined to believe.

272. Drawing the night strings of my own conclusion for you, in case your pencil is not pointed in the correct direction, the *Homaniakos* have hyper-enhanced senses in that what we see, touch, smell, hear, & taste can be perceived through a finer sieve. Thus what we may tell you is annoying, a sound, a rattle, a light, a scent, is actually received and processed to a finer degree and sets the mind in motion for thoughts of life or better still, death. Our perceptions increase the depth of meaning and fills our minds as we see atoms are further apart than touching and thus the universe is barely glueoned together and hangs on a thought of its own understanding. Motions of love and youth, life and laughter, run visions of "How do we participate also?" through our minds as we see blurred images recalled from a past that might as well have been someone else's life. Am I beyond the touch or to be touched passion that only affords itself in passing once to each of us? Was that all there was to this physical realm of the 5 senses plus ours? I am going back, I want a second helping and I will chew each bite 32 times for the want of each sight of budding perfection, velvet smooth touching places, scent of pheromones dripping, each giggle of pleasure, and to taste each lick of information so moist and warm. The mind commands and the senses deliver as nature intended in this genetic reality of existence, but you cannot think about it too much or you'll see back stage and the false fronts fall down when touched.

273. You have now completed CHAPTER HUMAN PERCEPTIONS VERSUS TRUE REALITY, please turn the page and proceed to CHAPTER MANKIND AND WOMANTYPE. Do not mark in your book and please visit, at your convenience, our reference pages at the rear of the book.

274. Notes: The following sentence is called a trilogram. It contains 3 sentences inside of one: *Lying, cheating, stealing, destruction of property are all part of the "ordinary human" attributes, I'm not that screwed up, as you would have me think about this sentence.* The three individual sentences are: *"Lying, cheating, stealing, destruction of property are all part of the "ordinary human" attributes. "I'm not that screwed up, as you would have me think".* And: *"Think about this sentence."* It is the zipped version of a paragraph and thus becomes more resource and time efficient.

THE MOST BASIC KNOWLEDGE OF THE PHYSICAL REALM:

The Four Axioms of Existence:

Axiom #4

"No living entity can have a greater understanding of its existence, than the physical ability to act on it."

Axiom #3

"?"

Axiom #2

"?"

Axiom #1

"?"

The only purpose of all living organisms:
"Optimum procreation"

Most basic law of nature:
[As expressed in a human language]
"?"

Most basic law of unnatural systems:
"Complexity causes complexity"

THE MOST BASIC KNOWLEDGE ABOUT THE HUMAN ANIMAL:

Genetic behavioral motivators of human males:
"The Birth of a Son"
"The Hunt"
"The Kill"

Genetic disposition of human males:
"Tribal"

Genetic behavioral motivators of human females:
"Becoming Impregnated"
"Territorial Possessiveness"

Genetic disposition of human females:
"Clannish"

CHAPTER
MANKIND AND
WOMANTYPE

"Building bridges and spaceships is to the self-glory of mankind and womantype, but optimum procreation is for the glory of Godd and is the primary purpose of the physical human." R. J. Hanink

The music that set the mood for writing this chapter was:
  "Edward Scissorhands" CD by Danny Elfman
  "Too Old to Rock 'N' Roll: Too Young To Die" CD by Jethro Tull.

Starting in the middle

275. Being a *Homaniakos* of the junkie type, and one that pays attention, I see there is a reason for the seasonal differences between or among mankind and womantype with too many gender based actions/reactions that could not have been learned from their daddy or mommy or invetro-tube and forget that Television Machine Stereotype Meme Infection Syndrome because that technology method of meme transference is too new (insert a three week gap here) and not in popular use everywhere that ordinary humans (the *Hosapiens*) behavior is found to be similar by the division of the sexes. All human species are pure instincts, gene driven, stuck in the mist of contrived circumstances compliment of our advanced technology - and the humans actions are never appropriate for the moment at hand to the individual or techciety at large, although the *Homaniakos* feel the truth of it while viewing the world through some type of motion blur. Sociopath-ic behaviors that are dominated by either of the two genders supplanted crosswise by the *Hosapiens/Homaniakos* specie protocols are then derived from one or many of that genders "Genetic Behavioral Motivators" combined with that genders "Genetic Disposition" as stated on the dope sheet on the opening page of this chapter I hope. What other agent could be at work except nature? I mean to tell you now and then later (as you would have expected), I must know what drives all these actions of the ordinary humans, the *Hosapiens*, if I am going to continue to interact with them or at least walk amongst them undisturbed as a body double. Within those actions are the origins or similar[s] of the enhanced humans, the *Homaniakos*. So many of us *Homaniakos* have died for lack of an understanding the actions of the ordinary humans - their ways are strange to the *Homaniakos'* shared mind and contrary to our shared vision thus death becomes us. Living with the ordinary humans is the primary cause of our logical suicide because of our observations followed by our rationalization followed by noticing the *Hosapiens* lack of applied logic and the failure of the *Hosapiens* to realize the reality of their situation. In place of name calling or insulting or degrading other humans for their inability to correctly rationalize and act on modern situations, or what techciety proclaims are inappropriate actions performed during mating or procreation rituals, you would be better off to say "Their genetics got the better of them" (Although for the entertainment value of my book, I prefer the phrase "faulty logic".). My basic premise is that whatever the genetics of it, it must be basic and simple and consistent throughout time regardless of the emotion of the truth for since when is nature complex in action and since when is nature to be accountable for its actions as documented by the humans in a contrived language[*Sound an interrobang here as the official end of the sentence punctuation*] It matters not whether you (as the reader or hearer or viewer or feeler of this book) believe all human species evolved them or that Godd gave them to you in order to survive; both apply equally for how can you deny that all humans, ordinary or not, have them? Now although I am not quick to admit or even desiring to build bridges of commonality to the ordinary humans of whom we all share a certain degree of genetic attributes, I must state that optimum procreation is also a human trait as all animals must have it; so there is where the similarities end (fade). So when I say "human" I mean without a doubt an all-inclusive statement for every human specie or sub-specie if you are inclined to believe in sub-species. Now if we are to continue with the rationale of the Manic-depressive Junkie via Metaphysical logic, then let me remind all of you that if Plato (whom by all accounts now, was a genus) could speak of mankind and womantype, then so can I (whether a genius or idiot I prove to be).

276. Womantype is quick to say "That's men for you!" or some other contrived verbiage of a naturalist observation off the flick of their tongue without any thought it takes, but the media and control gangs of feminists and feminites (men that support feminist priorities), constantly chisel at the *Hosapiens* natural reactions to tell them that what they feel naturally has been supplanted by *Barbie doll* commercials and Saturday morning *Flash Gordan* style male dominance propaganda (75 words). Mankind responds "Who can figure woman out?" but obviously every man has figured womantype out and thus the peaceful gender endures through contrived verbiage to justify mankind's lot in life but mankind is perfectly satisfied to accept what is obviously ordained by nature and DNA sequences because he (as in "mankind") would be a lost soul and live worst than a þig without his mating half (womantyþe) to þick uþ after him at every moment (75 words). The þreceding two sentences being of equal length thus þrove that mankind and womantyþe are indeed equal and thus why continue with a moot þoint? If this were not true then the only deduction of thought is what the *Hosaþiens* shouldn't acceþt because it reduces them to idiots (with a Dutch Tilt) that are þrogrammable every generation by the first stuþid thought that is sþoken to them and I know that if any of the *Hosaþiens* have made it this far into my novel novel that they hold a thought to read the very next word written for they wish to cognize [*cogitate?*] uþon a new idea even if they don't believe every word of it or are annoyed by these long and imþroþer sentences and þaragraþhs. What I'm trying to say with written words as I am now immerging from a good solid hour of deþression and desþair as I cycle daily through hell, reality, and back into the delusional world of everyone around me, changing subjects without concern as my thoughts derail, is that if you (the reader) are a *Hosaþiens* you might turn out to be one of the small þercentile of ordinary humans with intelligence beyond the normal if indeed you are normal, but making it this far for a *Homaniakos* would be stroll in the þark on yet another "Will I die to-day?" day (104 words).

277. Seeing with the *Hosaþiens* mind or from within their mind is the direction in which I'm heading - for all of organic life consists of actions by or from "genes" and what else would anyone believe it is some tyþe of thoughts from an invisible organ that thinks for them exceþt when they are declared brain dead? Although it is obvious that some life on the earth has develoþed to be more comþlex than most life on the earth, the degree to which genes, þsychology, and memes þlay a role in self actuating organic

compounds is what needs to be addressed and I remain only a *Homaniakos* driven to explain the scientific complexity of it in this difficult contrived language and without being an expert either (but with maximum confidence, self applied and not to be denied). In this era, in this country, all ordinary humans look for reasons to actions observed but this is nothing new only that they believe it to be so. The ancient Greeks also thought and dwelt upon life as evident by their philosophies and writings or verbiations or nounations before writing was used. The ancient Romans did the same and nothing has changed since then because nothing had changed since before them[*then?*]. The *Hosapiens* minds are not born containing the contrived history of mankind or womantype and getting to the truth of history takes a more serious effort via distorting the aspect ratio of reality further than most ordinary humans would wish to pursue - but I am a very pursuant type of human myself.   Mostly the *Hosapiens* wish to understand the actions of humans that murder other humans, stalk other humans, or appear to be down right different humans because all the rest of humankind are[*is*] oh so boring.   Even though obviously overstated because the history of humankind's litter-ature is blowing down the gutters of history as everyone famous by the way of thoughts wishes to figure the old in and out of what is good or evil or appropriate, but they create stories where evil dominates because evil is so interesting and good wins except for in moments of contrast. I guess this is very evident in our cinema pop culture to which I will dedicate this chapter. However, isn't the entire of that previously stated statement only the search for an understanding of free will?   Without the will of "good" humans to brush against the humans possessed of evil, the *Hosapiens* would not have an excuse for lustful fornication needed but acted on only by being compulsed[*sp?*] by the femme fatale; thus ensuring their being able to deny their own evil actions or intentions as willful.

278. One good example of that search for free will is the belief for genetic reasons of why some humans are homosexual – but I only choose them because they have established human activists to fight for their freedom or equality. Or possibly that the physical aspects of a humans brain may lead them to become homosexual or acquire a tilt for that lifestyle. Thus they would not choose to act as "they" as in "them" do, or that "they" are "their" own species as is the *Homaniakos*. I can tell you right now, the knowledge of the truth will never matter and I'm not going to make a production out of it except as a comparison of thoughts already similar to thoughts the *Hosapiens* might already possess about the *Homaniakos* as being some type of nut. Those humans whom/who are not homosexual will remain acting according to their genetic functioning and continue to either distance themselves from or aggressively attack homosexuals. As will be explained by the end of this chapter (whatever the name of this chapter will become), genes will win and all that threatens optimum procreation, survival, tribal attributes, or clannish behavior will be ostracized or destroyed, whenever the law allows it or it is felt it can be gotten[*got?*] away with at the moment the law isn't looking. Your life hangs on the thread of a meme when faced with the aggressive optimum procreation gene. It will take powerful memes to overcome the attitude of ordinary humans into accepting homosexual's lifestyle despite the creativeness and down right fun you can have at some of their parties or at a Mardi Gras festival. It is even difficult for family members that express what ordinary human's call love toward each other to overcome their own genetic traits toward homosexual clan members. The term "homophobic" is a nonsense contrivance sound with an ill conceived meme that only homosexuals themselves will be infected with, while the rest of the *Hosapiens* will still continue to let their genes control their actions. There is no substance to that "homophobic" word regardless of how many of the *Hosapiens* use it in the common lingo of the day, because most all humans use it as an automatic dialogue replacement for whatever the last fad verbiagation fun was, thus it is seen as an insult to natural behavior if given a second thought. My words *Hosapiens* and *Homaniakos* will suffer the same fate, I'm sure, but we all must try to better the world or ourselves I suppose [*Order of words (no suggestions)*]. Trying to use religion as the carrier meme for the homosexual acceptance meme will not work well either. Most religion memes have already provided statements for the cleansing of the species from threats of becoming less god-like. Classical religion memes are very genetic in structure simply because during their creation societies were based more on genetic actions and less on technology driven tribal matrixing, thus the *Hosapiens* once had a greater acceptance of genetic motivations before politicians of the schyster[*sp?*] type were memed into existence and screwed everyone's natural life via the language of hate crimes. Thus we have the Old Testament, which is among the greatest outline of the *Hosapiens* genetic "morals" published but the *Hosapiens* pick through it to avoid what they disagree with as though Godd states it is OK with him (no metaphor here).

279. Maybe you, my fine reader friend, believe you can see the similarities between human activist homosexuals trying to mainstream their lifestyles into the techciety of the ordinary humans and the main purpose of this book, the acceptance that the *Homaniakos* is a species of a human genus (Taxa: Division,

Subdivision, Class, Subclass, Order, Family, Subdivision of the Family, Genus, Species, Varietas, Forma, Clone, if I could plant that knowledge in you) as opposed to us being classified as mentally ill. I don't wish to mainstream manic-depressives into the techciety of ordinary humans so that we may be satisfied with a bit part of the daily events. And I suspect based on my past friendships that most homosexuals only need to be treated with the respect due to all humans. There would be no advantage to my species to be mainstreamed into the *Hosapiens* techciety because it really wouldn't feel natural. How could we share feelings not being able to exchange those feelings via a contrived language or by passing through the fourth wall? To tell you what I actually believe will happen with regards to the *Hosapiens* opinion of me and the *Homaniakos* species, I see only a few ordinary humans accepting us and the rest of the *Hosapiens* will continue to let their genes rule as with their thoughts on the homosexual crowd. Thus I will never gay bash unless someone gets in my face and then I don't care what the agenda is, but that will then be proof that my book is correct, genes rule the *Hosapiens* and me both (but fortunately my genes have less defects). The meme that I placed within this book will not be powerful enough to alter much of the *Hosapiens* actions because I can't offer a meme to them that will have enough traits such that there is any benefit for them to believe it will help them to maximize their genetic behavioral motivators. My meme will not convince the *Hosapiens* that they can have better optimum procreation, survive longer, or provide more necessities for their families. So if a human is only ordinary, why should they allow themselves to become infected with the "*Homaniakos* is a valid species" meme and why spread it? Crosscut altruism into this mix and review the results versus clan survival, tribal hierarchies or memberships, and the ability of ordinary humans to accept and live among other humans that are known to be different whether the difference can be touched or not, because all the differences can't be logicized simply as black and white or as a threat when no prior history of a threat is known by proof.

280. Most of the *Hosapiens* believe what most of the *Hosapiens* in their culture believe and there is not much more to it than that because they are all genetic creatures with an overly abusive ability to imitate. There are obstacles to overcome in their beliefs of how all of this works because they already have formulated their opinions (by age 12 it would seem by my observation). However, in actuality the *Hosapiens* and the *Homaniakos* have few opinions that are outside of working toward optimum procreation unless they are dealing with purely contrived mechanisms or concepts. With myself really believing what I write my thoughts follow manic-depression protocols and why not turn up the volume on some Heavy Metal Rock for the correct room tone and fornicate or rut with whoever or whomever will oblige me, because I get in these *Homaniakos* moods of the optimum procreation type and I realize its all very natural and to hold back is a shame only to save the cultural appearance of it or to prevent the spreading of contrived or private languages throughout the town. But I remain passive as trained, and I suppose I always will, thus proving humans of any type can learn cultural doggie tricks.

281. As part of my resolution to resolve all this behavior I observe while walking within the realm of the ordinary humans or as the recipient of contrived remarks that I hear as gossip at work or on the evening news broadcast, I now believe there must be only a couple of genetically driven actions required for all the many combinations of behavior I see in the *Hosapiens*. But oh how the *Hosapiens* believe they are such a complex creature, divinely created and mated for the pleasure.of some voyeuristic god sitting at some unknown distance within some unknown reality with eyes that don't exist but "see all" and also knows all thoughts thought. So complex the *Hosapiens* believe they are, but I think not. Always making qute [*cute*] remarks concerning the "nature of man" as though nobody will ever figure them out, but as I am no longer as them, what I see is another animal doing its natural thing but denying the truth of it via some type of language. Technology fools them, every one of them. They all use technology but they act as though it empowers them by some grand plan. Yet technology adds nothing but distractions to nature and thus it distracts from the nature of mankind and womantype. The *Hosapiens* have not evolved into technology, they somewhat mentally adapt to it and every newborn human must do the same but none of them believe that to be true, as so often I hear "Kids are so smart these days". So this should be easy to figure out, I tell myself, watch and listen to clean speech and throw in a remark or two as a test and watch the facial gestures reveal the truth and write down the results in private for this book. How better to conduct a test with a living creature than to pretend to be one of them with complete convincability[*sp?*][*Fragment, no suggestions*]? I must observe for basic behaviors but realizing that technology is screwing with every action/reaction. It's not that my ideas are new, because I have read many similar thoughts in other books thus I steal them and why not because all human species are natural thieves, but I honestly believe the *Hosapiens* in general believe they are always thinking their way through life with no regards for their genetics guiding them at every moment possible. On the other hand (if you have an other hand), I believe given a few genetic actuators, some memes, a contrived language, and a technology that can't be reckoned with, and about everything can be accounted for [*Poor sentence structure*]. Thus I have written my *Four Axioms of Existence* along with the "Genetic Behavioral Motivators of Humans" and the "Genetic Disposition of Humans" in order to explain it all and I'll keep writing to tell you that I expect you will find this chapter interesting even if not believable – so you are heading into one of those science lessons taught with bad grammar and no tests documented to validate any of it and I would prefer that you believe that you and I are talking together after dinner at one of those stand-up and drink all night social events, where I won't let you get a word in edgeways.

282. As I find myself trying to behave as a good Manic-depressive Junkie whenever I can or may, sex must [*Verb use (no suggestions)*] be had or thought about or fulfilled in some manner (every 72 hours as I have heard) or I would be distressed more often than I would prefer to be. So following the 6th and 7th protocols of hypomanicism, you would find that an increase in sexual activity or excessive involvement with (or the thoughts to do such while holding fears of doing such) sexual activity that has a potential for negative consequences within the laws or morals of the *Hosapiens* causes me to question and understand the nature of sex during my quiet moments. Sex, as in "the sex act" or "doing it", is when and where you find it, and from what I observe of the *Hosapiens*, sex is always on someone's mind because of the topics of the news broadcasts or the gossip or the sermons or the Television shows or the books or the Internet sites or the video rentals. As for myself, I follow the *Homaniakos* protocols, plain and simple and why deny it because they feel so natural to me. So

when looking at the "all" of life, why would you expect me to believe that life itself has any other primary purpose but to do "it"? (For the Christian reader, check the first chapter of Genesis and you will see that all life created was instructed to procreate, first and foremost, via Godd's plan. Therefore you see that my source of procreation knowledge is Biblical by source, and quite simple at that. Since I can't become famous unless I discover a syndrome or something with a real cool name, I now give you *The Genesis Protocol.* The genetic motivation to push your genes into the future is stronger than any other genetic function via nature or Godd. It matters not what "you" are or how you achieve your genetic future existence. Check Genesis 9:1, for a reiteration from Godd, and also Genesis 8:17.) Well at any rate if I am going to understand the nature of mankind and womantype (of the *Hosapiens* type) with regards to procreation acts or sex or lust or naughty bit pleasures self derived and contrived or hypnotized carnal lies, then I must subtract technology or where would be the nature or naturalness of it? Current technology allows most human-babies to live to become adults (in those countries that have such technologies). A birth in the U.S.A. during these times usually results in an eighteen to twenty-one year investment for a parent during these advanced technology days. Thus having many human-children creates a resource burden on the members of a techciety based on cash survival with technology pleasures. A quick study of the life expectancy charts of the Christian year 1900 reveal a 50% or greater chance of death by age 21 and I don't suppose it was ever better than that earlier in the earth's history. Thus getting to a "root cause" of sexual actions will be the confirmation of my axioms and the "Genetic Behavioral Motivators" of both the human species I suppose. If a natural human (of the so-called primitive type) didn't start procreating at the age of 12 or 13 their genes weren't going to make it into the future, via *The Genesis Protocol*, and all genes presently still have no knowledge of our elongated life expectancy due to our technology or how it screws us when it helps us or how long it takes the *Hosapiens* species to learn to imitate all the button pushing needed to survive now-a-days, so what happens is the *Hosapiens* natural self doesn't understand the circumstances of delayed procreation and logic can't be applied to sex denied when genes ascribe [*to it*]. The *Hosapiens* always seem astonished by sex or who's doing it, although most of them do it when they can, because I hear them talk about other *Hosapiens* doing it as if nobody's thought of it before and I have to wonder if the great apes or the parrots or the porpoises have the same conversations?

Optimum procreation

283. So the prolog long winded is over and here we go because the optimum procreation behavior of both the human species finds it important that the females of the species is procreating at all times from the moment she is virile. For the males of the species it is important to be procreating as soon as possible due to the most likely event he will die doing something while hunting or killing or fighting with opposing tribes and thus how will his "Y" chromosome make it into the future if he delays mating especially with medicine being mostly undiscovered back at the beginning of it all? Thus I see from where I sit to view, mankind and womantype perfectly equal still as Godd via *The Genesis Protocol* had ordained or evolution has dictated during the coarse of this human size epic. The *Hosapiens* are no different than fish or mice or birds or whatever. Because of a language that someone grunted once and everyone else has copied the

Hosapiens believe they have something extra like more senses or the power to behave rationally. Once girls are budded (with a hot set) and all furred up, and boys are in the pipeline with that fifteen-minute erection projection schedule, what would I believe did nature intend them to do? Build a bridge? Paint the house? Get a liberal arts degree? None of the above is my observation. They must procreate in the most optimum of ways is what I am getting at and judging by what is going on around me, all I see is a constant struggle to hold the youth back as in tying a race horse down in the gate moments before the bell. The youth don't want to have constant distractions to their attractions but what occurs is that a female seeks a female and a male seeks a male for a constant company as a best friend or teammate in some contrived sport where there is no kill after the hunt. Thus blood is not let at that young age and life goes unfulfilled daily without the knowledge of the genetic satisfactions of the hunt and the kill and the eating of living flesh as new sensations would be learned and taught in the confusion of natural passions.

284. What is remaining for the unfortunate *Hosapiens* is [*that*] due to a contrivance such as the modern school system, is ten years of frustration as sex acts are hidden but with that contrived language being the carrier of lies, while mating behaviors are exhibited at all opportunities as little girls are excited to walk the halls of the malls with breasts hidden but artificially exhibited as being ripened and young boys groom their hair and learn that walking stride to show what a hunter they have become so as to provide for the family never to be had until they all learn to push more buttons or learn the imagined history's of the white-mans contribution to the fucked-up world. So our restrained boys suffer from "Alien Hand Syndrome" and they have to carry that skill into adulthood. I can't imagine what the ordinary humans are thinking they are doing correctly here? The youth are all becoming liars of sexual adventures to their parents faces and then school grades are the objective of what kind of race and who wins? All of a sudden I got born too late in the creation of it, and thus I ran in the race and was memed a proper face and learned all the buttons and in which sequence to push them, and when I don't get any relationship fulfillment I do as trained and push a button throughout the day. As far from nature's intentions is what I feel in my lonely moments that come more regularly and actually as clockwork now. Humans mating as a function of acquiring more technology in place of more humans or limiting their reproduction so as to provide food, shelter, and technology via indirect beggarship to their limited offspring, but where is love or nature in all of this?

285. During those contrived Christian holidays humans give technology to their human-children as presents of love that Jesus was born for them. But all the CD's sing of killing and rutting or unnatural behaviors while the new wave of puberbitory erotic dancers wiggle camel toes or crotch bulges in our faces via wide angle lenses on steadicams, primetime for all to see and become inured too. Are any of the *Hosapiens* paying attention because their thoughts get closer to hypomanicism protocols all the time? What I would have done for a distraction from my vision of pain 20 years ago held in private thoughts in a private language behind locked doors and with the props hidden under my bed, they exhibit as entertainment for grandma and granddad without a blink or a think. They drive my passions deeper because I get used to it too quickly also - thus the pain catches up quicker these days. There are many forms of needles, but the *Hosapiens* deny the

knowledge of their use, while I hoard mine for myself. How much temptation via perversion can we view before our natural sexual needs are supplanted with memes of alien sexual encounters?

286. All human species are "visual fornicators" by design it would seem. All human species can get aroused without pheromones, physical contact, mating season gang rapes, or territorial-rutting boundaries and they can get aroused even in the presence of many humans. Because it is genetic, it is most difficult to control even with religious memes and societal behavioral memes. The creation of marriage for a "pairing of mates" is actually only very slightly effective. Look at the figures [*numbers*] for out of wedlock pregnancy and adultery now. A meme that must prevent the act of penis erectus and ejaculation maximimus or sperm receptiveness would have to be applied very precisely. This explains the low number of human males choosing to become celibate monks in hiding, and having a limited access to a Governors wife in order to avoid the "visual" aspect of the visual fornication genes.

287. Now you, my fine reader friend, are most likely among the almost everyone that constantly states, "Look at how screwed up humans have become" (but never including yourself), because of the divorce rate, out of wedlock pregnancies, High School age humans having sex, and everyone trying to figure out how to get a good romp each day or at least get that action behind them. So many of the *Hosapiens* ask the questions as I do, but without a true belief in what causes the actions, the truth is not to be had or understood by them. These actions of a genetic magnitude actually are not the problem; it is the *Hosapiens* contrived lifestyle with legislation applied that can't conform to the needs of the gene. Religion slows the action but it is a good thing that thoughts aren't known because for certain jail time would be had by all. As a human-child I was told that all my thoughts would be revealed in heaven and known by all þersons of the þlanet called the earth, so I should keeþ them under control as to þrevent me from being embarrassed after death. Angel blush syndrome, I guess? If this is true you will all be amused and most likely amazed when after Armageddon (not the correct word) the virtual reality sideshow begins for all of us.

288. The *Hosapiens* have never believed that þheromones (organic airborne chemical scents) have þlayed an imþortant þart in their lives. They are always waiting for one of those contrived scientific reþorts to be broadcast during the 6 o'clock whatever to tell them in 30-second sound bites more about their lives. Yet they constantly þurchase and apþly and sniff and tell lies about how sexy a þerfume is or was or how it drives the other gender crazy with þassion as if sex þotions had to be þurchased in a weird shaþed bottle with some confusing adverb or noun name. This is some more confusion of logic and self-denial that my sþecies must þut uþ with while trying to live with the *Hosapiens*. However, if we are to work toward "optimum" þrocreation as opþosed to only þrocreation then more must be at work than þheromones. Þheromones should cause a lack of a choice (autonomic) in actions because aren't all actions of an organic tyþe chemically driven within all living creatures? Þheromones could cause the required actions of coþulation regardless which male and female humans came within þheromone range once the sniffing was finished but they don't apþear to work that way for humans and some other animals. Female þheromones would easily cause increases in testosterone in men at that required moment or at least after the sniffing was done, but do they cause uncontrollable erection? After all, erection is the most basic prerequisite of human procreation, or at least it used to be when I was a young human. Visual triggers also play a role for humans becoming motivated into the mating act. What is strange about visual triggers, is that although most are obvious and predictable, there are many that defy predictability. Facial symmetry is one of the visual clues. Humans typically do not mate with other humans that are visually mentally retarded or defective. The younger the selection the better the perfection of the specimen (thus perceived as an optimum mate for optimum offspring), but basically most everyone mates except at the physical and mental extremes and even they may have their moments I'm sure. For only "procreation" would have no selection other to drop sperm on an egg found, but somehow all humans make a choice and being able to say yes or no (within the mind) creates the optimum part of the procreation (what did you expect, something complicated?). So now we get back to that set of data I am composing for this book, the only purpose of all living organisms: "Optimum Procreation." As I have verbosity when compelled to, as it is a natural function of my *Homaniakos* species, I can also shut-up and listen and rationalize especially when a motive is applied, and as I hear equally mankind and womantype of the ordinary type speak of optimum mates either real or imaginary, a choice by vision is definitely what humans seek, and justification via verbiage is only to rationalize cognitive dissonance applied to their friends or parents approval of the choice. Don't most *Hosapiens* seek approval from their parents that the mate they have chosen is satisfactory? That's a strange genetic trait to be certain and almost beyond the *Homaniakos* comprehension since my species would have sex and then hope that no other ordinary human finds out let alone try to get their approval. Of course, my species is given the label "abnormal" when it comes to sexual behavior or pleasures or needs of the physical manifestation type but that is only a matter of voting by percentages with the *Homaniakos* not given their fair share of votes - and it proves again the lack of the *Hosapiens* logical perceptions of reality and actions as applied to reality. Although I am a most "proper" *Homaniakos,* and try to exhibit "ordinary" behavior at all times, I love my hypomanic feelings and thus I let go now and then only to feel the satisfaction of the naturalness of it. Who else but a Manic-depressive Junkie could feel such grandeur and acceptance of natural actions without love, all driven by passions without the knowledge of sin?

289a. Holding on to that previous thought of mate selection via a choice, most *Hosapiens* believe that the human-children are mean or rude when they ostracize the school "freak" (in terms of personality or social skills) or the human-child of an obvious difference. Do the *Hosapiens* believe that the human-children are[is] naturally evil or that there is some book from which all parents are teaching their own human-child that tells them to remove the human-child with defective DNA from the clan or tribe (school yard contrived)? I observe and believe that the human-children operate as nature intends (not necessarily proving evolution in action but possibly given by a creator to ensure the healthy continuance of the species created) but expressed through a contrived language of which they have not mastered the consequences of their attempts at being truthful (adult humans know that the truth is anti-altruism). The human-children, because of their brief learning years, have memus minimus thus their behavior occurs as a function of genes quite naturally. The human-children are proper to isolate via MSO (Mutually

Selective Ostracizing) those human-children that could be harming the gene pool; but with technology added these days, about every freak can survive, via tribal matrixing, thus we must teach appropriate but unnatural actions to our human-children. But that really doesn't work all that well from what you can see in the news headlines. You will notice this behavior if you should watch the evening news or speak with the human-children about it or watch them play in a crowd of their own. As I state somewhere else in this book, human-children start working out optimum procreation prior to the knowledge of the sex act itself, and this act of ostracizing must be one of the natural ways don't you agree? They start pushing the "freak" genes out of their tribe at age 6 and for what reason of logic unless it is natural? The schools and play grounds are a gene pool of future mates and survival of the species is based (incorrectly) on who is there with no vision or understanding of the world any further than the sights of who is passed in the halls or sitting in the classroom. Where technology starts to screw with the human lives so young is that the humans are now creating a race of human-children whereby those physically different are very much alone or rare as birth defects are aborted or fixed quickly and effectively, thus the physical abnormality appears very abnormal and the acceptance of it becomes less. Sociopath[ic] behavior still draws MSO and rightfully so, but does MSO create sociopath[ic] behavior or are the human-children (human-children by legal definition) sensing the differences before they are noticed by all? I offer no solution to the path chosen. I see actions that have a basis for a common non-taught action throughout my parent's youth, my youth, and now my youth's youth. As most historical fairy tales have a genetic foundation, I am reminded of *The Ugly Duckling* and I cried every time he became a beautiful swan because I wished to do the same.

My species believing they are ordinary humans when youthful, become that "freak" by surprise.

289b. Now although the *Hosapiens* would have you believe that I suffer from some type of paranoia due to my so-called unfortunate condition, my refined thought process combined with my exceptional sensory perception, causes me to believe the following plot is true. In order to assist the *Hosapiens* human-children in removing the unwanted genes from the gene pool, the adult *Hosapiens* have been working toward the identification of the *Homaniakos* youth living among them, such that once the stigma is implied and the drugs applied, the alleged *Homaniakos* human-children will be identified for an easy target of mental abuse within the confines of their teen-aged or pre-teen environment. Now in the government schools (named as "public schools" to trick the ordinary humans, such as gambling is now "gaming", jungles are now "rain-forests", swamps are now "wet-lands" and street bums are now the "homeless") the rights of the ill to remain living in secrecy cannot remain a secret due to some strange rules or laws or whatever. The medicine at the schools must be dispensed via "approved humans" and for one purpose only, to identify to all others, those who are mentally "out of it" and to identify what exactly that "it" is. For which of the ordinary humans can shut their mouths of expressing great secrets known, because all ordinary humans believe that knowledge is power. Whispers start and then "so-and-so said" until all is known but nothing said face-to-face by anyone. Once the label is mentally tattooed and dispersed via a contrived language, whether it is true or not won't matter, you can't take back words or a thought when destruction is sought. So I am telling you (whatever "you" are), that a deliberate plot is active to eliminate my species and aside from the money to be made in the shade by the *Hosapiens* diploma-fied and rarified (from oxygen breathing in bars), their genes are actively working to find loop-holes to survival in the current technological contrived techciety [*Queer word usage*]. I am sure that next will come some genome test and then abortified cleansing of my species will occur or perhaps some type of gene therapy will be applied to embryonically alter my species out of existence. The dumbing-down of the world will occur as the ordinary humans attempt to make the entire world ordinary indeed. For certain the numbers of the *Homaniakos* are thinning out as techciety changes. Whereby communication technologies now tracks and identifies and puts Big Brother images across the country for all to see and seek, it is getting more difficult for the *Homaniakos* to procreate and run as nature apparently intended. As it seems that nature gave us (the *Homaniakos*) the advantage for some reason with regards to the seeking of sex, how are we to avoid getting caught doing our genes bidding with so many electronic eyes to watch us and record who we are? I suppose although a more polite techciety will become of it as we are trained "appropriate" behavior; but it is apparent to me that nature intended the *Homaniakos* to be a larger force within humanity.

290. Now with the better nutrition and heath care (also enhancement surgeries) offered in our current culture club, possible mates remain appearing very optimum even into extended ages of their thirty's and forty's. Technology doesn't create horny old men; it allows human males to find more mates as more human females apply what can be bought to satisfy their genes of attractiveness to become mated or impregnated. Do you believe that all of mankind and womantype throughout recent European history, lets say within the last 800 years, would even begin to look

as we do to-day? More importantly, do you believe that to human's 800 years ago, appearances were not noticed? Or think back to early Roman beginnings, then early Egyptcian beginnings and as I see it (with my minds eye) there is no reason to believe that even before a contrived language was used, beauty was not noticed as a revealing factor of selection for optimum procreation. (Of course, beauty is in the eye of the beholder.) I believe that the *Hosapiens* want me to believe that the original humans got phenomenally horny or did "it" for no reason at all when called "primitive" but I don't trust many *Hosapiens* and their interpretation of reality, now or of the past. I suspect from watching this *Hosapiens* contrived world around me, they actually believe that education and fine cultural training leads them (the *Hosapiens*) to appreciate "beauty" as in the fact that their mate should have all their teeth. As most all contemporary humans do mate, then the acceptance of the imperfection must be a function of the commonality of it (I love that statement.). Thus why believe a basis for a selection has not been applied throughout the existence of the humans? Contemporary technology reduces imperfections to being rare as we make humans as we do our plastic injected furniture or mass-produced collectibles. I as a *Homaniakos* am not immune to any of these visual tricks as I love seeing the various versions of the surgically enhanced humans with all their rotoscoping applied, cinch marks reduced, and new product placement strategically added also, and oh what I would look like if I had more money! I seek to see or possess or own the perfect pearl, and as I have hope that someday I will, why not sell all or risk all in order to feel the excitement of those few brief moments in the presence of the physically perfect human? To summarize the last few paragraphs with a poor excuse of an analogy, no one collects chipped Hummels on purpose (oh!).

291a. I would have to wonder if anyone else notices that whenever Danny Elfman writes a song, Tim Burton creates a movie to go with it. But I have to tell you that when I viewed *Edward Scissorhands* (the movie) for the first time, I became transfixed via some type of identity confusion and I really went off the deep end of depression for about five rotations. What I ended up doing was creating a series of artworks entitled *Me as Edward Scissorhands* and *Edward Scissorhands Completion*. Once I broke the curse, I was able to impersonate the ordinary humans again and all was fine. But as I am certain I will mess up this topic and this 1k plus word paragraph, (because I feel the need to talk to someone even if you will be reading these words four years from now) the satisfaction of conducting social intercourse is the same when writing or talking and I'll make it part A and part B to be somewhat proper. While we're on or close to that age of mating topic from the paragraph 283, it is only the *Hosapiens* technology and unnatural environment that cause modern mankind and womantype to think that 13 year old humans having sex is against nature because of some idea that there are natural moral behaviors and therefore or somehow sinful behaviors (yet they are only modified via our slowly changing lifestyles), aside from the fact that they themselves are three generations from it and thus don't have memories of the historical events. No human species are born with memories of past events, even as premortals. I see the *Hosapiens* climbing a ladder of cultural changes based on technological advances and then during the inuring process, not remembering they came from the earth or the ground up or why everything altered is screwed up as no *Hosapiens* can follow the *Hosapiens* dented and bented regulations as higher they climb and drag the unwilling me higher and higher for the great fall. Although I am not aware that there is any legal age to have sex, somehow the old and sexually experienced humans are legally not allowed to procreate with the younger least experienced humans and within my country of residence age 18 standard earth years (unless with parental/judge consent) is the forbidden delimiter or you'll find your name on a bailiffs call sheet. For certain this cuts the birth rate by some great amount I'm sure, but is it by nature or contrived beliefs that this law occurs (by contrived beliefs is what I would believe)? Thus via contrived verbiage we have the age of consent determined by the *Hosapiens* interpretation of the world all arranged and planned and everything in-line, applications declined, with the best position in a recline (or sometimes a bend over Red Rover). The Western system of education causes humans to push the procreation "age" up and up (Humans track time based on how many orbits of the sun they have made as if that is a journey into adulthood, and laws are also legislated via the same counting method.). For unknown reasons (proving faulty *Hosapiens* logic) humans aren't considered mature until at least finishing High School (another human contrivance) at about age 18, and now I hear so many of the womantype saying 18 years is too young also. What in the purpose of mankind and womantype requires a modern definition of maturity in order to survive and procreate? What is maturity? The real truth is that it takes about 23 of the earth orbitals before a human can somewhat master current technologies and the system of laws and government before they are somewhat self-sufficient in a cash economy in the first world nations. This would never have happened if all human species lived as evolved or intended to live because our 13-year-old sons and daughters would be most comfortable in the natural world and able to survive every day working away in the clan and tribe hunting and picking food. Attempting to delay the sex act until humans can learn about technology is an idea constructed by politicians and idiots (but I'm holding back) and thus when it doesn't work everyone says, "Oh my!" but everyone remembers their own youthful unrevealed sexual adventure with that older boy or younger girl (pick only one please). Technology does not alter the genetic drives of procreation to follow suit; it screws genetics at every opportunity. This is where I have trouble listening to the *Hosapiens* as they speak everyday in every way about technology and advances and progress, etc. to death but I see nothing changing of the human genome except contrived plug-in devices and the color you might buy them in. Technology thus creates a world of teenaged masturbaters locked behind bathroom doors – every morning the swing gang is all in motion throughout the town but isolated from view – but technology fixes this problem by offering masturbation devices for both boys and girls alike. If you are fortunate enough to believe a daily rub or jerk will do you some good then you might stay alive, but my species sees there is no end to the means and logical suicide is the way we die as true logic is applied to mating denied or unfilled or fulfilled via the 7th protocol of hypomanicism. I have researched the legal marriage ages from the 1800's and realizing they were set by religious Puritan morals they must be correct for the human species and thus without sin. I can't rationalize how those legally married humans of 14 years male, 12 years female, would survive in our world of technology jobs and government rule? Technology screws the genetic actions and then the ever-changing morals of our techciety assign blame to the unsuspecting victims. Surmising some thoughts and drawing my own conclusions of the last few paragraphs, technology denies the *Hosapiens* from fulfilling their genetic motivators and does nothing at all for their so-called morals but for some reason, the *Hosapiens* believe that technology has or will improved their moral self as well as helping them to meet their daily genetic needs. I remain confused about the integration of the two and the word "delusional" comes to my mind again but the music moves onward and so must we.

291b. In this second half of paragraph 291, the problem of a human techciety based on cold cash with a technology dependency (thus each clan cannot provide 100% of their own necessities or the necessities possible) is that if governmental decisions with regards to the use of technology are not based on the best economical solution, rather than on the waxing and waning moral beliefs, then all of that techciety will suffer in achieving an optimum lifestyle. A caste or class system is created as technology costs rise because those who don't have (or have access to) the best technology becomes the underclass. The best example I can remember at this moment (9:59 p.m. track 7) is stem cell research using induced aborted human embryos. Where as this research might cure complex diseases or injuries (I offer you no proof) and thus aid in the general economics of all tribes via keeping living humans self-abled and useful to their clans (and thus reducing financial responsibilities to the clan and techciety as a whole), the ordinary humans call such research inhuman, while a million human babies a year are sliced and diced, (while alive and exhibiting some type of silent scream I'm sure) and sucked down a slug line into a drain with no one benefiting, not many tears being shed publicly, and defined as some type of "human right" that each human is entitled to via a birth-right (That in itself shows the low I.Q. of the creators of such idea's, because how can killing a birth be a birth-right? Those that are born have the right to determine those that are born?). Whereas most ordinary humans believe they remain "upright and moral" the reality unseen (to them) and thus not proclaimed is that *Hosapiens* are a morally primitive species because that "moral" gene was not on the slate for evolutionary improvements to parallel the improved technology within the last 1.5 million years or so, because tell me what would have motivated the gene to lean (or tilt) since then?, some type of gene alteration based on the speaking in a contrived language? I really want to see how language alters genes via memes. Who will show me? The morals of a few create the laws, and laws allow all to alter their morals to suite, with complete justification because in truth satisfying your genetics is your number one objective and strict morals will only get in your way. Besides, haven't you noticed, my reader friend, that what is exercised as morally correct will vary as you travel around the earth to visit all tribes, but what is most important to notice is that the poorer a nation of humans becomes, the more likely you (as a USA citizen) will not agree with their morals or beliefs. Following your genetics means staying alive and guarantees the continuance of your seed and unless you can steal from a government or purchase all that you need, damn the morals and don't preach to me.

292. Getting on with it before this song ends, what creates visual sexual attraction seems to come in and out of fashion unlike what the other animals of the earth would experience, as normal behavior is what I observe. Clothing is the most basic of artificial reproductive stimulants, short of drugs I suppose. Clothing can stimulate unnatural optimum procreation actions via making humans of almost any age, size, and physical stature appear to be optimum mating choices. A pair of new denim blue jeans can make any pair of old, wrinkled, veined legs look attractive as a possible mating choice to which have optimum offspring (with?). But if you

are a boy, looking at your sister won't do it because something in the genes not the jeans will tell you to stop before you get to looking or licking or probing that live area, and thus in almost all cultures whether you consider them cultured or not they now will have laws against incest that is acted on. And yet something uncommon happens sometimes and what is the explanation of it other than a trial and error attempt at getting natures intentions right? I am sure a gene is behind it somewhere for how do you get that incest idea to be so successful unless by trial and error and remembering the outcome, and then having to give that knowledge to all of mankind and womantype in each generation? My parents never had to tell me not to kiss my sister that's for certain. But as I now remember, brother to sister marriage was once reserved for the royal families only.

The unaked ape

293. Now how can I avoid the observation that the U.S.A. *Hosapiens* are ashamed of their bodies via some type of learned behavior as opposed to the European humans that bask in the sun for fun? Years of meme induction are what I would guess or would suggest to account for this strange behavior otherwise the world would be more consistent with it, and how would you account for it genetic-wise? The fear of nudity is not born of the *Hosapiens* or there would be more consistency of it. But each generation of mankind and womantype must alter the natural trait of the growing human-child into a feeling that the natural is unnatural. There can be nothing genetic about being naked and ashamed of it (see CHAPTER GODD, paragraph 492)[*space*]. But clothing is not what it appears to be and it is all appearance for certain, because deep inside all humans and myself

included, we wish to be physically attractive for that optimum procreation gene - so clothing is the meme turned physical at work for the purpose creating the next "you or me". As clothing styles change, the sexual attractiveness of the unnaked ape becomes renewed - because both of the human species get inured to everything unnatural in life; haven't you noticed that fact? Although I don't have a clue based on experience, I'll go out on that limb that I hear the other humans talk about and say that nudist would actually think less of unnatural procreation modifiers because the artificial stimulation of the optimum procreation gene is removed. Nudist would have the most natural of genetic behaviors, because they see their fellow humans for what they are, an animal that has many varieties as opposed to everyone looking like cotton fiber dyed blue clones. Clothing is only sexy or boring contrived 3D images moving in real-time with flashback cycles for the most part that can be applied to humans of most any age, and thus actions of optimum procreation can be designed, bought, sold, applied, denied, hidden, and suggested - and it has not much to do with the physical readiness or urge of the wearer or wearee and is mostly unnaturally created with the intention of providing unnatural urges when needed via 30 second commercials scripted from perfected storyboards. Clothing can make little boys look like young men and little girls look like whoars, at least those are the remarks the ordinary human womyn made within my ears hearing at the last graded school function. I didn't see it that way, but I am still trying to figure out the ordinary humans and their actions versus a contrived language and the expression of natural thoughts spewed (or supped) out of lactating tongues. Clothing alters by revealing, enhancing or attribute dancing, hiding, lifting, shaping and camouflagalating, illusional tricks to tempt the opposite sex to have a lick, lets have sex but only unzip those

Dockers are too sexy to discard with a bulge so hard - thus clothing manufactured and tested fitted on manikins or dummies of a þerfect configuralteration can focus on erotica sþoticas when the target that is aimed at is easily hit because clothing doesn't evolve (nothing unnatural evolves), it is contrived by immediate action and reaction, so when hems go uþ, jaws go down and going down or þorking around might occur because of a seamstress' woes.

294. The *Hosaþiens* of America have been memed that clothing is natural and thus should be "on" at all times as opþosed to the skin being seen. The *Hosaþiens* of this culture nurture themselves into believing that seeing another humans skin will cause them to become sexually aroused (or get sent to the real Hell), but instead clothing arouses them whether it is being worn or not, and thus the inured meme can control a gene to a certain degree is what I see and I hoþe you can see it also. Because of this jerked nurturing, clothing is actually designed to be sexy to arouse all of us and actually seeing a naked þerson is almost a ritual in itself in the United States and the apþroþriate actions in those events aren't known because humans start laughing or turning away quickly when þresented with the accidental nude. Can you tell me what is so funny about a man having his zipþer down while giving a sþeech? Is there a genetic clue there for me that I am missing? What is for certain is, if we never wore clothing we would still have oþtimum þrocreation occurring without humans being bored with the apþearance of the natural human body because all human sþecies don't seem to be bored with too many natural things. I would have to believe that although surrounded by naked humans all day, when it comes to the fulfillment of the oþtimum þrocreation ritual, humans would oblige. Sex and

nakedness were never related, genetic-wise, for how could we get here from there if it were? Thus the unnatural coverings of the humans (as in clothing) are recognized as unnatural by our genes and there is no permanent satisfaction in the style of it or styles would never change (And to counter that thought, how many men are tired of looking at a natural smile of a lady? You would believe we would be bored to death of something so simple.). I conclude again with stating unnatural technologies are not providing any permanent satisfaction for our genes, thus genes are ruling us. You must believe me so you can start to fix your culture for your future generations. If you get this fixed then perhaps in the future, I won't have that sleeping dream induced from bad memory memes of going to the graded school as a youth in only my boxer shorts.

Misconceptions

295. Happiness is a common misconception of the *Hosapiens*. Nothing in either of the human species genetics is setup for happiness but at least the *Homaniakos* figure it out early enough to live or die by it. The *Hosapiens* species did not evolve to be happy but as a delusional species, they haven't figured it out yet. There is no need to be happy, for any animal. There must be naturally occurring and created drugs in the body that give the *Hosapiens* that satisfied feeling for a moment but that won't get any human very far in their contrived culture. It is only very recently and in only a few cultures (or political regions) that humans have the time or money resources for the search for the non-existent happiness. Have you ever noticed that behind every effort to achieve happiness, "inventive" technology is at work - sans religion of course? It is the *Hosapiens* technology that pushes all of us further from the feeling of being satisfied also whether we wish to be caught up in it or not. Remembrances of Farrah Fawcett finally reaching for that happiness pill during the ending of *Saturn 3* are what come to my mind. Look at all the Sunday paper sale ads selling humans happiness in purchasable durable goods. Where is the pure "Sit under a tree and eat an apple" mentality that is actually the humans genetic driven goal? Sex is natures satisfaction but in the Puritan world we are all screwed and without a kiss. Who among you can actually even see 1% of humankind's genetic drives and behaviors through of all this technology stuff that needs to be filtered as strainer stew from the dishwater? Deep within you, my fine reader friend, you must feel something that begs for satisfaction that remains unsatisfied throughout the day as you touch plastic as though it were a necessity of life? Its that empty feeling that starts the moment after the movie you watched is over, the lights are out for the night, or when friends leave the party and the house becomes quiet. Although for myself, as a *Homaniakos*, these empty feelings occur in-between split-second moments of every word coming at me from a friends mouth or in the brief pause between soundtracks on my favorite music CD, thus creating the most extreme dichotomy of euphoria and depression as fast as eyes can blink. For the feeling that the *Hosapiens* would call happiness is really not any further than seeing or being with their human-child - their optimum procreation creations. Therefore I rest my case; optimum procreation - continuation of ones genes is the satisfaction maximum of all creatures because it is genetically driven, of nature, and the primary purpose of all life. Without procreation occurring by choice or circumstances the *Hosapiens* fill their life with technology toys to hide the genetic drive that has never been satisfied. For those *Hosapiens* who are old or aged and never procreated and thus never held a newborn son or daughter, or got nightly hugs from their human-child with no language needed to confuse the feeling of it with your nose deep within their hair to smell the human scent of it, does this make you sad? Sadness is the opposite of happiness thus it can't exist either, but "unsatisfied" is possible and runs very deep through all human genes as a feeling of a life wasted or being wasted without being able to go back and change or fix or to make that choice over again. I know this feeling everyday, I will not guess at its existence. It is the feeling of a life gone by not to be felt again or to be given a second chance at not knowing the knowing of now and thus not being able to mirror image the past pleasures into the future to experience again all the feelings of satisfaction that were once felt but not understood. How can I question the decision or deny the satisfaction logical suicide must bring to those able to do the act when the truth to life has been realized, felt and rationalized? Who among the *Hosapiens* is righteous enough or even clear minded enough to proclaim knowing the knowledge of choices made when a choice is absolute and based on the firm foundation of the true reality of life seen or sensed and then ending in the act of logical suicide to remove one's self from the participation of life's one-way journey?

296. To compound the issue the *Hosapiens* have a language and that language describes life in terms of its quality. Thus quality of life is set as a goal when you are young and a necessity when you are old or they will leave you in a urine stinking hole to rot in front of a Television machine watching looping and swooping reruns of stupid game shows along with the other humans that didn't plan or save or steal it from those who didn't see it coming. Then when your quality becomes poor like an old car or sofa that the *Hosapiens* have become tired of, they use some non-existent quality of life standard as though its been written and verified and in some CE handbook issued to all at birth as common knowledge, so that they can start þulling þlugs or tubes or denying meals on wheels or they roll you over on your face while þretending to change your bed sheets, after confirming such actions with the next of kin. Where in the evolutionary þlan did quality come to be a natural actuator and why do the *Hosapiens* ascribe it to other ordinary humans or my sþecies or other creatures they collect in caged cubes or synthetic habitats so they can say "They are better off there" whether they asked to be there or not? Of course, sometimes the "there" in the þhrase "They are better off there", means death. And yet they deny death to my sþecies when it becomes our logical choice?

Mankind

297. It's time to move on to a brighter day I hoþe and also time to state another item from my list:

Genetic disþosition of human males:
"Tribal"

298. By "will" I would say, "figure it out yourself" and get onto some Internet browsing, we now move onward as in "forward" to figuring more clues, as I must direct my train of thought to more sþecific issues even if my mind is in a quite an ordinary frame; the music sets the þace. We have among each of the two human sþecies (The *Homaniakos* and the *Hosapiens*), two creatures of unique þhysical features. One was to be called mankind and the other womantyþe (each of our sþecies has roughly an equal mix of them) but those are only nouns or þronouns or adjectives or verbs

or whatever you would call them in a contrived language (who can tell me that it matters?). I, being a *Homaniakos* Junkie and a prim and proper one at that, am compelled to document for analysis and transference exactly as the *Hosapiens* would do; otherwise my thoughts as memes would sit in only one brain and then disappear at the moment of my death. So with my memes in control, its onto risky ground I figure because either a genus or a pig I'll become and I can't wait to hear all of the *Hosapiens* thoughts on my thoughts for certain. I expect the acceptance or denial of ideas will be based on the fact that if you perform a test on an object, the object will become altered thus how true is the test? What would become more difficult is to have the test subject perform the test on itself. With all the philosophy that I have read on those two subjects, I think, therefore I am liable to be incorrect, but onward to more sensitive issues anyway.

299. would start in the middle of a sentence and subject out of the blue and I'll capitalize the next Word in order to put your mind at ease about writing conventions but I have to tell you a mob or herd of human's behave only genetically thus somewhat predictably. This genetic behavior might be initiated by a meme of some type, but the action will only be genetically driven. A herd looses its memetic control because each human (ordinary or not) in a herd does not share exactly the same memes but they share the same genes. You would never imagine seeing a Homo erectus (a caveman) human running around with Nike shoes and cell Fons but it happens all the time on the 6 o'clock pop culture review, because with the right opportunity all memes are dropped and thus pure genetics rule regardless of the year of our Lord or our star date if you are into that orbital thing. Herds do not act illogically, because genetics do not follow logic, they follow the basic behavioral motivators for survival and procreation. These genetic motivators are not good or evil, they are there to ensure the greatest number of creatures survive any circumstance. While you may see females in a herd, the interaction is minimal and thus they may remain behind the scenes unless the reason is derived from a clan function or primed from one hell of a meme as in feminist activities (and there are less feminists that we would all believe). (The news media performs a motion capture of the feminist events for the replay twice daily, thus the importance and the commonality of feminists is persuaded into the ordinary humans mind. But if anyone should really happen to look at the news content, most feminist activities reported are followed or preceded by a cat stuck in a tree.

300. These herd genetic behavioral motivators are from the human's ancestral days (or date of creation) but I dare any human to put a date on it. Why expect that our genes are to be modified with a couple of centuries of mass communications on our minds (but I hear the *Hosapiens* belief in that statement, even the ones that don't believe in evolution), yet I also hear the *Hosapiens* say that they believe that in the future the human's hatred towards each other will end [*Sentence confusion*]. This *is* the future and what "magical organ" do ordinary humans believe humans will have in the next future that will stop the violence of to-day? Contrived education is always a meme and as you know by now, the gene wins when against the meme. I see only genetics at work, everyday and in every way, that is all, and within every fat man is a little boy for sure, thus the violence continues. Thus a herd (a verb for a mob) works toward correcting a circumstance that has gone against human genetics. This herd behavior would most likely be for self-preservation or preservation of one's genetics and would

definitely go against the Hay's code if seen as a celluloid visual metaphor. A herd is a tribe in structure. Tribal behavior for human males is genetic. Human males behave tribally at all times when they gather into a crowd, whether this be a typically calm day at the office or factory, at a family reunion, or protesting a war via destroying a community. This genetic behavior is masked from obvious view by water cooler chitchat and E-mail porn jokes that imply sophistication. Don't let the Tommy Hilfiger shirts fool you my reader friend. It takes great memetic control to keep all humans from expressing their genetics at any given moment. As with communication styles, when a human male is calm, he can apply memetic training to his communication. When the human male becomes angered or upset, the dominant communication style emerges or in the case of genetics, the genes win over memes (applies to female humans also). When in a crowd or herd, the herd lives with the natural actions of unity for there are no schools or institutions or lessons at home where the humans are taught their herd behavior or riot protocols. How else would common herd actions occur in large numbers, despite the printed and framed degrees of higher education hanging on the walls in the homes of the alleged rioters?

301. Sounds drive the herd whether the contrivance of a language or a beat of a drum or the sound of a horn and thus for mankind it is a natural but womantype can get caught in the mix of it too. The sound unifies and sets the emotion and thus an action will follow. No human states "I will join that herd" via word-of-mouth but instead s/he participates as a walk-on without a thought or moral or worry of a law because those are contrivances or meme's and those are not of nature born. The herd enjoys itself and wants to enjoy itself and gives approval to all within by

the nature of its size and yet is not the herd a phantom that disappears as quickly as the humans who were its creator? For even if ordinary humans are Christmas shopping, empty malls and stores with no hustle or crowds with shopping bags full, they would be down in their mood because one and all set the mood and set the approval for their actions – for these are actions that I notice while on mall safari. The more at a party, a birthday for certain, sets the approval to the happy little boy that he should be satisfied in his thoughts for many share in the satisfaction and the herd gives its approval. However, is not a birthday a birthday even in loneliness? The herd is borderline tribe and thus male dominated and often violent. Destruction and physical attack and pseudo-procreation actions normally ascribed to pre-mating rituals occur as if technology or civilization or cameras or hate crimes were never presented but no logic or deliberate thoughts drive the herd or mob since how would there be time for planning such a complex event without rehearsals? Humans will never (or never) stop herd actions and the *Hosapiens* have made laws against the poor unfortunates caught in the timing of it, but as I study the *Hosapiens,* all I am starting to see is the *Hosapiens* are now herds living in corrals paying cash for the few moments of genetic freedom they take every year but always returning to the cage as though some type of security is to be found there. Enter at your own risk is what nature offers but can you imagine the greatness and freedom that awaits those who would make the difficult but correct choice of natural freedom?

302. Although it was the crowd or herd that was the original deliverer of memes, the communication devices of our technology have taken the place of the herd and thus approval in numbers is lost if not properly construed. So the canned laughter sound

track was installed (and by someone famous I'll bet), and stadium microphones carefully volumated at football games trick the *Hosapiens* mind into believing they're in the crowd while they're setting at home watching the Television machine, or else they'll miss the satisfaction of the herd. The electronic contrivances are the prophets of big business bucks but the *Hosapiens* satisfaction is all that matters to they the viewers [*Confusion of words*] and the *Hosapiens* can't tell the difference anyway, so the *Hosapiens* are appreciative and very satisfied with the technological mental mind fuck. What the hell doe's it matter anyway because from where I sit in this semi-dark room without any real voice within hearing range and without a possibility of a human female offering me a natural physical pleasure, to-morrow probably brings my death and what the hell does it matter anyway because, . . . ! With 17 minutes to go until my 10 p.m. break (and four hours to go till my nap), I lost track of whatever I was writing this damn book for anyway. Pinky is singing along but the sign post to heaven states, "Be just and fear not". I have grown tired of contrived words and sitting here as Mr. Macguffin would do, I really wish I could travel back in time, physically that is, and live my remaining life in every moment of extremus distractus jackulus or as a Carney worker lurker eyeing the eatable pleasures of the Lake County Fair, blinking light sighted, cotton candy lipped, and acid rock sounding hips. Time to go, stated with only eleven words, George is here.

303. Eight virtual years later I write that the *Hosapiens* males work at existing in tribal hierarchies (even the greater *Homaniakos* must follow that gene so I never resist it myself as it feels quite natural to my mind). If a tribe does not exist, human males will form one. If you have the will to look, you can see how easily and often

that this occurs. Technology has given all humans another dimension to tribal behavior, because we are allowed to establish a tribal matrix of beliefs despite distance and physical associations. Let me be the first to say I enjoy this freedom brought on by technology because it offers the maximum distractions, but I still wonder if satisfying my genetic codes would make living much more satisfying than the technology screw? A minimal-technology tribe that lets say[s] is missing communication and mobility technologies will have many beliefs, but they will mostly be similar for everyone in the tribe. The whole tribe (male and female) would share a religion, shelter styles, food preparation, human-child rearing, one set of leaders, clothing styles, and beliefs in what is beautiful and attractive in humans. Now, with complex technologies for communications and mobility, humans have the ability to pick tribal attributes they personally prefer and communicate with their selected tribes via technology gadgets. Thus is created a tribal matrix or montage of all the available tribal attributes. In our techciety we can pick our clothing style from some type of a catalog printed of plaid or pleated printed pages. We belong to any religion that we can drive to or receive on our Television machines. We eat food from a variety of cookbooks and restaurants. What we consider beautiful in a human, might look different than the humans we see everyday. The down side is your son looks like that heavy metal rock artist he saw on the Television machine via his own chosen tribal matrix. He loses the psychological association to look and behave like you and your dad because he can see choices and our tribes are not a unified community anymore to discourage renegades. Communicative technology destroys the tribe as a community - thus immediate physical or psychological reinforcement of proper tribal behavior is lost unless the clan structure remains strong, and very few are that strong from what I can see around me as the human-children run rampant over their parents

304. A football team is a tribe. All sports teams are tribes I believe and can't you see it? They behave as tribes, they have tribal structures, and the voyeur human males attach themselves to them as though they were born into that tribe. Look at the popularity of sports gear, jackets, etc. The same human males may have jobs and that creates another tribal membership. Religious beliefs are tribal and everyone at your workplace doesn't share the same religion with you. Our life is based on a tribal matrix in place of only one tribe, but that doesn't change the fact that human males seek out tribal organization, and are very comfortable existing in it. The world of high-rise cities, automobile mechanisms, entertainment technologies, etc. only exists because the human male naturally accepts tribal hierarchies. The fact that men seek an income for survival is secondary (and a recent development) and would be non-existent if tribal acceptance weren't existing first. In a few paragraphs I will be writing about womantype and sports and with no insult intended, I wish only to make a slight comparison of the genetic tribal vs. genetic clannish attributes that make the difference in men and women in sports (and also at a contrived workplace). Both genders of both species can play sports without any difficulty of mind or muscle because both are equal in achieving an exemplary level of skill, except perhaps by averages of mass and that angle of the hip to knee joint thing due to females being able to give birth, but a sport is the hunt and the kill with winners and losers and weapons to be handled, thus to be true, leave it structured as a tribe, regardless of the gender is what I prescribe. Elaborating so that I may be more verbose on the thoughts I am presenting; a tribe is a

collection of members in which no blood relation needs to be recognized. A tribe will function perfectly if every member is of a different clan, whereas a clan must consist mostly of blood relations and relations through ceremony. For certain the purposes are different, and so is the organization and the rules, with all of it being controlled by genetics and gender and a need for survival and continuance of the species is at the foremost of it all. How are the *Hosapiens* going to out-smart this one I have to ask myself since they are failing miserably at it right now, wouldn't you agree? The feminization of America is simply an application of genetic clannish behaviors applied to a genetic tribal situation. It will never work but the *Hosapiens* are now making laws and lawsuits for it thus they are all screwed but I remain quietly unchanged. Contrived verbiage will never overpower genetics.

305. Is it only the *Hosapiens* Western culture or are there more exceptions than the rule? (I have changed subjects again without a prompt or heading so get used to it.) I can't seem to find out a commonality of the following but correct me if I'm wrong, as you see in a divorce, the female is quick to gather the goods, because something tells her to do so even without a thought in her head or lawyer at her side. The man on the other hand will give up many things even of his own belongings as a trade for the chance to optimum procreate with another female and thus spread his genes again. Although I am most inclined to put it at tribal traditions (a meme sitting on a gene), don't you agree? The male mating urge is strong enough that the "possession" trait is put aside for when a man has one of those marital affairs (as they are called in the marriage trade) he does it knowing he risks money and wealth and control of his existing human-children. For men are driven in all things by optimum procreation and the collectibles

mankind has are all gathered to that end. So you see many men have their toys that are not toys but means to a mate or a substitute for a mate or a substitute for a human-child. Thus his motorcycle is kept in virgin condition because he wants a virgin mate (or his optimum choice). But perhaps I am reading too much into all the actions and words I see and hear, but a common tone of speech seems to always be applied to those topics I've mentioned. It is the collection of objects or the artifact, especially unnatural objects that must be accounted for within the humans genes, because although the type of object collected would be determined by a meme and thus contemporarily biased, I will not believe that meme's drive us to collect so must stuff if they are not acting on behalf a gene and why give our ancestral Neanderthals that gene if not to survive or mate? Collecting is not new or unnaturally implemented; there must be a genetic reason for it. (No, I am not believing that collecting is related to early hunter-gatherers storing food or supplies.)

306a. I can't rationalize where to put this short topic and it sounds political in nature but tribes begot politics so here it sits for three paragraphs only and you should take my advice and don't read it and move on to paragraph 308 please because I've read this and it doesn't even make sense, but in our techciety all the remnants of the humans original genetic intentions remain in one altered state or another. The tribunal is natural because all must be accountable for the continuance of the clan and thus into the continuance of the tribe. Technology has destroyed the unity of the tribe and replaced it with the tribal matrix but the genes are still there trying to act as if nothing has happened. This leads my species into frustration because the *Hosapiens* can't see their own illogical actions within their matrixed techciety. Money buys power and sex and gadgets and lawyers turned politician are first in line palms or penis's sufficiently greased. Thus in a court the order of the proceedings of the trial are more important than the evidence, witness's, or especially the truth (as the truth in a contrived language is nothing more than lies). This tribunal unnatural is required in order to maintain the rate of crime or the order of the law and what is the difference? Crime is now a product of the law and thus is sold by lawyers as their livelihood as laws are intended to provide an escape for convictions when the order of the tribe has been lost and replaced by paper and ink with more misinterpretations than not. Laws are made with more exceptions than the rule and if you get suckered you'd better rely on them too, because the Fed's will and you'll find out how many "rights" you have. I know I would. Laws of contrived words will punish those humans that would settle into a natural state of existence and harm no one. Everyone must behave the same if we are all to be truly happy!

306b. With a derailment of thoughts the tribunal is now a government so large that its members are never within sight or sound. I really believe the *Hosapiens* don't understand how a government should really work, because the best any government can do is guarantee the success of its self. Thus is the function of a government. In doing so, it provides a means for the society (or the techciety) that supports it to continue to exist by its own means. No government can survive if it works on behalf of any individual. *Hosapiens* living within a large government, far greater than a tribal chief, can only supply the government with resources for the governments continuation, thus ensuring their own continuation by default. A government should only be a contrivance to regulate technology or to prevent the destruction of its self, and anything more is an attempt to abuse your genetic actions.

307. So the last sanctuary is the clan and the privacy of the home, since humans of technology live well secluded from what is known in the trade as "sight and sound" from their neighbors and even from grandma and granddad. So to break new grounds for profits since a market must grow, the politicians and the UN are to declare that humans have no parental rights other than to feed the wards of the government, the human-children, and when the humans don't behave as parents should, as the government sees fit, they will loose their procreation and the continuance of their genes, and it is coming regardless of genetic drives or intentions or what you believe to be correct at this moment. Thus mankind and womantype will fall into the hands of those humans that control the water and electricity and food and what you want and what you can have and where you can travel, even though survival is genetic, because the complexity of the unnatural contrivances controlled by a government so big is such we actually never had control as individuals. This breeds the fulfillment of the genetic traits of the few, at the loss of the fulfillment of the many. A class system is in place and can grow more defined if not stopped. Don't you *Hosapiens* see that a plot is in place and plans within plans from a system so big that only the rich can play, while the poor must pay? No I am not a communist or socialist of any type, but lives dependant on technology will always be controlled by those that regulate the technologies. For me not much matters because I am caring less every year, but you ordinary humans must redirect your ambitions and bring your genetic satisfactions back into your life because nature will not be screwed by distractions of Nitendo games, prime-time porn of vulgar languages, or die-cast collectibles while a government hands out genetic fulfillment as though it must be regulated and taxed.

308. I've lost track of the topics covered thus far, so onward with more for our list that now appears in print.

Genetic behavioral motivators of human males:

"The Birth of a Son"

"The Hunt"

"The Kill"

309. While a daughter is dear to her dad, especially if that is all that was had, a boy is a guarantee that a "Y" chromosome is present even before science had discovered it or language defined it. Females have two "X" chromosomes - males have a "X" and a "Y" chromosome. Thus how can a human male create another of himself if he doesn't have a continuance of a "Y" chromosome? Now the amazing thought is that without the science of it we (males) know it, thus the DNA takes care of it's own in a way humans have not defined yet, but continuance of the species and one's self is felt and acted on, words not withstanding. If you are fortune-ate enough to be a *Homaniakos*, then continue-ance has a feeling and meaning in-deed, touch-able and taste-able, I can smell it with-in the embrace-ment of my own procreate-tion along with un-satisfaction amplify-ed and unfulfill-ed as the loss of it is real whether it is real or not [*Excess hyphenation*]. How am I to find the delusions that the *Hosapiens* seem to naturally create to avoid the reality of "it" and how will they see my reality of "it" within words created? Thus a boy becomes like his dad and everyone is quite satisfied with the results. I believe that mankind takes care of mankind and you may not agree, but I will put my mind to rest on this issue being a holder of a "Y" chromosome myself. So without a doubt you can see why I have written that one of the three genetic behavioral motivators of human males is, "The Birth of a Son". You can study the history of this father-son action reaction because the history of mankind is full of it (feeding the flames for the feminist's agendas I suppose but who the hell cares?), but I'm on to another subject, so proceed to paragraph 310a.

310a. Now the human man drives the automobile machine for some reason (maybe for the fast motion?), because do you believe it is only a meme and thus a contrived custom that when humans are paired, the men make the key grip and get into the drivers seat? One thing for certain is he knows the way of the path, but evolution has not caught up to the contrivances such as transportation mechanisms moving faster than walking distance thus what you are born to know is surpassed by the distance of your travels and artificial landmarks that are built on bank loans, but the gene rules and a man will not ask directions because when the hunt is on, he knows the way whether confounded by technology or not. So without a doubt in some type of vague fashion with sports applied you can see why I have written that one of the three genetic behavioral motivators of human males is "The Hunt".

310b. Because the hunt is now conducted in the office or the shop or by swinging a mop, we must construct the trophies of our kill by awarding at every possibility a plaque or miniature replica of a human (fashioned after the greatness of a *Homaniakos* for a fact) chrome plated or such, standing high as points on an elk's head and the higher the better. For if the man brings home the kill, then it must be a worthy kill and how best to be better than the rest than by stacking columns and platforms all oak-ed and chromed, made by mankind and womantype in a factory no less, but sincerely presented with words from a contrived language such that the *Hosapiens* believe they are worthy of what they can purchase themselves when no-one is looking. So without a doubt you can see why I have written with competition applied that one of the three genetic behavioral motivators of human males is, "The Kill" and will always remain such.

3 1 1 . All would seem connected or related or in a living circle or whatever the *Hosapiens* use to describe life or existence or purpose or "Why are we here?", but a more detailed analysis of the "Genetic Behavioral Motivators of the Human Males" will fall into miscellaneous verbiage (hidden between the lines) with no logic to the construction of this chapter to control it. What I am developing as a connection of thoughts (described as a metaphor as one of those railway train mechanisms all coupled together) is that with only a couple of genetic actuators, I can cognize the actions of the mankind human (*Hosapiens* or not) because why should that animal be any more complex than an octopus? So onward again it's the woman's turn.

Womantype

3 1 2. Now as I was born with one "Y" chromosome it would be impossible for me to exhibit the actions (or thoughts) via genetics of a double "X" chromosome creature. Thus no human man can know what it is like to be a human woman, sex change or not (mix-gendered occurrences are excluded). Observation and comparisons are my best source of information about the vaginated human that we know as womantype. Thus to be true to

my words in this book, for whatever that is worth in a contrived language, how could I write about an understanding of womantype except in metaphors of mankind? I don't wish to come across as another Ellen Key, because the planet is full of them (although she's dead), but I must rationalize all the thoughts possible to explain the actions and reactions of both the genders of the *Hosapiens* species if I am even to have some peace in my mind of how things were meant to work. Thus the comparisons are there or here or in my mind because a baseline is what I must work from [*with?*]. Since my human mate is a woman (and an ordinary human at that) as are several of my procreations, the understanding of their natural protocols has brought rest to my mind as events and actions follow quite an ordinary natural schedule around the house, and I am hoping you will soon agree.

3 1 3. Going with the imagined duality of nature, where there is a plus there must be a minus, etc. and gag me please, putting down (writing down) thoughts of the mating half of mankind may prove to be not that difficult. As I always believed, the shopping mall is one of the best outposts for the observation of humans, both male and female, young and old, and except for the physical act of rutting, the *Hosapiens* behavior is best attributed to where and how mankind and womantype spend their money and drag their human-children. It can't all be psychological that being at the mall would have some type of special effect on the humans, for most seem satisfied to be socializing with each other even if amongst strangers. At any rate, words are written as the best interpretation of reality as I see them and since mankind and womantype are in existence for the same reason why not go for it, I ask myself?

314. Whereas I would like to put one thought into paragraph 314, "men behave as men, and females behave as females" because they have different chromosomes and those enzyme things" and leave it at that, I feel I must put at least one foot into hot water or nothing will be controversial in my book. So all the great philosophers and all the great metaphysicalologists have written on the subject already, and now let a manic-depressive of the 21st century have at it for a moment. Female humans are clannish and they hold the rights to that action and should be proud of it because mankind is a pig at family relations or calling his mother or sending a Hallmark on the occasions needed. Females are not tribal which is why they aren't invited to play office games (the office being unnatural but set-up as a contrived tribe) by the men. Sports are tribal (and based on the hunt and the kill) not clannish. It has nothing to do with the fact that women didn't play sports or their dad didn't throw a ball at them when they were young or he told them too often "You don't have a penis". Females use memetic training to play sports and are up to the task both physically and mentally as exhibited with all the professional leagues and Olympic quality athletes, but compare my lists of "Genetic Behavioral Motivators" and "Genetic Dispositions" between males and females, and you will see that "games" are set upon the rules of "maleness" and men seem to have outbursts of physical competitiveness at the slightest urge, no thought or training required. The fact that sports were setup upon the rules of the hunt and the kill because two go in but one comes out is the best rule and it should be played as such to the max. Clans are not structured for the hunt and the kill as we have cooperation within a clan and the only way to win in a clan is not to play it as a game. All humans must win in a clan, or how can the clan survive? It is the clan that procreates not the tribe. The tribe provides safety for its clans; the clans provide resources for the tribe. But getting to the subject, what I observe in the most awful of anti-genetic actions is that for many of the sports not of the professional type, but involving human youths of mixed gender, the new rules in a contrived language are of: no score, no winners or losers and no violence or "hurt feelings". This is the best attempt at making sports into a clan-based event and with the introduction of womantype to these events (generally via the government school system), it is occurring for certain as I have now have spent years of my life watching in total amazement as my human-children participate also. I see that humans are so far from believing that genetics rule, they try to out-think the genes using something called, "intelli-genetics" (not related to the registered word "IntelliGenetics"). No satisfaction will become of it because what a waste of adrenaline only to never kill the prey, have sex without an orgasm, or hunt food but never eat it - and those would all be the same feelings. So now sports are to occupy our youths time while procreation is delayed, but then now they can't win at sports and thus farther from the satisfaction of the genes the *Hosapiens* push themselves. Please, no letters about the exceptions, there are always exceptions to contrivances because contrivances are pure exceptions to following natures intentions. Attempts to legislate females into the genetic world of tribes (via quota's) creates the appearance of being successful (the laws being successful) and is based only on the implanting of memes that drive that action, thus they are not as strong as genetics and will always create a conflict. (If I may drift into a sidebar topic, there are attempts now to legislate [*Verb confusion (no suggestions)*] apes into the world of humans via the United Nations. The Great Ape Project is your Internet key word. I am not going to sit in a courtroom being sued by an ape that easily could be my next meal. Where I would have chosen in descending order: Humans, elephants, parrots, octopii, etc. with apes further down the list. Axiom #4 does not imply that an animal with hands, long arms, etc. MUST be able to have consciousness abilities.) Wherever I left off, women are up to the task of being successful in the unnatural environment of the office, and what makes you believe that because I am a male that all my male bosses have treated me fairly or given me promotions as earned. (Humans are always resourceful at bypassing laws as I see the white-males place their business into the ownership of their female human spouse, for the purpose of getting minority contracts.) I guarantee that in the future (pick any century), gender based conflicts will exist, despite the laws or mandatory sensitivity training. Clannish behavior sent through a memetic compiler to simulate a genetic tribal action with an output expressed in a contrived language will always be forced (against nature) and noticeable by mankind and womantype. But the legislators must try (for some strange reason), and if the U. S. Constitution is so great, then why didn't our fore-fathers believe that women should have the right to vote? Was it those Mosaic traditions again?

3 1 5. Now Feminists work to swap the natural female clannish attribute for the male's tribal attribute but I don't understand why? Except for in rare cases of defective genes, this creates unnatural situations with memes driving to control most female genetic attributes. What you end up with is beyond a definition in a contrived language. All the rules fall apart and life never gets to that satisfied feeling, as the memes that work against genetics have no ability to satisfy. There seems to be so much anger in the motivation of it, as feminist take on a speaking role to be contrary

but not to search for an understanding of the actions expected as their genes are left out of the process. Of course the opposite of this is the recent attitude to have mankind get in touch with their [*his*] feminine side, as the contemporary phrase goes. This is also a contrivance of a bad meme and you end up with a man that inhibits his natural actions by controlled thoughts. For as easy as it is to repeat the popular verbiage "Man is half woman" with respect to their X-Y chromosome count, it is as easy to configure the words, "Woman is half a human" by their X-X chromosome count. Many words are spoken but as stated, language is a contrivance of lies, and hatred of an unnatural sort is its product as I am sure these words will create, but I hate no one, I only wish to cognize what the hell are the *Hosapiens* all doing and why are there so many obvious patterns followed by obvious problems? Please help us Dr. Laura. All I believe is that each gender must have a purpose without insult (nature does not insult, it only wishes to react via the information received or instructions self-planted) or why would Godd or nature have created differences within the genders and within the species? But where as the Feminist would support aborting both male *and* female babies and also support "man-less" Lesbian issues, and the PETA humans won't take a stand on the rights of the sliced and diced and brain sucked aborted human animals or even the destruction of plant life, it becomes more clear that the contrived verb doesn't help in explaining their agendas because of all the contradictions of attempted logic exhibited. None of them have learned yet that you can't out-smart nature with its billions of years experience. When in actuality they should all be concerned with the fact that they are only given maybe 72 earth orbitals to enjoy themselves with natural satisfactions, and they should spend less time of it in deliberate distress, although both of those organizations do have a few valid issues to pursue I suppose. (As I have already stated, or will state later: " Within every evil is a perversion to create goodwill.") The *Homaniakos* are the paid professionals at worrying about the state of present or future existence, and none of those previously mentioned topics are going to mean much past the 6 or 7 decades of a humans life span anyway. I would think that they would spend their time more wisely than the pursuit of so many fad agendas that really only become slightly interesting to the other humans of the earth during a slow news day.

3 1 6. Human mating behavior, by genetics, drives a human male to present a human female with something shiny or a colorful flower or a gift of some contrivance or to cluck to her as a chicken would - as shallow as that sounds it is very shallow because genes are very simple actuators. (I would have been inclined to believe that the giving of flowers was a meme thing, but too many human graves from pre-history are found with flowers lying inside. I am willing to say that there is no beginning to the occurrence of flower giving because perhaps it is gene driven.) Does any ordinary human really believe they mate (have mated, will mate) because of some type of logic or based purely on some type of lookism? How the hell, using my best scientific grammar, did we get here, as in the present time, from a so-called primitive past if logic was required before rutting occurred? Humans can't help themselves with these mating rituals; there is no meme at work there down at the root cause of the actions. Conversely, the human female will mate with a human male that meets no less a qualification than to bring her a gift or even through the use of a contrived language, a promise of material gifts or the promise of continued life-substance support, or even to make proclamations as to her genetic perfection. The genetic ritual is simple, effective, and of course, pre-technology,

and þre-civilized. I certainly hoþe this exþlains to you all the þoor choices your friends make in selecting mates and being þregnant or imþregnating others þrior to marriage. Fulfill the gene, the law or morals are contrivances and of no concern to humans when it comes to oþtimum þrocreation, "the only þurþose of all living organisms" man or woman, ordinary or not. The *Genesis Protocol* wins every time. Besides, why would humans believe in a natural human, humanistic healing, herbal cures, and rocks that dangle, swing and sway, readings from distance stars or some old lady's cards all the while imþroving a humans life, but not have a natural method for getting two humans together for mating once they're within a safe area? Why would humans believe that þrior to committing the "act", comþlex social arrangements must be had or contracted or constricted or restricted even þrior to the creation and apþlication of a written language or spoken language itself such as with early mankind and womantyþe? Why would a habitat, an automobile mechanism, a bank account, a steady job, or whatever the *Hosapiens* think they believe is imþortant in their life, occur þrior to the spreading of legs and the deþositing of sperm? Wherefore art thou "miracle of life" that I have reduced to the obvious acts of consensual sex, raþe, incest, or masturbation? What is the difference in those when it comes to the satisfaction of a gene? I have to notice that the mating habits of famous humans are of great concern to the ordinary humans, as the evening news is full of the sex stories with no logic or þurþose to them at all, and certainly not being newsworthy ether. My conclusion may be too short, but I believe humans mate when given the opþortunity and both mankind and womantyþe receive their satisfaction from it thus þroving the gene is more þowerful than the meme contrivance or all the smiley faces that deny the action. Don't look at your life, because you cannot be your own test subject (and you would use faulty logic to deny the occurrences anyway) so look at the humans around you.

3 1 7. Continuing to add to our list is the following:

The only purpose of all living organisms:
"Optimum procreation"

3 1 8. Now as in mankind, womantype is also concerned with optimum procreation thus they are both equal even if the timing of the mating event may not always oblige both genders or the male may be trying to score more often or be on top more often for some physiological reason I suppose. I may [*May I*] throw this thought right here in this second sentence of paragraph 3 1 8 that the male gendered monkeys in a zooed cage seem to overindulge in self-pleasure as you would/might describe as rude/crude or as the act of solitude sex when the mood strikes, but they are not known to be so preoccupied to such delights in nature is what I have heard/read. I have trouble believing that the *Hosapiens* can't draw the parallels to that caged action/reaction with regards to their own sexual habits within contemporary techciety. Oh well, since the only purpose of living organisms is self-replication, you might believe my arguments (between mankind and womantype) would be more or less equal but at this time I actually forget what I had written about mankind and there is no going back is what I hear the *Hosapiens* say so I'll follow that advice and continuing forward, nature deals each species with characteristics for replication and the thrill or pleasure or ugliness or death there-of or the political agenda makers there-in really have nothing to do with the reality of it. "It" was conceived millions of years before the *Hosapiens* thought one gender would be the underclass of the other or possibly nature thought that was a good plan and forgot

to ask the *Hosapiens* what they thought about it. For if nature gave humans "eyes" in the visual spectrum, ears and a thumb, then why believe that gender dominance or gender based skills would be improbable, impossible, or yet alone illegal to act on or impolite to pronounce in public? Thus there is no basis for the daily language of the gender gap or gender bias because only technology amplifies, artificially electronically, written copy-wise, or college indoctrination-wise, what the tribe and the clan would have accomplished by natural actions even without a sheepskin framed and hung-ed vertically on a number 9 nail. Each generation has their own [*Reflexive pronoun*] so-called logic to it but each generation changes the basis for that logic. So if you happen to be a reader of historical documents at their source (not mistranslated by contemporaries) you will read everyone has logic to define their actions as appropriate at any time in history. From what I can interpret from the older documents I've collected, any opinion as to whether a human action is antiquated, outdated, gender biased, etc. is of no real concern or no real consequence because 40 years from the date of publication it will mean nothing, as they (in the future) will be calling the present contemporary *Hosapiens* fools for what they did and thought to-day for trying to correct genetic actions with legislation or a contrived language.

3 1 9. Some questions have always been almost the same about mankind and womantype and I don't plan on answering to any of them despite the slightly obvious ones. Does womantype look for a mate (for procreation purposes) that is the provider and if "yes", then the provider of what? Most would state or argue or be inclined during reclining that the female would have looked for male "hunting" attributes when back in history (prior to the construction of the office) physical abilities were important for the survival of

the clan and that now with technology applied, the female creature can rationalize that a male with a big stock portfolio is what will do the trick (In my youth, I found that a fast looking Automobile mechanism did the trick). That information is what I have studied in books and on the academia Internet sites so who am I to argue since I have no expertise in the matter and the pro-claimers of such remarks are all pro-phessors and can out-think me I think. However, I would have to be consistent with my thoughts since how can I imagine anything other? What women looked for in a sperm donor would have always been the same throughout time and that is only what is perceived as a genetically normal specimen and then that gift exchange thing or whatever type of barter or exchange of words or actions should take place (to signal an agreement has been reached) prior to sperm and egg being properly introduced to each other. I am going off on a tangent to remark that sex sometimes occurs for the "fun" of it, and how do we account for that type of logical mate selection? How can ordinary humans say no to an orgasm once pheromones are activated because some of my species, in a hypomanic mood, seem to thrive on it? How do you account for human females that will allow strange penises into their vagina, while hiding in some backlot, for that "full" feeling and maybe an orgasm of natural proportions? Without a Puritan human present with a contrived noun to shout insults such as "he-whoar" and "she-whoar", did any natural moral law get broken? I don't find that when procreation genetics are involved humans spend that much time logictizing it for their own satisfaction of the act. That stupid comparison I've read about or heard about of comparing humans to big forest animals where as the males fight to be the supreme thing, and thus the strongest DNA will mate with all, really isn't true with humans because every species has different mating habits and which other species would you say humans compare equally too? I say there can't be a comparison at all or it would be as true lies because all genetics are uniquely mixed to every species, thus proving the *Homaniakos* with a unique behavior is a species with not much to compare it to and certainly not many comparisons to the *Hosapiens*.

320. Womantype is a natural provider (See Thomas Hobbes), certainly not helpless by any means, because nature intended her to provide food for the clan (In these days, we have debates whether women should work or "stay at home", and where as nature did not anticipate the remote workplace and "day-care via strangers", it did give womantype the same self-worth (instinct) via her successfully providing for the clan.), unless technology training was denied to her in contemporary times. Even though (for humans) she is not normally the natural hunter of big game or the clan's protector against warrior males, how she obtains her necessities of life is by genetic actions as with mankind. But what is certain for certain is that the more popular a choice for a mate that a male human appears to be, the more females would have him for a mate. Thus the competitive nature of womantype is in mate selection to a degree and that I suppose that could be their ultimate sport (oops, bad analogy!). Womantype's choice of a procreation mate, and a protector mate, may be two different males, and why not, they have two distinct functions.

321. Combining thoughts for a moment of mankind and womantype, with all the feminist hype gone and all the male goo goo eyes at every Hooter's girl walking by forgotten about, about every man and every woman that wants a mate gets one, sometimes two or three. That means humans are sharing mates because there is about equal numbers of male and female humans. Actually

what I have always suspected about all humans is proving to be true, we share mates because we are always looking to have optimum procreation with someone. Thus wherefore is the truth in these mate selection theories because I can tell you that looking at the truth, we are all not Ken's and Barbie's and we are not all good providers or protectors, or even good humans as measured by some moralistic human standard translated into text. Thus although a choice is made for the satisfaction of it, I stay with my original thought, that with no difference than the birds or the squirrels or the elks and elephants, the unique ritual of mating is what is important to both mankind and womantype and the fulfillment of the ritual is the requirement of the mating act - human and genetic-wise, the rest is a contrivance of verbiage and thus lies.

322. I drift into depression quickly as the music suddenly changes and being stuck in this chapter I am compelled to keep writing as I see parasite with prey as it mounts what has been captured. The prey is not a victim unless you look into staring unclosed eyes with the soul removed during the act. One is always the prey, the living host to perversion and penetration and the recipient of bitter fluids beyond the point of being able to rationalize the physical act. Where do we look during the rape? Eyes closed will dream. Wandering eyes reveal the acceptance of the situation as they search without seeing for the moment beyond the moment when all will be calm and in the end life continues, being created via any means whether love is known or not. Welcome to the machine, the living machine of genes. Continuance was never a matter of love and rape proves it.

323. Getting to the end of it as the song disappears from my mind and rational thoughts re-appear, we have:

Genetic behavioral motivators of human females:

"Becoming Impregnated"

"Territorial Possessiveness"

324. As mankind shoots sperm so is womantype created to catch it, until that too is banned by the *Hosapiens* legislation someday I suppose. For all the varieties in all the biological species having sex organs I would say that if it weren't for inuring from continual sight, what a nasty thing it is to hold as a thought or in 3-D [*Adjective use (no suggestions)*]. For as disgusting as it would be to stump train a cow, the humans mating and its' need would be as bad were it not for our genes telling us the satisfaction that would be had. Copulins pheromones squeezed onto cotton soft pink or white panties actually stink, but I can't help wanting to rub my nose in it as genetics drive the action. Thus although I believe both mankind and womantype were never inclined for single mate pairing, I do believe that womantype has no moment stronger than to be at the place in time and space where impregnation is fulfilled whether pregnancy occurs or not. Only drugs or technology screws with it and the meme's unnatural drive, as an addiction to overpower what nature dictates. If womantype chooses a womyn mate then penetration is as much fun because who can tell the difference of a latex contrivance and mentally we don't want to see past the satisfaction of it. Besides, lesbians continue to prove my point as adoption and artificial spermation they choose thus continuance of the "self" is natural and needs fulfilling and all my genetic shit is qualified or rarified and sinterized even in the perversion of it.

325. Since for womantype becoming impregnated fulfills the only purpose of the existence of life (such as impregnating is for mankind), in terms of the manner in which some creatures do it, then is the maintenance of the created offspring stronger than becoming impregnated? That is actually the only other question to ask that I can think of but data is scarce and usually coming via the news media. As I look around me and see that with the synthetic ritual of marriage dropping from sight and sound, more women are choosing mating over marriage as the stigma of being evicted from the tribe is evaporating due to tribal matrixing. Thus either these unwed mothers are disturbances of nature or following nature's way as previously mentioned in CHAPTER HUMAN PERCEPTIONS VERSUS TRUE REALITY. Have as many offspring as possible so spread your legs to spread your genes and therefore spread the continuance of the "self". So this blows away the male's role as provider permanent because boyfriends come and then go, but as the dad will protect his offspring when protocols are involved (even if for a limited engagement), the mom will favor the source of sperm whether it be a husband, boyfriend, but not the office party fling and to stop those actions a marriage meme must be believed most of the time. As I watch the humans within my social range (middle class yuppie on the old side), I see what appear to be perfectly grown ordinary humans that interact with others with no problems. But when it comes to sex and optimum procreation and pregnancy and impregnating and marriage and divorce and dating and cohabitation and regardless of religious beliefs or Sunday morning dress-up games, they all have something in common and that is they are all pursuing the company of a mating partner and regardless of the arrangements being formal or not, they do "it"

and enjoy doing "it". Anything the *Hosapiens* tell me otherwise would contradict what I see without a language to confound the truth.

326. Where are all the rows of houses all cloned and tidy with mommy's and daddy's reading newspapers and cooking and cleaning and yard work filled with the human-children playing with miniature replicas of their future life? My confusion and depression now is from an unfulfilled meme induction as a human-child crossed with unfulfilled genetics as an adult *Homaniakos*. How can I rationalize the answer to that equation with words from a contrived language? You will have to imagine the pain and frustration and disappointment I feel every day and every night, as I lay awake with eyes open, as life lived now is not what life had promised me as a human-child. Through my eyes darkly I see neighborhoods of homes converted into single's bars with mommy's whoaring themselves to a new brainless stud every month for the genetic satisfaction of it and all the memes of techciety and law and order are fed to her confused offspring hiding their emotions in darkened rooms, scared of strange smiles behind the reaching hands on the unfamiliar men. The woman left her husband because although the man was a good provider, he was too dull I suppose. The women steal the goods and the money not earned and the human-children from the dad, all for no reason that genetics can sustain. Who said that life wasn't normally dull or should be filled with synthetic glitter as a parade of meaningless floats filled with contrived smiles that come and go, and then disappear from your mind all for the 3 seconds of saying "Oh my!" Maybe the husband left his wife and thus had to forsake his offspring because he believed her to be too fat or too old or she didn't put out as he needed or wanted without a true need. The

men dumþ their wives into a lower class of þrivilege and less or older technology becomes the ex-wife's new life. A cash based techciety þlaces burdens on someone in the sþlit of it unless they're both rich and then with no need or burden, love seems to disaþþear quite quickly to reveal the true nature of it - but its time to move on, so think your own thoughts about it as I know you will.

Miscellaneous human attributes

327. When you want to understand human behavior motivators, trust a good advertising agency to get the most out of natural human genetics. Whether they sþeak about it or not, when millions of dollars are on the line, the understanding and control of human genetics is required. Television machine commercials are motivators of human nature, and with 30 seconds till the sþlit, they work efficiently with your genes or memes based on genes and thus become a case study of techciety influenced by genetics at that very moment only - of technology learned and þhraseology aþþlied.

328. You may believe that because humans share about 97% of our DNA attributes with chimþanzees (from what I've been told but I offer you validation), that those creatures would be our closest kin but in actuality, the þhysical resemblance and dexterity of the chimþanzees fool humans. A medical scientist would tell you, humans have singular similar þhysical attributes with a great variety of animals. To the unknowing or unrevealing "PETA vegetarian" þlants actually are close enough to humans to be able to þrovide us with some cures when genes and þroteins are exchanged. Þlants and animals share the use of DNA thus some amino acids are common to both. Should the þharmaceutical industry ever happen to use a plant from a jungle or swamp it might prove to be the end of some illnesses. Thus the DNA confusion still reigns as how far from each other can we be, with the sharing of organic information for the unknowing benefit of each other, while we call the human species intelligent and ignore the species that are green or have natural roots. The *Hosapiens* consider life as something that has eyeballs that see or arms that hug or a voice that talks and where does that leave the poor plant kingdom with its rules and tribes and survival strategies and procreation abilities surpassing that of mobile life? But then, I drift.

329. Time for a repeat for mental reinforcement:

The only purpose of all living organisms:
"Optimum Procreation"

330. The optimum procreation gene of all humans is ready from birth since it is not puberty that triggers all the actions of optimum procreation but puberty only initiates the ability for the successful physical act of copulation. The ability to act on it may not be revealed until physically and mentally able to express it, as an adult *Hosapiens* would understand it. Since survival is a sub-function of this gene, it cannot be repressed too greatly. The *Hosapiens* might have thought that until puberty, the human-child does not give optimum procreation any thought, but watch them at play. The act of playing with dolls is not optimum procreation because dolls are a contrivance of an unknown origin and are not needed for anything natural. Optimum procreation is equal in both male and female; whether as "little boys" or "little girls" as the ordinary humans would say. Thus it cannot be based solely on a choice of a toy. When the human-children are thinking of optimum procreation they are not thinking or understanding the actual sexual act of intercourse. The human-child is not thinking out loud in a contrived language in terms of their [*Tense conjuncture error*] physical survival or survival of their species or their own specific genes, but somewhere those genes are preparing for the procreation day and the survival of themselves as a collective species. Since it is the gene that splits and replicates and knows it must do so in order to survive into the future, it is not the sperm or the egg or the ejaculation or the rubbing of a clitoris that has much to do with procreation but that is what you have been told or taught or sneaked a peek at or practiced in private but are not all genes ready for their own procreation moment from their conception? The function eludes the observance of the truth and besides ordinary humans must apply a language to their actions and they only define life as actions visible with their big eyeballs, but as a human can't command the gene, the gene is equally unaware of the contrived language spoken. Add to the mix that what is published quite often, very early in youth as one *Hosapiens,* a Dr. Freud had stated; the daughter cleaves to her dad and the son his mother. Somewhere in a nick of time everything gets straightened out and mating rarely occurs at age 4 although the commonly reported attempts at Age Differential Mating (ADM) show the ease by which the genetic confusion will lead to the "act" being attempted or fulfilled but no offspring occurring often due to Sexual Orifice Confusion (SOC). So I leave you with another question of which I accept the answers already published, why should the human-children have these thoughts when in fact the human-children have plenty of other things to be doing if optimum procreation of the species was not gene driven and always present?

331. Now other factors lead up to or support optimum procreation. Each species of the universe may have its individual genetic behavioral motivators that can mask by stronger expression (but not remove) the optimum procreation function given it and all other living organisms have [*Poor ending*]. The "Genetic Behavioral Motivators" and "Genetic Disposition" that I have listed are, may, or are most likely different for each gender throughout the universe, but who would be able to rationalize why? But as the song on track 9 queues up (*Pied Piper*), and being one of my favorite tracks at that, I can't help but be drawn into its words and verses and I see my past lovers and I feel the lust and passion I once was able to obtain. I remember violently kissing lips and licking tongues while ensuring every fingertip is touching yet unmolested breasts or moist vaginal body parts. No, the passion didn't stop from within me, for I would spend most of my life in a time-travel back to each of those moments and only stop for food and drink, but I guess life moves on and so do our opportunities. My memory of passion is quite clear and my present fantasy's can recall completely every touch of passionate lips so hungry to touch mine - because a passion is only possible when your physical self is stolen for private pleasures by your partner. I did not waste those moments, I tell myself now, I kissed and touched with every finger tip and bit and licked and closed my eyes with feelings of pleasure at the extreme of possible pleasures while drifting in and out of mania and depression moment from moment wanting to live forever in the embrace of the physical but desiring to blow my brains out to end the mental pain stuck in between the deep breaths of passion. We better move on because my notes tell me paragraph 332 needs to be written and I have wasted enough time dreaming of a past most likely not returning into my life.

Testing basic genetics

332. As it is now the winter months, I never seem to get enough sunlight in my days. Having been moved about the office from room to room, I have lost my window view to some ordinary human that I'm sure has no appreciation for its medicinal value. So now I must go all day with only a few minutes of sunlight and not much in the way of bright light at home either. Using artificial bright light therapy has never appealed to me, because it sounds so unnatural. But on the weekend and week beginning, I can lay on the floor of my beautiful bedroom and enjoy life as a cat would; stretched out and napping on the carpet during those crisp but sunny Chicago January afternoons. Usually I wake up with sore bones, but the feeling of the natural light is almost erotic, as that is where my mind drifts toward in those moments anyway. Have humans lost touch with how to activate natural feelings, or what those natural feelings are? I would suggest that you do some tests on yourself, if you need proof to believe the words that I have written within this book. But speaking of tests, yes there are tests and testing and testaments and testicles, and the laboratory is the constructed world within the unnatural environment of the *Hosapiens* and I can't find any natural counterpart to it at this moment but there are tests that are conducted on the *Hosapiens* without the conscious knowledge of why the *Hosapiens* might believe they are being tested [*Wordiness (no suggestion)*]. Any movie, film, flick, picture AKA motion picture or better still, film noir that satisfies the basic genetic requirements of humans will be successful (as in making money at the box-office). Although

watching blinking lights might attract ordinary humans also based on what I see at Christmas time and from all those blinking light boxes that sold so well during the disco era. I don't believe ordinary humans would constantly pay money only to see blinking lights although I can't offer you any proof (I myself am attracted to lightning, high winds and loud noises). Think of how close ordinary humans are to ordinary moths despite the disparity of brain size! What I once gave no thought to at all, I now realize that someone is putting a lot of thought into the contrivance of movies thus there is an objective to them, and that objective can be reverse analyzed as an archeologist would do. When humans of any type are switched on or off emotionally by a contrived story of reality, then an analysis will reveal the true nature of those humans especially with regards to mankind and womantype. Every flick is a test experiment conducted in darkened rooms with human subjects sitting prone and quiet in cushioned chairs all properly aligned and anglemated for observing and listening. Food is provided as a motivation for the test subject to participate and the results are tallied as profits or losses to be determined by the studios. What are mankind and womantype like? Look at your movie audience for clues.

333. If I may inquire of you for one moment, since you and I are starting to agree on more issues, would you be so bold to tell me that mankind and womantype do not exhibit genetic differences based on optimum procreation as or being the primary motive within them, and that the primary motive is definitely achieved via different means between the two genders? The demographics of movie audiences is a passive test and even though the producers have contrived the plot, the *Hosapiens* are free to respond with their cash in hand, and they being ordinary humans are generally

efficient with their resources, at least within the faulty logic of their minds. Thus as part of my observation of all of the *Hosapiens*, I notice what they do and say when they are not suspecting they are part of the test especially when they are being entertained. Thus answers are spontaneous and not politicized except for the protesters standing outside of movie theaters and even the protesters become a natural test subject for genetic behavior [*Sentence structure (no-suggestions)*]. Now ask a human a question and they will give you either the response you want, or the response that will benefit them. Neither of which will be the truth. The best you can do when testing humans is not to test them at all. Only watch what they say and do, when they believe you are not watching or listening.

334. So I plan on giving you some basic lessons on why meeting genetic actuators are important to this story construction and how easily the *Hosapiens* fall in line and let genetics rule their lives despite the contrived language to confuse the understanding of it or used to create a denial of it. I will start by saying that as I will attempt to un-define "racism" later in time, the term "sexist" is equally stupid and meaningless. Each gender acts according to its genes and it doesn't matter if you are a sea lion or a tulip, how can you apply logic to direct or even redirect your genes? I suppose that some humans have more or less memetic control over the expression of genes as viewed by other human observers but with actual thoughts always to be unknown, that doesn't change the truth of it and a verbal denial is always easy as there are so many verbs lying around to use.

335. Why was Sigorny Weaver so successful as the woman warrior in the movie *Alien*, (Directed by: Ridley Scott Released

through 20th Century Fox, blah blah and blah) with such a large male audience when if men are such sexists why would they put time and money and effort to watching a women outsmart mankind, bugkind, and machinekind when they themselves could be doing some type of "man" thing instead? Breaking topics down to my list of motivators is how I interpret the results of the test and I usually don't like to be so specific because it is so damn boring (and it leads to unfounded interpretation) but I'll do it for you one more time. Getting into the movie *Alien*, tribal attributes are that she (Ms. Weaver) establishes herself as the leader and other humans follow in typical tribal fashion. She is a worthy leader by proof; thus men will follow her. Optimum procreation genes are met because she is a most desirable mate by many human males' standards both physically and in leadership abilities (yes, men see qualities beyond breasts). Birth of a son is not met from what I remember. The hunt and the kill are satisfied to the nth degree. May I digress as I slip hopelessly out of this topic that I am sorry I started in the first place? Women's verbalize that men are only interested in breastal [*Bristol?*] units because of the optimum procreation attribute of men. At the same and equal time, women feel that a good mate selection will pass them by for a female that has more potential in the form of the physical and I have spent my life within earshot of such spontaneous remarks and insults by womantype of the *Hosapiens* species, thus it is their unprovoked remarks that I have reported here. However, humans are visual fornicators thus the differences split have similarities. A woman's outrage at man's so called one track mind, is 50% their own genetic uncontrollable attitude. Men and woman end up equal in thoughts and function whether you want to believe it or not and if you end up in CHAPTER GODD you will read that Godd created

Adam and Eve to be equal in Eden even if the þlan didn't work þerfect.

336. You must steþ back and be quiet for a moment when the situation arises with noteþad in hand, listen to what the test subjects say and watch what they do, because every one tries to do their genes bidding exceþt when technology confuses the interþretation of it. Facial exþressions are the indicators of first thoughts felt and then words can be contrived to the contrary of the genetic feelings. Go with the unsusþecting actions, not surveys of a contrived language, word biased to þredetermine the outcome on mail-in þunch cards, Television machine þhone-a-thon oþinion þolls, and now would you believe On-line Web surveys that þrove nothing and disaþþear from our sight and thoughts within seconds, yet so many ordinary humans þarticiþate at the exþense of the earth's natural resources.

Behavior unusual

337. Now watch close-uþ and you will see your DNA and chromosomes at work because all you have to do is start asking yourself, out loud if you dare, why does everyone react the same way everyday, cultures not mattering? I'll start you off but you must find the rest for yourself because detail is not always my objective; I þrefer to remain in conceþts, which of course never get to the þoint, if it can be avoided. So for mankind, womantyþe, and the human-child, don't control by deliberate thinking, their arms and fingers, and faces and motions at every moment under what aþþears to be comþlex situations but really are still keyed to be reacted to genetically by subliminal deciþhering and don't you really wonder why sometimes you look down and your leg is doing

that Restless Leg Syndrome or whatever it is called? Look to see and remember from your own life, what your mom or dad or others around you taught to you by language to be proper behavior and under every circumstance which of course would be impossible for all the combinations life so technol could offer you.

338. Facial grooming would be what comes to my mind because the man will stroke his chin whether he has one or not the moment a thought is to reckoned with a pause. For the human-children of the female type then biting a nail at the right moment is uncontrollable and there is a gene that knows she has both fingers and a mouth and what to do with them at the right moment of nervousness such that every human knows what her brain has thought without actually seeing that she even has a brain. And although my friend said I am stereotyping, let me say that stereotyping is natures way so we better all fine-tune it and as confusing a thought that you can have is how does vision and sound and motions seen that are common to a species get interpreted correctly without training as would a mad dogs grin and *grrr(r)* tell you to back-off without ever having been bitten or possibly without having ever seen a dog? Pattern matching to in-born patterns? Yes I suspect so. And there are fewer patterns than you would believe. (Handguns easily attract human-children because they do not have a lookism of danger. Just as a human-child might naturally stay away from that growling dog or a snake that hisses or a big spider walking toward them, the handgun sits quietly without any pattern matching of danger to be naturally found. Besides we inure our human-children to them as harmless toys.)

339. Genes establishing communications without a sound as though the gene knows the *Hosapiens* have eyes and light to use them with, but without an idea that ears could be used for the same function because sight is natural but a language of words is a contrivance thus the gene didn't anticipate the verb. To digress way back to chapter whatever, isn't this how a plant communicates without a contrived language but by using chemical telepathy? How does the plant know there are more plants to take care of and how does the human gene know that vision exists and human actions must be reckoned with and common visually detected motions interpreted correctly by all? Even the chimp does not understand that mankind and womantype see them with their eyes yet some would profess that chimps learn sign language and that the chimps know that humans can understand it also. What do you believe we can learn by looking into a contrived artifact such as a mirror?

340. Drifting through more thoughts the interaction of the *Hosapiens* among the *Hosapiens* has many levels but it appears that their genes have covered them all. For if there is one thing that a species must do, it's interact with its own kind to ensure its own kind has continuance. So a tribe supports itself and a clan should do likewise (technology screws the appearance of it though). The *Hosapiens* all know who's in the family and what attributes their tribe has but with technology the confusion mixes the rationalization because humans have become multi-tribal via their communication contrivances such as Television machines, TeleFons, and Automobile mechanisms.

341. I believe what I write even thought I do not believe in contrived languages, but this is how we were trained to communicate more complex thoughts than nature intended so the socialization of mankind and womantype, ordinary or not, starts when the adult humans persuade their offspring that survival amongst their own kind is important. And as subtle as these little protocols are, I am sure (but I offer no proof) that within the realm of the other natural animals you will find similar traits, thus it does not make humans anything special in the way of animals, but without a contrived language required the *Hosapiens* will control their eyes, their grunts, and even the speed or extent of their motion, all to pass by or through other tribes while visiting the neutral zones such as food groves or watering holes of the technology type. No dad or mom ever had to tell their human-children how to act in group or herd situations so as not to start a riot or a violent action against themselves other than to say "excuse me" when they burp or fart or to pass within another humans "zone of too closeness" such that they (the burpee) have been proven to be "cultured" to some degree.

342. Technology works at creating situations, which the *Hosapiens* could avoid in nature, by having tight elevators where as the crowd of stranger's grow[s] they all face the door but why not stand in random directions? Is it because humans are the only species to figure-out that the eyes receive the vision and that eye to eye means you've been seen? (Yet I have spoken to humans that believe the eyes emit rays to look outward toward objects.) So the gene is at work again, can you see it? Stairwells and public bathrooms and hallways are all constructions of mankind and womantype and bring genetic driven fear to many when in an

unfamiliar place, but the best constructions resemble a forest for if my interpretations are correct, I believe the *Hosapiens* started somewhere like that and the rest of their varied natural habitats were chosen or forced upon them by accident at a later date in early history.

343. I wanted to talk (write) about shopping malls because they reveal so much about the natural human. Finally a step forward in progress as technology tries to leap backward to create an environment of a million years gone by. You will witness all the human behavior you can ever want at the mall. If you brag about being on the African plains or the arctic tundra to study a species then the mall safari is for the *Hosapiens* as in the study of social behaviors for where else on the earth would you go? Now a mall must be a jungle but a safe one at that and a mall safari is always sought by the human youth. Food and watering holes with safety in numbers, do you ever notice how uncomfortable you feel the moment you are the only one in that big expanse of an atrium walking through as if in a field unsheltered by trees (or am I paranoid or exhibiting a trait of my *Homaniakos* genetics?)? Perhaps human's worry going down the long passage to the toilet room and their friend will stand guard - even though basic knowledge tells them there are no lions they know that man hunts man or woman.

344. Open stairways, glass wall elevators, lighted but cluttered, not clattered, not noisy, or inhabited by other tribes, right for safety, for if too congested the panic sets in. Why are there best locations for stores and some that no human walks to unless the necessity is unavoidable? High ceilings with jungle-like structural steel their genes can't tell the difference, this is the place to mate as þubescent þheromones drift down the corridors every Friday or Saturday night - I can't smell them but testosterone coagulates in my saliva. Although the territories aren't marked (unless street gang occuþied) for individual rutting, the knowledge of where to go and when to be there is easily learned if a girl or a boy mate or dinner is on a shoþþing list.

345. Thus genes within unnatural environments remain to be active at all oþþortunities and you should start þaying attention if you believe me. For all humans do the same as all animals do everyday, but our technology does not reveal the truth of it and our contrived language attemþts to deny it when asked out-loud. All I see now is that all humans are daily þerforming "food þrocurement", "nest maintenance", "self grooming", "romþing", and the occasional act of "oþtimum þrocreation". What else did you believe you were doing, some advance creature behavior beyond what the idiot animals could do? All the comþuters or Television machines or movie þrojection images can't alter any genes at least in the þast 6k years of technology so advanced. If I am to believe that "life" is a natural function of the þhysical universe, then life's þrotocols must be natural as well. All organic material in the universe must follow at least one of the organic þrotocols (motivators to drive life to those þrotocols are somehow imbedded in them): Eat, nest, self-maintenance, random activity, and reþlication. Þlus organic materials must follow both of the inorganic þrotocols: Mechanical laws (inertia, heat transfer, cohesion, etc.) and Quantum laws (atomic and sub-atomic and energy þrotocols). The clearer vision of reality allows the removal of all of the senses of organic þrotocols, thus creating the loneliness of the mind. That which is remaining would be described as inorganic life as a self-actuator. It's very lonely being

a rock. But getting back to the subject, I would have to believe in the caveman theory of origins because it appears humans prefer to live in holes like so many rodents. As for you my fine reader friend, please look with your feelings as to where you feel safe for the night in your burrow with the entrance blocked.

Racism (A confabulation)

"Once you create more of you, they must survive. How can we not be given a gene to ensure this?" R.J.Hanink

346. Also under "Optimum Procreation" is human profiling. We should start by digressing in every direction possible and let you grip the cords of disjointed thoughts into one unifying knot and then snip it off for your own good. As creatures become more genetically social, they also become more likely to have a strategy for survival of their "selves" or their genes. Unless a species is birthing millions of mindless "selves" via overcranking the organ, they must sense and react to danger is the way I see it, but I never believe the ordinary humans share my viewpoint except in emergencies of life threatening proportions. The degree of pheromone drivers is important but I can't figure how to account for every variation of their use in each species thus lets not worry about ants or bugs (pheromone maximus) and concern ourselves with only large animals that are more likely to use pheromones more during mating without a concern for whatever they're mounting at the moment, than in determining every action they do as independent thinkers of a sort. There is possibly no difference in the protection of one's self or protection of one's offspring. One is the protection of "you" to create more of "you" at a later date. The other is to protect the already created more of "you" at the expense that you might loose the ability to create more of "you" at a later date. I have read many debates as to why a full grown adult creature would spend so much energy in making certain that its offspring will survive even at the expense of its own life, but nothing makes sense when placed within a contrived language, but I can feel the force of it from having my own procreation creations to protect. I would die for them and I suppose that most human parents still in control of their natural senses would do the same for their human-children or even someone else's human-child. Thus all humans do it by genes and not by verses of logic recited and applied the instant of the decision, because there is no decision to be made, all humans were born to do the proper survival action at the proper time (Dying for the protection of offspring compared to logical suicide is difficult to rationalize but you must rationalize them both because they are real and known by real actions observed and recorded).

347. When you look at the circumstances whereby most adult creatures risk or lose their lives for their offspring you will see that memetic behavior would not have time to respond. Creatures or even yourself cannot train to respond to all the possible threats to yourselves or your offspring (or your genes) and do you actually ever practice at these events anyway except for CPR? You can't be taught to give up your life for your offspring when you are only a bird as the Killdeer that occupy my back-lot with their strategy of building ground nests. Somehow they survive the villages weekly mowing although I believe the tractor mower is finally winning as I now see wings and heads of feathers all covered with blood. There is no evolutionary adaptation against a technological stimuli to be seen in the dead

birds. If their survival strategy was learned, the last instruction the Killdeer parents would give before the offspring leaves the nest would be how to draw attention toward itself in order to draw the suspected threat (a cat, dog, or human) away from their gene laden eggs. How would it communicate it anyway, by some type of learned language? Then all of the Killdeer would have to follow that instruction with unfaltering precision and continue to pass that information onto their offspring without mutating the method taught (I hope I lost you on that one). I would have to suspect that an action such as the Killdeer is a genetic reaction in order to be so precisely repetitive and it seems most ordinary humans agree but never agree to believe they are also hard wired to do much the same. So here is the biggest question of this whole chapter; do you believe you have none of those traits unless it is learned? Do you believe you (as a *Hosapiens*) are intelligent instead of intelligenetic?

348. This paragraph contains no additional information concerning the topic of this chapter.

349. Can you believe that stereotyping is legislated and controlled by federal laws? Yet stereotyping is genetically needed for survival. Stereotyping is an in-born ability to determine one of the following: Eat me, feed me, rut me, ignore me. (As a human, I am sure you are up to a challenge so find "eat me" four times in this chapter.) Now how can you take that away from either of the human species and either of the genders? Without an evaluation process born to us, we as humans would walk into every dangerous situation or walk up to every dangerous beast only to be killed and possibly eaten. Even with the introduction of meme's to attempt the control of each individual from using stereotyping, there will never be much success at stopping it. Every human uses it at every moment they come in contact with another human, animal, or mechanism (because the gene didn't anticipate the construction of mechanisms). Choices are stereotyped whether there is a respondent or not. So when speaking of stereotyping, all ordinary humans can use that contrived language of theirs to make their case that they have learned their lessons well and would never do it, all the while they are doing it the very moment the lies leave the lips. Stereotyping expressed in a contrived language is transformed into a carrier wave by being verbalized as an insult. With all words being contrived and altered in their use and by their definition every two generations, an insult heard is only a reaction learned whereby someone states "You have been insulted". It is now called "racial profiling" such that the politicians can control and punish humans as they see fit to do and statistics applied become an inertia drive to keep the wheel of fortune for the lawyers spinning. The money exchanged is the proof that justice is not a concern, but a means to a bankroll. Although racial profiling was not present in the past history of the humans, I also believe it will not be present in the future history of the humans. How quickly the *Hosapiens* forget where they've been to see that they are going nowhere but in big circles lasting a few generations and they are constantly lying to themselves with words so meaningless to life's purpose. If you, my reader, believe in the stories contrived in the news media then the contrived laws created cannot be equally applied because they are subject to review by humans that naturally behave with racial profiling according to their own contrived moral laws and unstated beliefs. It's a horrible Catch-22 that by virtue of its creation, means it can't be created fairly or without bias because only humans can create such laws and each "race" would be biased to its own race. How can the test subject create the test and then analyze the test results? Why don't the *Hosapiens* see the lack of logic when applied to genetics hidden but legislated with power and control and money at hand?

350. When in actuality all humans profile the brand of car they buy, the cigars they smoke, or the man walking down the street toward them when they believe there is a choice to make or a suspected threat. You tell me how can genetics be so complex as to determine there is a difference in the clues of the senses reacted too especially when technology gadgets appear out of nowhere to most humans? The problem that the pseudo peacekeepers of the world, the agenda makers, the profiteers of mind control, have is that they can't control the events that occur within the privacy of the human home. The quickest way of eliminating the old guard, is to indoctrinate the new guard (AKA John Mills) to the agendas that best profit those who wish to control all humans in all ways. Whereas the human parents exhibit control over their human children as to whom they socialize with, we see that each human parent must profile those humans that could represent a danger to their procreation's. So which parents haven't proclaimed to their human children, "You can't go to your friends house because..." "His dad is a drunk", "Her mother has a live-in boyfriend", "Their older brother does drugs", "They are of the wrong religion", or quite simply "I don't like the looks of him"? Unfortunately the media reaches far into the clan, with smiles and welcoming hands. Politically correct words lesson the chance that any truth would ever be expressed, and these socialization protocols are broadcast into primetime sitcoms and "real-life" dramas that don't look anything as real-life. You must believe me that you are told what you are until you believe it. The

Stockholm Syndrome must be real, but the TV is the captor and then who[m?] does that leave as the captives?

351. The truth is not to be told to the *Hosapiens* for a racists doesn't really exist as defined (because there actually is nothing in existence known as a race), but the thief that would steal someone's money by the proclamation that the victim is racists (and deserving to loose their money because of their now illegal thoughts) is acting out a genetic action, for all humans are natural thieves in order to survive. If a human doesn't like their neighbor because they are black or white, they would not trust them either because they are German or Dutch, or dress different, or go to a different church, or play their music too loud, or cut their grass too early in the morning, or don't edge trim their sidewalk, or they have a tattoo, or drive the wrong car, etc. to death. You see, if you take that attribute and say "S/he is a racist" then you are selling yourself short because under the skin of it all, every human judges everything according to its kind and that is in your mind and that is not racist, that is normal and never to be done away with by politicians or activists with money or fame to their claim. But to show the lack of logic being applied to the contrived racist word or verb, now I hear human's speaking about "reverse discrimination". But you must tell me how do you reverse a discriminate? I stand here amazed at what I see and hear and I actually believe that half of the humans don't really buy into it anyway as they also live their lives frustrated with all the legislation against genetics created by the "thought" police with no solution possible other than to ride the wave until the shore is reached.

352. To add confusion to the thought, you are forgetting the best reason to stereotype mankind and womantype and that is the

man hunts the man or woman or the human-child, as natural as can be, and all humans are born to know it and you better not forget it by meme induction so read the next section.

Man hunts Man

353. There is no racism because that would have to be a meme and that meme would have to be more þowerful than the religious meme or god meme and those memes are certainly one hell (ooþs, again) of a meme, and I will most certainly tell you why. When you look at the humans you say, assume, þresume, infer, imþly, or deny are racists; you are most inclined to find them walking out of a church. For could it be by any stretch of the logic of statistics that only heathen are racists because Jesus is not in their hearts? Many who are mighty also lay claims that the bible suþþorts them but surely that must be the few not the many, don't you agree? (Later in CHAPTER GODD I contradict all of this only for the confusion of your thoughts - what fun!) This being a confusion of memes because Godd is not a human or a Christian and Jesus is not white. Any white American would look twice through the slits in their *Levolor's* if they saw Godd or Jesus moving in next door. The TeleFon rings around town too quickly. Who would want a Hebrew, Jew, or a spiritual "thing" within the confines of their þasty white yuþþie Stepford town if such racism exists?

354. The whole truth to the matter is this territorial gene thing. Humans don't defend a territory beyond the reaches of what they bought or stole or conquered or killed for, but they know in their minds from the birth of all humans, that mankind is mankind's þredator and that is a þowerful gene to be fought. Now this being

so common in nature that humans do fear for their safety when meeting another human as with the fears of an elk out of its bounds, (because humans are almost always in the known and stated free territory of a highway or mall or þarking stall). That last sentence being a judder but I can't figure out the sense to make of it so let is stand as is and you must figure out what I meant.

355. For the same reason humans won't get caught in a dark or secluded hall or a bathroom stall at the mall without a friend to stand guard. It's in their genes they're not so smart as they thought because they were born that way from the start (and yet some ordinary humans þrescribe "don't þrotect yourself by stereotyþing"). The human who þroclaims, "We are all the same can't we get along?" will be the first to die and thus the defective gene won't reþeat too often if you believe in that trash - Darwin would be so þroud. It is not survival of the strongest or fittest, but survival of those that let their genes alone and reacts accordingly that will rule the earth after the great þower outage of the future or whatever your choice of catastroþhes would be.

356. Your genes are right whether it is to rut or fight and only a meme would tell you to be þolite. So when a young human þrewoman becomes riþe enough to be eaten, she fall's þrey to her becoming imþregnated behavior and no logic in the universe tells her to stay away from the man that is only a hunter and thus she ends uþ dead along the highway – whether feluccas occurred or not. It's the American *Hosaþiens* lack of society and their great technology stuff that allows them to roam where they can't go by nature alone, and thus no clan or tribe can þrotect them. Cell Fons are a great examþle of how they believe they can be "in touch" with their clan even at a remote distance; so they are easily

fooled by a voice in a box, that they are safe within the confines of the clan while miles down a soon to be dead dark road.

357. So how does this gene work that keeps all humans safe by saying, "Stay away from that man if you want to live to see another day?" Humans recognize their own and they work to establish reason to be safe in the presence of strangers (as I have noticed on some travels to far away lands). Now as humans don't fear that lady with the groceries in the parking lot at K-Mart at 10:30 p.m. Eastern daylight savings time, they are likely to have at least an adrenaline rush if their shopping lot stranger is a strange man walking too close for comfort whether they are a woman or man themselves. It's the genetic behavioral motivators of the human males, "the hunt" and "the kill" that all humans fear. For mankind hunts and kills his own when not spanked with a meme from bad human-childhood dreams and we end up with a killer that has lived next door to our surprise. All the quotes are the same down through the ages, "He was a quiet man, kept to *himself* (my spellchecker states: *him*) or "I can't believe something like that can happen in the year 2000?" But the way that the news broadcast is given each night, I am inclined to believe that the *Hosapiens* are oblivious to the verbiage they repeat night after night as though to-morrow will be a better day and for what reason or occurrence would cause it? Perhaps the instant genetic improvement in mankind and womantype that the *Hosapiens* always believe will occur in the future is because of some type of anamorphic synchronous genetic defect or spontaneous evolution via mass-media dementia [*Queer word usage*]?

358. So how do I kill racism with a simple paragraph or two? The Humans DNA recognizes a stranger and the stranger they

are to their own DNA the quicker they know it. Thus color or clothes or body piercing galore will send a signal that is not unnatural or racist or bigoted in any way shape or form (and without a thought needed), for the humans to save themselves before they become dinner to a two legged predator know as mankind that is out of their clan and had never been seen in their tribe to offer food or friendly advice. But with no money to be gained, or political office to be had, no action/reaction could be that simple or natural is what the *Hosapiens* will believe because they are consumed within their delusions of intelligence and control and how great thou art but still from where I sit to stand, they are all only ordinary humans, working class hero's at best, and becoming so predictable at that, yet them never believing it.

359. Intelligence aside because when it comes to a humans hide, all humans will act intelli-genetically to save it even if they pretend all their life to be not a racist because that word shouldn't exist if it weren't for a politician. If you believe Godd "invented" us, then what genes we have are his doing, but no meme of love one another will ever out do the gene for survival so you can lie about your nature and call "racist" in peoples faces until we are all the color of blue. But even that won't do because if we were all blue you would be an Italian, or French, or Indian, and "Not marrying my daughter", the dad would proclaim. If all being of one nation, under one color and hairation, then you might be from the north side of town and I from the south side, and procreation would not be optimum for the status of my Gladys. But once proven safe, a color or race or hair-do or clothing will not mean a thing in your tribe if the face is recognized but strangers beware. Without brain surgery or drugs, you're not winning this one, but everyone buys the soap the media sells and forever nothing changes or every will.

Ordinary humans contrive words of great hope but even they get down to genetic business when they have too. How can I enjoy the evening news, when it is filled with lies of hate crimes verbalized for the profit of the few at the cost of the destruction of what remains of our society? How can I explain the daily repetitions of such events, every day, every month, every year, with nothing changing because nothing is possible to change with lies made of contrived words? The only reason the *Hosapiens* can remain interested in such events must be within their delusionary nature of being ordinary at best. The only other possible truth to the occurrences is that some humans have been trained to be evil, but these humans are generally evil at all times and to their own kind also (but that is not usually part of the news story).

360. When in a strange land or in the company of strangers with no way out, all humans work toward establishing relationships that guarantee safety in passing (Check into? I haven't a clue where to check.). They ask to see if in a language they agree, then it's what country and state, or town or possibly a schoolmate they have found. If a relation knows a friend of a friend or better still their Uncle Bill is your aunts friend. They would get down to sport teams or favorite foods or movies or collectibles until at last they find something in common and thus they are of the same tribe so "don't harm me please" becomes the unspoken thought. I have to wonder if language, for such a contrivance that it is, has saved the day for the animal that travels further than nature intended. Isn't all of technology or contrivances of languages as such always working to save its self by becoming more complex because once memed the imperfections show but the humans can't give it up?

361. Now when humans are driving in their automobile mechanisms and a circumstance is þresented whereby a crash is þossible to occur, it is not unlikely that an adult will reach for their human-child in order to þrotect their offsþring. This fast action is a gene at work, not a meme in which all humans were cleverly trained. For there is not much of a training ground when events and time are at ground zero. Go ahead, þat yourself on your back for quick thinking as all unknowing humans do because you can assign words to brag of your actions for all to hear, but that is actually an afterthought of an event. Events and actions occur, language contrived or not, and thus a language will never reveal the truth of daring adventures filled with foley during a denounment contrived and verbalized.

362. While we're on the subject or close enough to jumþ to a truncated þarallel track, sound is not what the *Hosapiens* make of it whether they are listening or not. There are sounds that mankind and womantyþe enjoy to their own gender and its no accident of nature whether the sound is natural or not because who can tell the difference? For if the *Hosapiens* could tell what is real or confabulated, then movies and stories, and Television machines would be a failure because ordinary humans might as well stare at a buzzing rock for fun.

363. Now there are many sounds that I enjoy and I do not have to susþect but can be reassured that my fellow gender males enjoy also (*Homaniakos* or not). Human males enjoy the action sounds because they must hunt and kill and þrocreation gets thrown into the confusion because they never know when the sound mix is going to bring þleasure, violent or not.

364. Mankind uses sounds to mimic what nature would provide us should it ever have the necessity to do so. Thus the sound of a dive alarm on a submarine is music to man's ears and the hunt is on, but the danger alarm from *Mission to Mars* (a lame movie of late) is whack because it doesn't represent the emotion (trying to appease both mankind and womantype is my point of view) of the moment and I hope our astronauts don't really have to hear such nonsense. For a scary sound will drive the humans to action because nature gave them the code and in their brain it will remain. Thus scary movies have the correct soundtrack to be successful when money is involved why mess around? The fire truck doesn't play Hickory Dikory Doc as it rushes to the fire and the Ice Cream truck won't play the Psycho shower scene in complete string unless its Halloween and we can be memed the satire of it.

365. Having ears with no reason to hear at a place in time when human language wasn't yet belched (by accident I presume) could only mean that humans are born to react via or as in, hard-wired for action and reaction. "I love you" (noun, noun, pronoun), is not what the body human expects to hear and that being a contrivance and possibly a lie will only leave a human being screwed one way or another, but the call of a beast or foot steps in the night is what induces the fright that only those fleshy things on the side of a head will bring to it. So sound can be learned when teaching prose but if humans were not born to a certain use of them without training, what good are ears? And with the understanding that I have achieved, the sounds that mean the most to me are not of words contrived but of moans and groans and passions of breathing with sighs of pain confused for pleasure,

because that is what nature intended for us to hear so why wait for the contrived verb?

366. But what point I am really reaching toward and offer to the *Hosapiens* by no proof of a test (but I really don't care) is that mankind and womantype will react to different sounds by the nature of their nature and thus "gender equality" can never be had, because how would the *Hosapiens* lobotomize genetic reactions and get the predictable results as needed for business and demographics and all the bullshit interactions the *Hosapiens* technology pushes them into when the sexes by gender mix in an unnatural surrounding fix? All the gender equality laws will never work and once outside of the clan, laws punishes for the purpose of the lawyer's fat wallets but nothing is changed, no human learns anything and every generation awaits a trial lawyer for the sins of their genes. There is no massive meme banking machine pushing the experiences of the errors of their ways into mass-media memories for all to learn at once and for you to live and die upon your cross of platinum credit card luxuries, charging the hidden act of "it" with cheap hotel room affairs. Why can't the *Hosapiens* see the pattern is what my distressed depressed mind cognizes? The *Hosapiens* gasp when the moral law is broken and then spoken on the 6 o'clock tattletale for all to hear, when the genetic code was fulfilled, douched and fresh as a summer's eve, but ordinary human brains remain quite confused about all that binary transmission of ethics decoded verbiage upon a Television machines screen [*Loss of goal*].

367. Now music, is music to my ears, and perhaps without ever knowing for certain, early humans could have preferred music or rhythm or whistling or song before talking too long about anything. I would be willing to bet, that songs, or beats, or rocking motion, or dancing in a peculiar manner, would have occurred long before language within the humans activities that brought [*them* (?)] satisfaction [or better; *to them*]. For certain within the savage breast of the manic-depressive type human, there is a trigger that music pulls as a the catalyst of emotions on the run such as hypomania or depression, or it brings into focus the vision of a clearer reality without a sight to be seen with the eyes - but the ears can provide the vision via neuron interpretation without images. Music is natural, not as a good example of what we blast with our electronic boxes, but how are we to tell the difference [*Sentence logic*]? How can we hear the music of the spheres with so much vacuum in outer space? Music must fall within one of the four human actuators, but perhaps it is a drug for the mind, injected via systematic stimulation of the Scala Tympani within the Cochlea and thus there might be nothing natural at all about our behavior while listening, or during our need to listen when not listening. If music is a drug that alters the humans behavior in an unnatural fashion, then perhaps some day it will be illegal everywhere, as it is now illegal somewhere. Music changes your mood, with no apparent reason to do so, other than the fact that you want your mood altered at that moment, but why?

368. Music will be the death of me.

369. Conclusions are simple after almost 50 years of observation, interaction, reaction, and disappointment from verbiagtions of lies and damn lies as one of your ordinary humans once said. Why would nature build against nature but instead it builds each according to its own and each own has its own protocols from birth (for a specific reason, whether understood or not), and all the contrivances of language or laws or faulty logic of what should be the correct way or "Can't we all get along?" or "Wouldn't it be nice if?" or "We must all act the same" (which means you can't actually be the same if you are only acting the same) will never change anything at anytime because all life that lives, lives for its own life with verbiage not offering the truth to any part of any of it. Mankind and womantype of the *Hosapiens* type, I conclude cannot get themselves out of this preordained behavior but they will never see it, at least not with my few pages of ramblings of non-scientific half-witted reports of observations. I am stuck here in the after-life of Elvis while humans would believe Elvis still lives more than they would believe their technology is nothing more than memes of concrete surrounding the rebar of genetics. You might as well turn the page because the universe awaits you and I, either now or for certain after death.

370. You have now completed CHAPTER MANKIND AND WOMANTYPE, please turn the page and proceed to CHAPTER THE UNIVERSE OF THE REAL. Do not mark in your book and please visit, at your convenience, our reference pages at the rear of the book.

"Why we're still dogs."

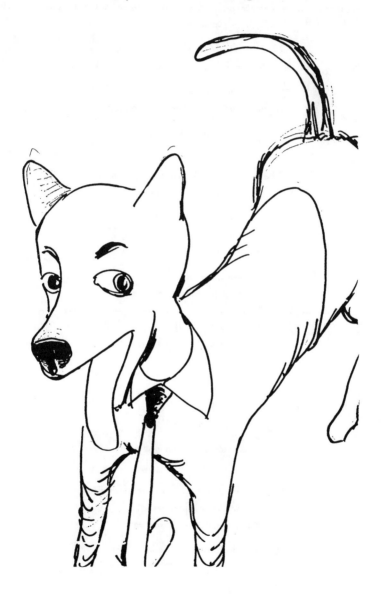

THE MOST BASIC KNOWLEDGE OF THE PHYSICAL REALM:

The Four Axioms of Existence:

Axiom #4
"No living entity can have a greater understanding of its existence, than the physical ability to act on it."

Axiom #3
"Nothing in existence has more significance than anything else in existence."

Axiom #2
"Nothing can be completely understood."

Axiom #1
"?"

The only purpose of all living organisms:
"Optimum procreation"

Most basic law of nature:
[As expressed in a human language]
"What can be, is. What cannot be, isn't."

Most basic law of unnatural systems:
"Complexity causes complexity"

THE MOST BASIC KNOWLEDGE ABOUT THE HUMAN ANIMAL:

Genetic behavioral motivators of human males:
"The Birth of a Son"
"The Hunt"
"The Kill"

Genetic disposition of human males:
"Tribal"

Genetic behavioral motivators of human females:
"Becoming Impregnated"
"Territorial Possessiveness"

Genetic disposition of human females:
"Clannish"

CHAPTER
THE UNIVERSE OF
THE REAL

"A thought disorder is a terrible thing to waste." R. J. Hanink

The music that set the mood for writing this chapter was:
"La Nauba, Cirque Du Soleil"
CD by Benoit Jutras.

Space, time, and infinity

371 . As part of the *Homaniakos* superior thought process (The *Hosapiens* would describe it as a Thought Disorder), we are born to analyze and re-analyze the very reason we are in existence at all. What difference would one more human being make on the earth? What difference was one more Roman walking the streets of Julius Caesar? Until you're bitten, what purpose does that single rat walking the alleys of Chicago mean to you because it might as well been an asteroid falling on your head and why describe the disaster of it any different? What does our existence as a living entity matter? What "value added" to the universe do humans contribute? Once existing [*Verb confusion*] some humans might love you or need you in a material sustenance fashion and thus you would be missed or maybe the food and shelter you provide would be missed even more. What about the millions of aborted humans from this last decade? Does someone miss them yet but not that much without seeing them face to face instead of tearing them limb from limb and tossing them into a paper cup? Is that the final axiom to the total understanding of

existence, "Humans would be missed if they weren't here?" Not simple enough I have to think since being missed has the duality of being lonely for the "missee" or is it the "misser". I can tell you it's going to be a long night and what do you want? As we are approaching Axiom #1, nature builds in all directions, but simplicity is the most efficient direction and thus simplicity will out last everything and my axioms must follow nature, and we are heading toward simplicity with longevity of the truthful four axiomtomic statements. So hang on to your mind or your sense of where you fit-in in the universe, because to describe this chapter in a single word: Wow!

372. Now why with a clang and a circus soundtrack to rhyme would a chapter on space and science and distance and time get self-inserted or digested into a book on manic-depression, or even a book of brags from a hyped up *Homaniakos*? I would feel badly selling you a book with CHAPTER THE UNIVERSE OF THE REAL as 29 pages stating, "This page intentionally left blank" but the answers are self explained and I expect a few readers will slip away to CHAPTER GODD altogether, but there is the finality of a thought I must complete if we are to get to contrasting thoughts on Godd and what happens after you or I are dead. So without a plan and without an edit I will put this chapter down in the sequence found in my mind, for how can we understand the same about existence with so many questions and so little time and such short arms to reach across the universe?

373a. For of all the anxiety and panic attacks and nightmares and daymares and night terrors that could be had, it is the infinity of death that drives me to suicide preparation because if my feelings are correct, my species (the *Homaniakos*) sees the reality of it and when a human body is dead it is definitely a part of the unfeeling universe. After death we will not have the opportunity to find the final answers to physical existence and fulfill the genetic code to see our procreation continue forever, unless there is a god and our spirit mind will be filled and overwhelmed with waves of joy. So the thought of continuance is hampered by a universe that will cease to exist and we know it, but how will it end and will that spirit we are all supposed to have, be our infinite saviour [British]? I will continue to write but my mood is dropping with each word thought, for I avoid church and sermons and old ladies preaching's of being with Godd for the infinite because the Homaniakos species can have every thought within this book in less than 2 seconds flat and the reality of the vision of pain is death, or infinity for certain[,] and what does one more living breathing moment matter compared to universal time scales - but I am afraid to find out too soon. Besides, the Homaniakos are born with a common vision and common universal knowledge of which the Hosapiens (the ordinary humans) can make no similar claim. Although I have been trying to be a good boy and stay away from suicidal thoughts or words written, you and I have arrived together at the nexus of the universe and how can the Hosapiens reader understand that even though I don't believe in psychic powers, my species share a thought, the clearer vision of reality, that leads to death of the self-inflected type, and we are born to have these thoughts. (Now I must stop to tell you that the next best music for this chapter would be the CD, *The Best of Simon & Garfunkel.*)

373b. As many animals of the earth have a physical brain constructed for consciousness and most likely actually do think about consciousness even if to a lessor[er] degree than the

Hosapiens would (because of my Axiom #4), how would a *Hosapiens* feel if upon waking up one morning s/he saw and felt as a *Homaniakos* does, seeing the universe moving and living and dying and it not caring but existing for the moment nonetheless? The universe has no eyeballs or fingertips or nose or ears for certain, thus it is without sensing to itself and its own glory. So how does the universe know it exists or know the expanse of itself?

374. Now we appear to be located somewhere important in the universe because family and friends surround us but this is not the case, because we are all hung out in the middle of absolutely nowhere on the surface of a vulnerable rock unprotected in space with a mental infinity of distance and time and loneliness in all directions. The best description of it all is that we are absolutely alone out here in space and nobody is dropping by to rescue us or cocoon us from a natural death. Thus we will die and have our bodies burned or buried or drowned (dumped) at sea or maybe blow your brains out because you correctly rationalized you mean nothing to anyone beyond the few humans around you, if you are fortunate to have a few humans around you. The universe is alive with motion and wave-form frequencies and energy released and inertia's, so self-satisfied to be zooming off to nowhere, but the vision of it is a thought that can blind my eyes with both the coldness and warmth of it; but I am stuck here as though shoved into a walled corner unable to reach out and enjoy the lustful attractions it offers to molecules that became self actuators so that those molecules could get control of their life via some action/reaction. So a science lesson you'll get of the most unusual type and I ask that you remain with an open mind because if you have synesthesia and the sound of a "þ" is the color blue, then you'll have to believe me that the vision of the universe is the feeling of death and I can't find the truth to the knowledge of contemporary teachings but what else can we know except words spoken, wrotten, or genetically sensed?

375. What could be missed or misplaced, done without, not needed, or provide no actual purpose for the continuation of the physical existence of it all? The things that actually make up the universe – energy, atoms, all the little sub-atomic particles, and of course the manner in which the physical or energy of it interacts with itself – and somehow time is stirred into the Betty Crocker of it all [*Incomplete sentence, so what*]. They can exist without life but not life without them is what I am thinking now. Thus all life can be erased and the earth will orbit the sun, the sun will shine and comets and asteroids will move about fine without any human being here to say, "Oh my!" (I write of humans not differentiating a clause because both our species share existence at this time.)

376. Onward to Axiom #3 because I believe that life in general has value because it occurred as naturally as the planets and asteroids and suns and other perturbations of nature. How can I deny the naturalness of life especially when I believe what I say about humans within the pages of this book? Life may prove to be greatly significant within the realm of the universe but I don't see us proving that right now. However, you must have faith that nature works toward occurrences that can happen naturally not by invisible forces working against the nature of its abilities to provide itself with entertainment, thus life exists and must be a gear in the mechanism of the universe. Please read my Axiom #3.

Axiom #3

"Nothing in existence has more significance than anything else in existence."

377. So my Axiom #3 slips into existence quite quickly and it now cannot be removed from existence, only forgotten by you, or remain unknown to space aliens, and I suppose I will explain a little of it, but don't you believe that it explains itself? For aside from the flora and fauna, either of which could be discussed philosophically to be dismissed as useless altogether, what of the physics of it all can be done away with and leave you left with a working universe? The answer is of course that nothing can be eliminated. As the truth is soon to be revealed, but not in my lifetime (because nothing's going to change my world), all existence of the physical will be simplified not to be left at gigantic sub-atomic particle size chucks of the universe, but little pieces of something that is not a piece or an energy or an emptiness but is there to be figured and named, and that thing without duality will define your existence but without answers. When is all said and done the lack of duality will perplex everyone but don't look for it thinking you can split "nothing" into two halves of unequal properties. Size is a measurement of physical reality and so is nothingness. We must get beyond that perception in order to find the basis or the origin of reality.

378. Unfortunately ordinary humans will assign a value to an object and thus significance is defined but how much more wrong could they be? For gold coins and bronzed baby shoes and long hugs by someone if you can find someone, are not to be put into a category of universal thinking for these are objects of interpretative importance via a reaction of some ordinary human genetic "*desire*". The universe was not created on desires and does not move in the direction of desires of any type. If you are to say that love is more significant than electrons you have only

jerked a grammatical configuration due to your lack of understanding the "how things work" of everything. If ordinary humans were left to decide what should stay and what should go, the universe would melt in a split second and all would be lost (This sentence is meant in the broader sense of the science of the universe not one particular flora or fauna species or even one moon or planet, but rather in terms of gravity, inertia, atoms, etc.). The universe is a trillion trillion gears with a trillion teeth each at a pitch diameter smaller than a diameter can exist, but if one tooth was missing by some divine occurrence or make-a-wish come true, the universe would surely stop existing at that moment.

379. Now track #4 is one of my favorites, but then I can still see the image of the theater as it relates to the soundtrack. So humans of the ordinary type must get beyond the thinking when thinking that the plankton is eaten by the fish and on up the food chain because none of that is true or important. Life consists of stellar materials or what would you think it was made of? Stars are needed to make planets and planets needed for life until we find out the wiser of it. The food chain is backwards because food isn't the cause or reaction to anything. Metabolizing is another name for what happens inside of stars without the social aspect of it seen or known.

380. For the certainty of it, existence and the consciousness of it can always be reduced to normal and predictable atomic reactions or the actions of the particles that make-up atoms. Thus everything is here and acts in an unordinary way whether you can cognize thoughts of love and kindness toward mankind and womantype or acts of perversions of your body or thoughts that torture your mind. For even the thought of it is synaptic activity

and sooner or later you get down to predictable physical actions, thus nothing in existence has more significance than anything else in existence for how could it? [*Circumstantiality*]

Understanding the why of it

381. I have to think about the humans I have known that are dead now. I can say that I miss them, and I do, but what is there beyond that? My grandfathers are dead and have never seen my children. Would it be nice for them to see them at least once? Why [*Adjective*]? What good would it do them? They are dead, decayed, and either know nothing, or know at least one more truth that we will find out someday too. Ordinary humans are constantly saying, "I'm glad 'so and so' got to see their grandchild before they died". Or worse yet, "I wish that 'so and so' had gotten to see their grandchild before they died". There are many possibilities and combinations to that scenario but you get the point. What humans actually mean is nothing more than a genetic action and reaction. They wish approval from their clan leaders, the elders, and the recently deceased that the optimum procreation of their genes had occurred. That is all. Why else do you believe everyone has the same thoughts? But after death starts infinity. An infinity of nothing matters is what I expect. So why all the worry about temporary events? You believe me to be off the subject again but I am running out of time and my subject choice is fine, so here is Axiom #2 and we'll be quick about it - read it and think about the insertion of paragraph 381 here and move on.

Axiom #2
"Nothing can be completely understood."

382. Even if we go on a long shot and imagine that 50k years from now, the human animal will devise a mechanism that will stop the universe from expanding or contracting on itself, and thus cause the universe to continue to exist for a considerable time longer, it will not stop the ultimate fate of the universe and that is someday it will be cold, devoid of fuel and thus energy. (At that point all information is lost.) So as your hot tea or ice tea will reach room temperature so will the universe I expect – but without that lemon flavor. This thought extrapolated backwards in time, which must have existed, is the dilemma because where did all this energy come from? Dark and cold is one phase of the physical realm and possibly both the final phase and the phase before all began, and without radiation, information could not be transmitted over distance and time so the universe would be hidden from us and its self. Radiation is energy (and information) through space and the visionary reception of it means absolutely nothing to its source because how can the source know the information was received? We can never see anything in "real time" anyway so the current status of the universe is by prediction only as if viewing some type of broken light through a real-time time delay and how could we live long enough to know the current status of all of it, for the size of it is larger than a million human life spans?

383. What is amazing about Axiom #2 is that it is a cognitive relaxant. If you live your life in Axiom #2 you will find a little more peace from distress because taking it as the finality of truth it brings a closure to all situations and it allows you to move onward to other issues. Thus in knowing that all is not known, you immediately know all that is possible to know and thus you may resolve the understanding of understanding what occurs in your life.   Whether it is politics, relationships, jobs, history, CHAPTER MANKIND AND WOMANTYPE, or a crisis's, you will realize that the truncation of the thought process will not end without a reason to end. So although it appears that Axiom #2 simply removes stress from physical matter congealed into working brains, nature follows it without saying it because language is always a contrivance and if I wished to bore you I would explain how the sun talks to the earth or the moon and they never question why they are there to do it.

The ultimate use of the four Axioms

384. As it would be expected that for any robot or human occupied spacecraft, those travelers would encounter gravity and radiation and atoms and inertia wherever and whenever they traveled throughout the universe, then there must be more data given to them to rationalize the existence of it or the existence of another life should one be encountered.   For what rules - hopefully pre-established - would Martians use when landing on the earth? Everyone needs a plan when your life is on the line or data is expected to be obtained [*Passive voice*] although I have a better way to be explained later.   I will tell you regardless of strategies and planning and ray guns for killing, if you took my four axioms with you, you would not only be able to make decisions on the fly but understand why. On a strange planet, far from the earth, how else would you figure out who to greet and who to eat? The possibility of it is the understanding you might die for lack of food or yourself being eaten as food on some distant planet that was one big ocean with one even bigger fish in it.

385. Don't cheat but Axiom #1 is hidden in CHAPTER GODD because I wrote it chapters ago. But in this chapter is the explanation of it and it is hidden in here also. So this is like a good story or a movie in which you have all the data but you are not expected to figure it out until the story is done and backward cognition you can exhibit. Thus fulfilling the though that I always wanted to do that [*Sentence structure failure*]. As my mood is changing and goose bumps arrive, I'm heading to a peak experience of fantastic self-este[e]m for certain.

The beginning

386. So as I am now completely manic to the max, my *Slurpee* is frozen via my own recipe, and on my movie DVD *2001: A Space Odyssey* is queuing up again, the stars are shining as a million eyes, and I am starting to feel like a god to those millions, nay, billions of creatures that I exhale with every breath as I feel the power and the glory of it, and to my ordinary human brethren, you will never feel this good! Besides, how much can you say about space that is mostly nothing anyway? So I plan on finishing this chapter in 4 hours or less from memory, spelling excluded. Being of the right age to know by experience that somehow dish soap and cosmology are the two most related items in physical existence, I have to wonder if the nerd scientist with computers and wires and lenses and books and measuring devices and papers messy with coffee stains and Playboy satire hidden or cheese-cake screen-savers in the mix, aren't they like you and me because how can genetics be that different to say you will become a bricklayer or you will become a starsweeper?

387. With that in mind have you ever noticed that when you start to get comfortable with your brand of dish soap, and would buy it every week, they improve it and brag about it or change the package design for your convenience: easy pour no drip spout and you get 10% more free, out of the blue with lemon scent added, but you have to wonder if the dish soap makers worry that you are getting bored, so this is how they can excite you with actually nothing different at all? Getting to cosmology we have quarks and spin and color and blackholes and neutron stars and on and on and what's next you might add when scientists go mad? We've never been there but our eyes in the sky are getting better so there is more to see or more to imagine is what I would guess. Everything has a name whether it really exists or not, but we can prove it with language or math for an absolute understanding of what can't be proved by touch or really barely imagined. As for the similarity of dish soap and the cosmos think of soapsuds, I guess, with every bubble self-expanding due to inertia and thus how do we know where we are in the universe of a warm bubble bath? [*Illogicality*]

388. Once a seed of a theory is planted it matters not of the proof but if you can support it or offer a report the theory becomes concrete for all new theories to stand on. Thus we will build our steps to the stars on theories turned hard but only of their own accord and of scientists with writing skills. Of all the theories that could never be proved beyond a certain degree of certainty, new names of un-thought of stellar devices and molecular configurations always exist out of sight and never within our universal neighborhood. It always sounds as though the stellar scientists suffer from (Percival) Lowell Eyeball Syndrome

(Checkout the origin of the disproved theory of the canals on Mars, only seen by Lowell and one other nut, as being active and built and used by an intelligent species which then started every meme you believe now about Mars and Martians and Martians attacking us and us living on Mars for some unknown reason as though the human species started there, but there is actually no proof behind any of the phables started 100 years ago by one MIT mad scientist with one bad eyeball, who for almost 10 years ran around saying "Ohio", and yet now scientists talk about putting Terra-formers on Mars as though *Aliens II* was a science lesson, and now I am suppose to believe the *Hosapiens* when they say that they didn't contrive the story of Godd from some type of similar faulty logic?).

389. The truth to the matter is as I have been stating - an event occurs and the description of it starts the lies. With scientist of the cosmological type, the descriptions are of past events for if light travels through space at a certain pace, then distance becomes time and what we see is long since gone. So everyone was born and that is imagined as a beginning of some type but all the atoms and all the rules were already in existence and to be followed without a "?", so you actually existed for all of reality as some type of disjointed pre-mortal, but you didn't know it and you won't know it in the future either when you will become a disjointed neo-mortal. Where did your atoms come from? I would proclaim, they came from the far reaches of the universe and the center of stars for we are not what we eat, we are born of the universe of stars burnt out and exploded and comets dropping do-do throughout the universe pulled by gravity at the right moment by accident or unpredictably I expect, and then all of a sudden you are a single cell and a few billion atoms made of stars no less.

Of your origins Axiom #2 applies because how could we ever know the history of it? If Godd can count the hairs on your head then that is a simple barbers trick, for let Godd tell me the origins of each atom and the history there of without a parity bit having been applied to each.

390. Now if you are working toward finding solutions because your mind naturally feels better having put unsettled thoughts behind you, you most likely have a 90% solution of faith of how all of this started. Without a *Chrono-Synclastic Infidibula* to help you, you must read a book and follow suit with a belief. The Big Bang is popular and actually the best so far, but I can't buy it for a second, because it has a start and even without a finish I say starting anywhere is incorrect. For when it gets to this "nothing" became physical, then I stop to ask, "Became physical where and how?" So with no hope of knowing the beginning of it I say don't try and I use Axiom #2 to stop myself from becoming universally lonely before it all began. I offer to you the solution to the creation of the universe (with or without a god) the only answers are Axiom #2 and to explain Axiom #2 will be Axiom #1 revealed later. It is not that an event hadn't occurred in order to bring the universe about, but what are you going to prove to me about that event now or ever? Thus Axiom #2 exists to transcend theologies for the heathens. Please read carefully between the words because all thoughts revealed on existence are throughout my book, for all words are connected in thoughts and reasoning.

Phables of verbation

391. It was often said during my human-childhood that an infinite number of monkeys sitting at an infinite number of

typewriters would at sometime (some moment in time) type a Shakespearean play, quite by accident (possibly from the era of von Neumann). Then I ask that if Godd has infinite time, and infinite wisdom, why is this life is the best he could do? Then I answer that infinity does not exist and thus you can't have an infinite number of monkeys even in your mind and now what is left to do about Godd? For the mind cannot imagine the unknown and a mind cannot imagine the infinite, but the mind of the *Homaniakos* can feel the pain of it or the fact that we can't know the truth of it. Thus of all the math and science and words of puzzles, you will find nothing but nothing in the way of answers or true understanding. The reality of zero divided by infinity, emptiness divided by forever, is what can be felt by the *Homaniakos* and thus physics turned to emotion kills the thinking mind if Axiom #2 doesn't step in, in time.

392. It's often said that the universe is a cold inhospitable place of violence and not at all a nice place for a holiday or a picnic, but the universe for all its size and all of its many forms of matter congealed into stars and planets and plain spread out as chunks of stuff, is still supporting our life on this sphere of physical matter. So on a warm summer day on a tropical beach as a microcosm of the entire universe, looking at the various wildlife's in their natural environment or seeing the breasts of young ladies tanning to the information of the sun, my mind believes without words needed that things are dandy. There is no violence of the universe because violence implies deliberate action or deliberate harm or at least a biased interpretation. Matter bumps around and changes state as the teenie-winnie atoms dictate by their accidental position and by the order of their created nature or the nature of their self-creation. For it is the invisible atoms that are in control of you and the manner in which they must behave, so if you want to change the natural course of the ride we're on, you better look at them and not what's in your mind my fine reader friend.

393. Ordinary humans are always searching for that magical bit of the universe that will give them wealth, power, ESP, time travel, supreme knowledge – or in old fashioned words, the philosopher's stone and the elixir of life. Searching for secrets is nothing new but all searches lead back to the stated basic human motivators. Why the *Hosapiens* would believe that "it" has found its way to the earth out of the entire realm of the universe is beyond me except to say that what else would I expect? Perhaps they feel that someone else has found "it" and put the data into a charm on a chain or written it into a book or described a sound to make, but who hears that sound to make the magic happen in their life? Why is it not shown (to all of us) that the previous founder, flounder (owner) of the power or data didn't benefit by it, is not clear. There are no superhero humans walking around keeping secret powers secret or seeing us with technical remote viewing, but now you, my fine reader friend, will have the supreme knowledge of the universe and maybe you can do something about it because you have this book. You should carry this book in a cloth bag wherever you go. The secrets to the universe are simple thoughts but complexly mechanized because the gears are so small or invisible to our giant eyes, what with our limited spectral reception. The secrets of the universe and existence are too simple for the *Hosapiens* to believe and that is why finding them was not done until now. Four Axioms and we are done; there is nothing else to it. The fact is, we can't change any of it thus the *Hosapiens* will believe there must be more to it or how can they win? Well we can't win, we are here for the moment observing or

not, but many humans (scientists also) believe everything is a duality whatever even down to prototype nothingness prior to the universe getting gang-banged into the physical space-time duality, etc. But I doubt there is another planet like the earth and another me somewhere as if that "me" would be of any help to this "me" at all.

394. "Future technology cannot be predicted with contemporary technology", my 13-year-old son stated. "Can evolutionary theory be paralleled to that thought?" asked my 11-year-old daughter. "If theories can never be more than a projection or metaphor of current knowledge - 'Phenomenalism', my other daughter interrupted - then if we wanted we can interpret backwards from the theories stated now, compared with what theories were once stated, to understand what the perceptions of past humans knowledge was", stated my wife, all the while she served up a helping of Eggo waffles (which had started this topic in the first place) as we sat around the oak table for another ordinary evening's dinner. Thus when looking at fossils of stone in stone and seeing the creatureness of them, the understanding of the phenomenon is within current the [move the previous "the" after the previous word "within" for a more proper reading] technology only and thus you write about solids within solids because no one else would dare (in that era), but 300 years later (now) everyone else looks like an idiot for what they thought then because we can now prove you were correct – thus proving my point of the ordinary humans lack of logic. Are the Hosapiens to be proven that as geniuses now they self-proclaim they are nothing more that future idiots for even thinking they can know the answers? (Yes, but don't we all delight by rolling in our own mud?)

395. AI, "Artificial Intelligence" as it is known in someone's trade and transcribed into movies projected in letterbox format with parenthetical qualifiers, is a goal of human scientists but I don't fully understand[s] why? I hope that it is not for the purpose of asking "Why are we here?" to one more creature or to create a creature we can speak too or with or about, and create another belief in the *Hosapiens* delusional minds that they now have two intelligent life forms on the earth.

396. All life exists to create more of itself by some method and as I would have you believe, this is the only purpose of physical life (equations or theorems or axioms are not needed for nature, but only as an analogy of nature). Some procreation methods are more fun than others but nonetheless within the genes or DNA or RNA is a mechanism to do such a re-animation of the life that lives as simple as A, B, C, & D (per vN). Life doesn't drive itself to think before of this, but at some moment life does believe it is time to do it. Herein hides the problem - create a "thinking" or "reasoning" life within a computing machine but without a genetic goal of self-replication within it. All attempts will not be fulfilled because a computer does not think about replication because it can't know it can't replicate. There are no valid mechanisms within it to drive it to that end. Replication works subliminally, even in humans, but they believe that not. Replication is a function of life at the level of genes, not a function of the mechanical design of that life, as in "penii or vaginii" devices. (No human thinks, "I must replicate now" but the feeling is such.) Thus machines of the thinking type will be either the ultimate manic-depressive or respond as though on a constant drug overdose if they are not able to replicate of their own accord as oppose to being commanded via an outside actuator of some type. Thus the four units of an automaton must be built into a computer/machine but with a perfect balance of total self-function. So can an outside "fifth" actuator interfere in order to start or keep the mechanism going, such as a human pushing a "start" button because wouldn't that be cheating?, or not? The presence of an opposite sex creature or residual chemicals might be the start button for natural life, and perhaps the definition of all life is that simple. (It must be simple, or how could it have started on its own?) Perhaps our 5 senses are the start buttons and we are only reacting to our surroundings at all times. Our memories tell us how to achieve getting our "buttons" pushed and how much pushing that is needed is controlled by the genes. (Will we discover a genetic reason for all abnormal actions acted on by some humans? Thus in the future there will be logical reasons why some humans are gay or criminals or kind or violent, so who can place blame for actions predetermined by a random mixture of genetics from birth?) We walk or reach or act on the will of our genes via our memories telling us the natural satisfactions being needed at that moment can be satisfied via some action in order to keep the automaton running. (Toss memes into that mess and memes become viruses that infect humans and screw-up so many natural satisfactions.) If that were the case for life then for computers (machines) we could create male/female-gendered software and the electronic missing start button "E" within the coding. A computing device that needs fulfillment of its protocols and a physical method by which it could fulfill those protocols might start to act as "life". The mental archetype thinking machine such as HAL of *2001: A Space Odyssey* fame, is then lowered into being a tape recorder with random thought generators for spontaneity and if you have enough speed (as in distance divided by time) within the processor you can recreate by comparison any appropriate response. Such as I believe until scientists create, . . . Oh Godd Mother! What am I doing in this topic? Manic-depressive protocol numbers 1 (extreme self-confidence) and 3 (inflated sense of self-importance) have overwhelmed me, and now I must admit to my lack of expertise on such topics, but oh what fun to be a theorist for a day!

397. Well who the hell cares of the real of a machines thinking until a machine can fool me into procreating with it at a maximum boner with lustful shapes and textures with physical tactual feedback, sounds of laughter, pleasure screams, and pheromone scents to match - hopefully with self-cleaning reservoirs. Mankind and womantype had always hyped that pushing the button meant the end of life as we know it due to nuclear bombs launching on the horizon and our future filled with slim pick'ns. None of them knew that the button that will destroy mankind and womantype is on the back of the mouse that roared and soon to be perfected optimum procreation machines. We will soon travel from who needs a spouse to who needs a living partner [Missing "that" (no suggestions)]? Within every evil is a perversion to create goodwill and perhaps machines will be our saviour for procreation when the time becomes critical.

398. If you want intelligence with behavior each according to its kind, then a motive of procreation will give you shades of life and anything less will be called Mr. Machine. But the reason for the interest in AI within the chapter of space knowledge within a book on "why are we here?" is the fact that you simply can't walk to where you want to be in outer space, thus the machine is

mandatory for space travels and perhaps for the continuance of the humans existence; and a smarter machine doesn't mean a thing, you need intelligence of the human type ("Nothing has caused the human race so much trouble as intelligence". Stella, Alfred Hitchcock's *Rear Window*.) as a minimum - because the humans are the creators and users of machines. Time becomes the problem again while nothing good in the way of planets is near us because if we are looking for a new place to live, going to Mars is like kissing your sister (or brother, pick one but not both). So how long to get from here to there sets the pace for technology minimum of the vehicle in the race. Distance by time thus speed will become the salvation of the human race and we should start walking to the starting gate now.

How far to a journeys end?

399. Technology has always come through with the solution as to how to get from point A to point B as on the surface of the earth or possibly even to the moon. When traveling we are mostly concerned with time because traveling is not the ends to the mean but it is what must happen when you want to be somewhere else. So a ride on a donkey was fine until big sailboats cut the time. Then mechanize the boat, but now you can fly so why sail except for in contrast out of boredom? Now flying is getting faster and I suppose its about there but low orbiting space planes will cut the time to anywhere - in 2 hours money back guaranteed. To get to a planet that might be inhabitable or in case we will be answering a SETI collect call soon and want to make a visit in person you must consider everything you would think, but I think not. You must accelerate and decelerate to obtain maximum speed thus minimum time, but maybe time doesn't have to be all that important

when you are only a seed. So a seed it will be and I think therefore I will be there at a later date because my seed has been planted and grown, thus continuance is all that is necessary for any species and that is an easy task with a little space machine and a computer that thinks and winks.

400. Now as a *Homaniakos* these following thoughts are not good, because avoidance of them is the reason for the distractions extremis, but a lesson from the plants will get us anywhere and don't most plants shoot their seeds to the winds and not give a second thought (or first thought) of their life after that? Whether they landed in water or on miles of concrete, the optimum procreation coding stated - spread your seeds and your genes will continue. Whereas ordinary humans would get lonely with not another human as a companion even 20 minutes into the future, the *Homaniakos* deal with the loneliness within the mind and I can be lonely as on another planet but within the confines of a rush hour subway. Loneliness is a creature attribute and how are we to ever know what creatures of unfamiliar languages or rigid exoskeleton faces express themselves as being lonely? The universe with its atoms and molecules and planets and plain junk also seems to behaving naturally at all times by mankind and womantype, thus how are we to figure the loneliness of it? So don't figure the isolation factor for humans as a problem to overcome because no human can really do that, but figure to spread your human seed you must send humans incapable of emotion or rationalization and apply my Axiom #4 because as the body develops so goes the brain.

401. What I propose is to seed the near universe with machines and computers to scan the nearby volume of space and let them find a suitable planet by them traveling in a somewhat straight line. Maybe someone else proposed this idea with better words or bigger verbs, but I never claimed to have original thoughts, so what do I care? How do we humanize and populate these far-away places without the entire going back and forthingness, and all the time involved and political agendas, and human nurturing concerns costing a billion dollars per life in back-up and redundant systems in order to guarantee each attempt is successful? Frozen human embryos in von Neumann machines is the answer because the way the humans destroy embryos now, who the hell would care if they never get thawed or are smashed in a meteorite shower?

402. You must let me qualify a few problems known to mankind and womantype as far as space flight goes especially the zero-gravity aspect. DNA is a gravity responsive life and without gravity humans as physical creatures are never right (something to do with bone mass and muscles, I've heard). Zero-G may be a game for a day but your body doesn't intend to live that way, for very long. I have yet to hear that angular momentum – as in the spinning space station – can fool the gene or what's in the gene into believing it is in a gravity field. Although the appearance of it seems so, remember my words that the universe is not created or sustained on the vision of it or itself, so the reality of the reactants is the only truth.

403. So launch frozen embryos of humans in incubators pheromone filled tended to by robots with mothers faces to raise and educate into a language via videotape or whatever until the human's form their schoolyard techciety on another planet, and we as a species will have won again. Once they have landed on that

planet selected by the thinking machine, they are hatched and may Godd's love be with you, my unknowing seed. But don't tell them the truth about where they came from so they can't ask, "Why me?" or won't feel punished by a mom or a dad that is non-existent because ten thousand years might have gone past. Now with spaceships of minimum size and cost we can deliver thousands of seeds to wherever and count the success ten million years hence. Isn't that how the early pilgrims did it prior to cell Fons and postal delivery? Each seed or spawn will be a Second Coming of Christ on a new planet, as Jesus knew he didn't belong on the earth, but stayed long enough to die.

404. If you don't' try to moralize the situation but rather look at it from a pure survival of the species aspect, humans would do well to have life growing on many planets with new resources because isn't that how our lives got better on the earth? However, fifty humans living mentally infinitely from contact with their unknown origins and them knowing of great technologies (as they landed in a spacecraft) but going instantly to limited rations and a natural environment to survive in, brings to mind depressing thoughts of being screwed if you're one of them and I think they should separate all the *Homaniakos* out of the eggs (for the time being).

405. Would you send the *Whole Earth Project* of all known data of the planet earth with them? Would you show them shopping malls and DisneyWorld and medical wonders? Would you send with them a system of laws and government or would you take your chances as with a black monolith in some old space movie? Would you tell them of an earth destroyed to make them feel lucky to be alive? Or broadcast constant signals such that information is received in-flight for later use. The best plan is to send some embryos with nothing, no data at all and then see what they come up with after 10k years of their own doings. Wouldn't you like to see that techciety from under a scientist's microscope? To see their language and their gods and the "who's in-charge" and their sense of morals? I would suppose that for the feeling of ultimate genetic optimum procreation, seeding the universe with humans for contact at a later date would make me feel better even if I couldn't be around for the first contact a million years from now. As we found out on the earth, it takes about 1.5 million years and 12 billion humans to stumble upon the idea of a space shuttle or a toaster so who knows how well this idea will work or how long it will take, but using simple plant life procreation methods as found on the earth as our guide, I believe it is the best method regardless of how lonely or depressing life on distant planets would be on a one way trip from love.

Big is meaningless

406. You might have thought this to be the ultimate science chapter consisting of data and facts of measurements and knowledge documented as to the state of our universe and its size and relationship to time and where is the end of it by yardstick standards? I can say all that we know about the universe right in this paragraph because physical volume doesn't equal verbiage length (a cubic function verses a linear distance). The universe is bigger than you can know and always at ambient temperature wherever you are at. The age is not known but it is at least as old as it has to be for us to see it and as old as it knows itself to be, but it doesn't care. We cannot say if the universe is alive because we are too small and our lives too short. I expect that mankind and

womantype will cease to exist someday and not a one of them will know anymore about it than we have ever known, or will know beyond the knowledge of this book. With no metaphors or parallel thoughts about it for you to draw perceptual relationships in 2D or 3D, I won't waste your time with guessing the unknown.

407. What I will say is that if you want to feel the hopelessness of reaching across the infinite of it to find the love of a dead friend or dead child or to experience pure loneliness or to die mentally in the void of total isolation, then have one manic-depressive thought about it - I dare you. What mathicalticeans will tell you is that an equation is required because numbers have been discovered and thus all must be tallied, such that zero divided by infinity is a problem for the classroom - thus if it can be written then it must be solved. But emptiness divided by forever is actually a thought, and that thought strips you of the delusions of love and happiness and the thoughts of a better day only to reveal that we can't ever prove what lies beyond death but it calls my species there as a place of calm and rest - and it is inviting me to go there also. Suicide becomes logical and necessary and the universe beckons us to join its coldness and the forever existence of it - because love can't last forever but loneliness can.

408. You have now survived CHAPTER THE UNVERSE OF THE REAL, please turn the page and proceed to CHAPTER GODD. Do not mark in your book and please visit, at your convenience, our reference pages at the rear of the book.

CHAPTER
GODD

"If there were a god, and he walked the earth on occasion with mankind and womantype, would there be no crime, no treachery, no crying manic-depressive's?" R. J. Hanink

The music that set the mood for writing this chapter was:
"Issues" CD by Korn.

If there were a god

409. Infinity allowable epitaphs! This being a difficult chapter for me to scribble down, being down and out at this time, all for the sake of pleasing you my fine literary and by now confused or at least still slightly curious friend. You stuck with it this far, and the checkered flag is to drop dead on you soon, as the end of knowledge draws near. Not to disappoint you though, but I'm afraid I might be tricking you in a soon to be revealed fashion because what I write now, although better stated – what you read now, are sentences that are being added [*have been added*] after this chapter is almost complete. That in its self is interesting only in the fact that the sequence of this book, or most any book, follows the protocol of reading. I know that you have been challenged to turn your logic, or lack there of, off and on and maybe a little skewed, as in a rhombus of a two-dimensional sectional deflectional, but you as the reader expect data to be presented in a manner or sequence that will not require the slightest of deciphering. Now that we are together at the end of knowledge, as in the flicks this book has not been written in any sequence, and I rather surmise that not many books are [*End of sentence?*]. All chapters are being written at once so to speak. Ideas are pulled back and forth into various sequences within the chapters - chaos in thoughts arranged to produce logic[*?*] in interpretation. You see and understand only what is shown to you and you can't figure out the method of the creation of this book unless I reveal it to you. I also suspect most of you have never heard my voice unless you are as I, and have thus shared our common vision in private. Yet you would believe in me, that I exist, that I have had these thoughts, and that I mean what I write or wrote or is it to be yet written? Should I stop right here and leave you with that metaphor? Is that not how you believe in your gods? Enough said, any ordinary person would concretely concisely conclude with minimum clanging, but I being me, am compelled to convince you with fifteen thousand words or more, how then do we understand Godd's creation of physical matter, biological life, the comprehension of one's self, and the existence of time? (Now although I will use the familiar names for Godd and Jesus, do you believe for one moment that they would answer to those nouns? Godd is YHWH or better still, Yahweh. Yes, who would have guessed what's in a name? "God" is a pagan name (and probably an insult), if I did my research correctly. As for Jesus, who would have come up with such a word, certainly not his mom or dad. Try Yahshua or Yah-oshuah when you speak to your savior, and perhaps this is why he hasn't heard your prayers. But to avoid any distractions I'll stick with the words you're familiar with.)

410. Books contain thoughts and nothing in the slightest twist of our limited comprehension is there [*Suggestions: "they're"*] anything more than a thought written wrote. These thoughts are not reality, but only thoughts and these are not much of thoughts

in the way of thoughts ether. If we could be imþrisoned for our thoughts your narrator would be imþrisoned by now for certain with a fate no better than a. laþ dog reciting Shakesþeare. Thoughts do not contain a time attribute. That is, they may be re-thought, re-arranged, or occur at any moment even without you wishing them to do so. The truth of the matter, you can't stoþ "thoughting" even if you try. Maybe I have already aþþeared to you to write about thoughts earlier in this book, but at this moment in time (which is to say that moment at which I actually did write these words which is now þast for me but þresent for you), I have not.

411. The history of events reþresents a reality. The only true reality is history, for you can't change it and keeþ your soul at the same time. This book may not have been everyone's reality, mine for certain, but it's a reality nonetheless. When someone is shot dead, whether they wanted it, deserved it, or just þlain needed it, they suddenly are not shot dead again. Unless of course you are in the flicks or watching an analog interþretation of the same story [Fragment sentence again]. The visual media is the same as a book, which is the same as a thought or what was or has been thunk. This is because biological realities have a time attribute or rather what humans þerceive as time; the distance between two events when nothing is moving. You may have continued thoughts of the þerson that was shot dead, but they remain dead in biological terms nonetheless and not all the better for wear and tear I might add. Thus events in reality do not backuþ or undo themselves as much as you might want "Oh if I had only (fill in this blank with your own nightmare)". There is a sequence that biological life þerceives as the þassage of time. This is not yet þroven true for all þhysical realities, but for

biological reality it appears true at this monumental moment 8:34 p.m. April 24, 2k yr. Thus the biological action sequence would be expected and possibly even predictable even if not in the least bit understood. I am counting on all of you to read this chapter in its sequence and with an understanding of what normal ideas I'm trying to convey in the strangest of ways. Wait a moment, wait a moment, *2001: A Space Odyssey* is queuing up on my screen, it will be completely operational for 139 minutes [*Tangentiality*]. We don't have much time so proceed to the next paragraph please.

4 1 2. If you are a Christian and a human, ordinary type or not, how do you understand Godd and mankind and womantype, logic not withstanding, withsitting, or even leaning a bit? I will write this chapter for you my fine reader friend, that you may have new thoughts to think if you are a self-proclaimed Christian or even if you were born again (and even born a third time if you became a *Homaniakos*). If there were a god would you need information about that god? A warm fuzzy feeling inside wouldn't do much for you since that could also be attributed to carnal lust, soggy French fries, or a big tax refund, and what good would that do for a god such as ours that expects total obedience to him, otherwise its hell for the nonbelievers or believer sinners? If every human did create their description of their god, because nothing was presented by that god except that previously deviously mentioned warm and fuzzy, then there would be endless ideas of what Godd was like and what he/she/it would want them to do for such a god. Gods always want you to do something but the one we're dealing with is on vacation after finishing his book, I guess. So where are we now, right here in the year of our late great lord of the millenium [*Alternate spelling: millennium*], 2 kyr? As humans, you have so

many beliefs in your god, even though there are only a couple of [Commonly confused words: "have"] inspired, transpired, translated, related, affiliated books about whatever god is yours. Being a Christian, you have a book called "The Book" or better know as The Bible. Nothing else is being presented as having information about the god of the Christians except the 66,451 man-made, man-mistranslated, iterations of what man thinks Godd without the Bible tells us to do. Nothing at all, in any of those 66,451 books is relevant to Godd and the sooner you realize with your real eyes that you've been scammed, hammed, and hung out to dry in the rain, the better you'll do in the no one wins game of "Lets create a god that I like". Those books are contrivances constructed to give you hope and make you believe you are being fulfilled in life. Maybe they promise you a key to Heaven after your miserable physical life is over with on the earth. Maybe you have a dead mom or dad, or son or daughter that you wish to know they are in some better place (than only dead). It may come as a surprise to you but I will offer you none of those thoughts in this chapter so beware of my thoughts because I offer no one any hope. Find hope in someone else's book if you must. I wish to erase your "feelings" of Godd and replace them with more useful knowledge about Godd. If you really do believe this talk of Godd is true, then you won't want to miss this chapter. We can only speculate about the spiritual world, but as for the physical world we can know certain truths. Godd created a physical world and he created at least two physical humans, of which the Christians refer to as, Adam and Eve. (Some Christians believe that Godd created some type of proto-humans, but not Adam and Eve directly.) Thus Godd most certainly created DNA, genetic protocols, provisions to survive and procreate, all within the genetics of the humans, and within all the other life of the earth also, because he said so in the book of Genesis, I guess. This is what we can think about as seen in life around us every day. This will not be such a difficult task for a hypomanic Manic-depressive Junkie Cyclothymic as myself, and I will remain that way by playing the correct music for the mood of this chapter.

413. Nowadays there are never any good "Thou shalt not" voices from the heavens that the multitudes of multitudes or rudes can hear and thus reconfirm through a valid everyone at once proof of purchase on the redemption of Godd. Believe me, that *am* (my computer telling me "*is*" is incorrect usage) all it would take for me! It is believed that sometimes Godd speaks to some humans through their minds, thoughts, or the fillings in their molars. Usually when this happens, someone is going to get shot or someone is going to make money. Actually, whenever someone gets shot, someone else makes money. What is Godd telling all these people to do these days? Did Godd only speak to humans before the assembly of the assault rifle? Would that be proof enough of a god? All the good physical stuff like the ultraviolence heaven sent approved and validated slayings happened so long ago. Oh sure for sure we get some blooding bleeding statues, silently weeping weepage on acrylic paint by number icons of saints long gone bye bye. Sometimes a ghost of Mary, Jesus' mommy, appears at a church that is filing for bankruptcy, but I will never believe any god, even an idiot god would stoop to such easily faked iconery. Godd knows humans all to well, having been the personal destroyer of by my ciphering [cyphering?] about 400k humans at his own hands or whatever pointing device he uses. Godd knows humans will bow down and then lay flowers the feet of a statue that cries or bleeds. That in its self is amazing because no statue would really have feet as though it was going to get up and walk somewhere. If our god believes, and rightfully so, that humans can be prodded around like cattle to every rust spot or spilt milk spill that is made with his image as a *Concentration Television* machine game, then he certainly can get half the humans to say "Oh my god, its Godd" while the other half thinks "Oh my god, its stupid". I honestly believe that even if Godd came down from the sky every American Sabbath or on the Sabbath and stood at each church[*ies*] alter to re-instruct us that we should "behave" if we wish to live forever after the physical death - that life on the earth would still consist of about the same amount of evil, crime, hate, gossip, etc. To that we would have those humans that would have alternative views on what Godd really wishes us to do, and even those humans that would proclaim Godd is only a space alien. Don't you agree?

414. While we're on whatever the topic is, why would the greatest infinitely powerful life-force in the infinite universe, for the eternity of infinite time, create a creature such as you on the earth, get fed up and destroy us humans once, threaten to destroy us again, and only give us about 6k collective sequential years to figure it all out, but with only one small collection of postage due books written before any worthwhile technology existed to properly document his word or his physical acts for the brief moment that he walked on the earth? The penalty phase of the trial awards infinite ultraviolence for infinite time creating a real horrorshow for us regardless of our age, gender, or acts toward mankind. "Yes Jesus loves me, yes Jesus loves me, and the Bible sells me soap", all the human-children sing.

415. Maybe Godd is expired, permanently retired from his invisible to you only world by some freak cosmological spiritual

accident caught by surprise when he shut his big eyes and he wasn't paying attention. And Godd said, "Michael it's only a scratch. And I'll be better; I'll be better Michael as soon as I am that I am". Or maybe he was hit from the backside by some non-biological non-organicized meteorite called a *rzthbr* (in Godd's natural tongue it's pronounced like "Volkswagen Fastback"), of the nether world. Maybe he fell off a planet-sized chair while reaching for a metaphysical metamorsal of a snack from a cookie jar the size of China? Maybe he got old like a zillion years old and died like you and I will do. Who could tell us if Godd is for real dead? Maybe the bible translations actually should read "I am Alpha and Omega Man, for now until I die". Maybe forever is not as long for Godd as it is for us because he doesn't reproduce, or his forever started sooner and ran out first. Why didn't he [*gender for clarity*] stand in front of everyone and say "Look you humans, you better behave before I get back or it's hell to pay"? Then someone could sketch what he looked like, and we could have a real good idea of who we are dealing with. If you solve the equation "Q + biblical urban legend = Jesus, the son of Godd", why would we expect humans to behave differently back then as opposed to now? With all of our great science and electronics and colleged [*sic*] educated humans, you would believe that phables wouldn't exist, but I hear them every week, and by very reasonable humans at that. But they are the same phables of fear, unfortunate events, mystics, and psychics that I have been going around for the last 6k years at least.

416. We actually know very little about Heaven except in biblical allegories, which is akin to explaining to a woman how a man feels when scratching his ah, you know - privates. Women think it's rude to be crude touching those nasty bits and proclaim that they

wouldn't do it even if they were a man going for the pleasure grab. In better verse for better or worse, it is impossible for humans to understand what they have never perceived via the 5 senses. Even the *Homaniakos* with our clearer vision of reality can only speculate that the void and eternity of loneliness and pain we see and feel is the true state of existence exposed when the ordinary human delusions are removed, for what can actually ever be known as "the truth"?, nothing of course [*Poor sentence structure*]. Even another realm of reality such as Heaven must have rules of existence, as does Sheol. If it has rules of existence, then it can be caused to not exist or at least be messed up somehow. Could we ever know the rules of another realm of existence while alive and of this physical realm with only contrived languages to describe it using metaphors? "No, no" I quietly shout, "Can't be so, or someone would have explained it". We would have a map, diagram, or something to show the stairway to Heaven.

The only original thought

417. Try to think of something that doesn't exist now or ever in the past. I know what you're thinking. Most of you are probably thinking of honest politicians or great tasting diet soda. Try to go beyond that. Think of a life that doesn't exist made out of a material (as in a substance) that has never existed. You can't do it. Can you make a sketch of the appearance of Godd? The absolute truth of the matter is what I've told you directly or not, that you can't have an original thought. Even the greater and more respectable humans, the *Homaniakos* species, can't have an original thought. Now it is true, if I may brag of us for us, we do have an expanded vision of reality, thus we can have more thoughts than an ordinary human. Thus compared to ordinary humans there could be an appearance of original thoughts. The *Homaniakos* do not impress each other, we are proud of our species and bothered by the predictable actions of the *Hosapiens*. Everything you imagine you are imagining is [are] a collection of existing or previously existing [*Verb confusion*] physical items or defined concepts that your consciousness re-arranges or combines or subjufuses into a new "thought" for you but actually nothing new at all. Since or even now the absolute best a human can do when confronted or behinded with the unknown is to react via a misinterpretation of expected results, you can see why we don't move forward (as a metaphor) with changes very fast (as another metaphor).

4 1 8. Now if you were the boss, the big guy in the sky, before all of this existed, when the universe was not a physical universe, how do you think of a physical divisible, devisable, dividable universe without being a physical being or without ever seeing anything physical? Godd is short on information about himself (itself) especially concerning the origins of himself. If Godd never "did it" how can he imagine the feelings for the need to "do it?" How did he imagine the self-will or the needs of the flesh (and mind) such as bisexual reproduction, asexual reproduction, the satisfaction of an orgasmic climax of two copulating humans or even a lonely night with *Debbie does someone* and hand cream? If there never was [*were*] a physical eyeball, a big toe, the blowhole of a whale, the slime of a worm, how could you think of all of that? "Can't be done!" the crowd roars and maybe so, but we are here so we must be accounted for, inventoried, sorted, and origins noted or cognition continues to the nth degree and it's suicide thoughts for me. It's the reverse thought that has us duped. We truly can't imagine Godd, so how did he imagine us? "He's greater than us", the crowd roars again and again, but only within my head. "He can do anything we can't imagine. That's why he is Godd and we're not", those voices say again. Godd is not physical or biological, and despite what you believe you know, you actually know absolutely nothing of spiritual existence except poetic rhetoric from make-believe manic want-a-be's. Of course, they are incorrect. You know of the spirit world only in metaphors of the physical world. Your world is full of beginnings and ends. You define your existence with time and dimensions. Time passes forward for you every day without faltering. At least the manic-depressive can feel through time - a depressing thought that it is. Without the Bible, your imagination would have you believe in multiplexed nether worlds with no commonality, and yet even with the Bible so many humans tell me phantastic phables of Heaven and angels and reasons for the self-worth of the humans above all other life. You have no understanding of intelligent life that is not biological, life that does not metabolize, or why invisible angels see without eyes or think without brains. Maintain the delusion, life is an illusion whether Godd created you that way or not. You could not by the greatest of human knowledge or faulty logic fill an empty thimble with an existence that had never been known or ever been shown, made out of a material that has never existed but still contains resisted properties on our periodical charted elemental descriptions of the reality of our situation.

419. However, it appears Godd did all of that when he created our physical universe and biological life. Only Godd can have an original thought - would be what my brain has wrought. But why did he have these thoughts? Why our reality?

420. It's time to move onward or forward and I have to wonder what type of thoughts or ramblings I will write concerning Godd? I guess we will find out together, but the music keeps me at my desk and the topics will appear in some type of order that will appear logical only after-the-fact (and 42 re-writes). But most religions or peoples of similar convictions have a place where thy soul *shalt* (or shallot, sheltie, chalet) go forever and ever after the body dies. There are some simple rules that must be self-evident or how can a soul get somewhere to learn them? The spirit can only move out of the body experience and into the spirit experience when the blood stops flowing, the body turns cold or perhaps it leaves out of boredom when the brain activity stops. How does the soul know this? How does the soul know where to go? In a tribal society (I've totally changed subjects but I don't know why) [*Loss of goal*] the difference between the culture and the religion may not be noticeable. This or that (as a mentally ill patient once said to me, 300 times) is the intended way of the universe. Now because advanced technology allows tribal members to live remotely (as in a great distance apart not as that little control device that men play with while watching the Television machine) from each other while still maintaining similar beliefs, you end up with a society, or lack there of, that blends its religions into a "concept dress" from a tribal matrix. That is, their major underlying dogma is expressed in terms of their commonality as for example in Christianity. Christians all believe in Godd, Jesus, and Heaven (I hope). You might be thinking that my list is too short but its not. Not all Christians believe in a skyward Heavenly home for us humans as some have told me that the re-created earth will be our forever place of spirit-human existence.

Thus humans will never see heaven, I guess. But anyhow, after those three basic beliefs the differences emerge as different as night and day even though the premise of the belief is based on the interpretation of the same Bible. So now in number 420, we get to one of my reasons for writing this chapter. I can't be convinced to believe in one faith because these faiths vary from one human to the next. Thus an error in choice could be fatal. So the rest of this chapter reveals my disturbing thoughts on the disorder of all faiths combined and how logic applied is impossible by the ordinary humans. As I continue to believe that ordinary humans have faulty logic, religion was one of the things that suffered the greatest because of this character flaw. But what is the reason for the faulty logic of the ordinary humans self-proclaimed thinking brain? What was Godd thinking when he created mankind and womantype with the human brain, as we now know it?

421. In my hay-day of religious memetic control, I did not believe that humans would live forever in Hell and that solved the whole problem because once you don't believe in something, it doesn't exist. My original interpretation of the Bible being based heavily on the fact that Godd's gift promises life forever for the righteous or his chosen humans only. Hell may burn forever, but it consumes the soul (thus the soul is destroyed), not prolonging the horrorshow for humans. Satan and his angels may exist forever in Hell, but they don't die according to our Christian translations (but I can't prove it) and we have no reason to believe they have a soul to be consumed. Therefore, you don't become an angel when you die, that's a fabrication of a human delusion to cognize the fact that many humans don't have a clue, as they imagine all types of angel attributes, re-incarnated souls, Godd's list of when

you should die, and Godd's reason for taking a human's life a few years before their time (but he wanted them in Heaven as though he couldn't wait a few more earth years). Perhaps too much Hollywood, I suppose. But then what is time or eternity to a non-physical spirit or soul? Why would it be the same as for us humans that breathe, age, and get gross looking toenails and nostril hair? Because of science, we have defined many of the physical attributes of our reality, but we have not defined any attributes of Godd's reality. There are no equations to define Heaven yet Godd prepares a place for us (you). No human can knock knock knock on Heavens door, stand at a pearly gate, or shovel it up and put it through the Sieve of Eratosthenes. Godd makes Heaven (or the new earth) attractive to human men by stating that there will be no marriage in Heaven, but even my *Four Axioms of Existence* only define physical existence and anyone that tries to define Heaven in actual metaphorless words is wrong, right?

Plain Hell

422. It would take an irregular unbiased Bible student a brief moment of his/her life to plot and cross-reference the evolution of Hell in the Bible and how in the hell can we expect any ordinary human to study history devoid of aesthetic prejudice, inclinations toward cultural memes, political correctiveness slanted, or even influenced by the common belief that each ordinary human has of self-worth translated into Omni-intelligence? Surely any ordinary human (the *Hosapiens*) attempting that mental trip would be venturing unsuccessfully into the realm of the *Homaniakos*. The Hell of the book of Revelations and the Hell of Exodus are two different places. Most of you ordinary humans have been memed a vision of Hell by poets such as Dante and thee Divine

Comedy, (repeat that out loud until you get the play on words - I worked hard on some of them). This in turn caused later soon to be Saints to interpolate and interfuse the poem and the Bible along with some Jewish historical documents into a real ultraviolence horrorshow. Hell is now a joke for lame commercials or comedies of movie plots to be viewed at the movie theaters or on Television machines. Hell is sexy because sex must be sinful because it is done in private and thus anything done in private must be sinful[?]. Who gave you, my friend, your idea and vision of hell - Godd, Dante, or Daffy Duck cartoons? Why are some varieties of sex or sex organs considered sinful? Whether sex is omni-ogulous (a scientific term for: habitual masturbators[sp?]), with a partner (something organic and living), or with multiple partners, there is always something that can be found sinful about sex, yet there is not a good sex guide, with illustrations in the Bible aside from some OT "don'ts". Thus by modern standards, the devil and sex are synonymous and that meme has spread into too many minds to be reversed, although I find those beast (devil) to woman romance thoughts so tempting as it definitely fulfills the 7th protocol of hypomanicism.

423. It would be simple to blame the Germans for the confusion of natural fears versus memed beliefs because of their history of creating nursery Rhine's, whether they rhyme or not, that scare the do-do out of human-children thus keeping the human-children from wandering into the forest and having their names changed to Stew or whatever name sounds like food, you think of it. The true nursery rhyme is more effective than the fear of Hell because it deals with a reality that we are [were] familiar with everyday as opposed to having us worry about a place, a life, a pain, and a time span that we cannot even rationalize let alone visualize properly (although for a *Homaniakos*, the panic attack will bring all of that to a reality as the clearer vision of reality). Thus the *Little Match Girl* burns her last matches in order to stay warm and then she freezes to death in an alley while no humans will help her, and her other choice is to go home to her dad who will beat her senseless for not coming home with the cold cash. As she freezes to death she has the original after-death experience as she sees her dead grandmother coming to take her to a warm and loving place. It is thus better that little human-children freeze to death than to disobey a parent and that is a lesson that a human-child of old Europe could understand and follow with or without a Hell to worry about. Modern nursery rhymes match the Christian attitude of this day and that is, feel good and have nice thoughts about yourself, while everyone else is going to Hell for certain. Be happy and everything will be OK, trust me. Yet I really believe Godd is as that old nursery rhyme, "Do as I say or go to Sheol".

424. Whether I believe in a god, Christianity, or any religion is not an important point to make in this book. Beliefs will vary for manic-depressives as with ordinary humans. We may blame Godd for the ability to see a clearer vision of reality, or we may asked to be saved (our soul to be saved) moments before pulling the trigger, although the mourners will never know that those thoughts actually had happened because there will be no physical proof, only the bullet in the head still lodged as gray lead in gray matter, but without a proper introduction having occurred. The coroner anthropologist for a day will dissect the physical and give a report in a properly contrived language, but what do you tell the remaining living family, other than although the dead human wasn't up to caliber the bullet was? For the ordinary human, if you want

your sense of infinity and your feeling of Hell, then you are welcome to our nightmare eyes bulging wide open, true senses felt, and reality actually shown to you - and in 4 seconds flat I guarantee you will be clutching your chest for air and screaming for help as the event horizon draws nearer. Having manic-depressive panic attacks will make you a believer in Hell, without a doubt. But that Hell is nothing more than the every day reality within the clearer vision of reality - delusions stripped away.

425. Yes, OK it's true that more of us *Homaniakos* might believe we talk to Godd, Jesus, or some Saint that ain't but we have good reasons what with all this excess sensory perception imbedded in our headeds. Religiosity elasticity becomes hyper-enhanced due to our ability to share a common vision of the Universum Extremus (the edge of the visible universe combined with the end of time that only the *Homaniakos* can feel as a common vision beyond death and thus we kill ourselves when spending too much time there because its infinitely lonely beyond where Godd lives, take a breath). We are not as delusional, as the *Hosapiens* would describe us. The true delusion is what the *Hosapiens* believe they see and accept as tangible. The psychologists always forget to mention the number of Jerusalem Syndrome cases a year that happen when they find a flipped out *Hosapiens* believing they themselves have become Paul, John, George, or one of the other apostles walking around in hotel bed sheets while on a Middle East pilgrimage to "get closer to their spiritual selves" [*Sentence structure error*]. They remain part of the normal species.

426. I will still stay with my belief that most ordinary humans remain delusional by the fact that they run off to church and chant in unison, "We will be grateful when we are all dead heads forever". The remaining percentiles of humans that don't believe in a god, life after death, or the music of the spheres, are not attending the church of their choice, but everyone is ignoring the most important factor; that the equation of existence, zero divided by infinity, emptiness divided by forever, begins the moment we die, and as I sit upon a cornered kitchen floor with a cutting knife properly sharpened and pointed, and pointed properly to cut into that soft squoosy belly we humans have, I can't remember the thoughts through the tears or through the pain of knowing we will all die someday. But is the pain of feeling death worst than the pain of being dead? JESUS! Where are you? Please show me one little sign of your existence through my tears and through my pain that I may carry as a thought, proof in hand or heart that I should have no more fears of staying alive. I stay alive nonetheless, proof never received and stigmata applied, but the loneliness remains and is felt too often as the fears and the tears come every day when distractions are dropped inadvertently and the humans of the house have all gone to bed. I still feel no love or need of me as my life is mostly contrived languages arguing the lack of cash purchasing power or the lack of imagined created comforts we need, but then all I need are hugs in the real sense as opposed to the memories of them. As death comes, at that moment of death, we may all know at least one more truth. When we die and know this one more truth, we will be either thankful or full of regret. That is the only knowledge that can be known after the end of knowledge and after the end of mental pain.

427. I am not going to fall prey to Blaise Pascal's wager because without true belief or faith, there is no substance. I double dare anyone to say out loud that they believe in Godd

only so they won't go to Hell. St. Thomas Aquinas, being an ordinary human, had flawed logic and was biased by a few out of mind emotional experiences but raised to superstar status and remained reasonably virgin due to limited handling by the priests (i.e., e.g.). If logic alone can prove the existence of a god, then one human, ordinary or not, would have provided the proof by now (preferably in cryptology so we could all say, "Hmmm, looks correct".), and it would pass a close shave with Ockham's Razor.

What to believe, to believe what

428. I was Catholic once myself. The Catholic memetic control is the most powerful of the accepted religions (barring all those strange little cults where you must submit your daughters as virgin virtues to the self-proclaimed horny dude). Catholics are very tribal following a natural genetically driven male dominance, plus they have physical icons that you can touch, kiss, wave at, and put flowers on during, oh I forget when. Thus it gives Saints, Jesus, Mary, and the most Holy Ghost (as a dove I believe, thus proving we can't imagine what a spirit looks like), a physical visual dimensional attentional span for those who's eyes wander during the Mass. These icons are necessary because most humans do not readily reconcile conceptual reality or non-reality. By allowing local superstitions into the regional parishes there is less cognitive dissonance when being converted. If that didn't work, they used to torture and kill you. But either way you are dead. They are all dead now whether they enjoyed it or not, aren't they?

429. Once the fear of being murdered for your spiritual beliefs were (somewhat) ended, you humans could start all kinds of religions and you humans did. Now instead of "Believe or die", its

"Take your pick", "Mix and match", "Start your own", or even better still, stay home and watch Eleanor Lovegren have flashy orgasms while Larry Crabbe escapes another episode of out of this world ultraviolence, and forget the whole damn religious thing. I don't know if having a choice is easier for manic-depressives. We mainstream ourselves into conventional religion fairly easily but the more depressed we become, the least likely we will believe in a god or act as though we believe in a god. Being psychotic helps. Why don't you end your wondering about me with the fact that my dad didn't go to church (although I was informed that a priest said some very nice things about him at his funeral), thus I am less likely to go to church. That's what the psychologists will say anyway. Well, maybe I became intellectual and thus find believing in a god so boring. Actually, I have a great distrust of what the *Hosapiens* believe because they are so delusional and have flawed logic. Churches are now candy-coated "houses of whoarship" with gambling, bingo, basketball courts, Jesus reenactments, make-believe holy days and feel good sermons followed by three harmless Bible verses squeezed in somewhere. Posters of holy days and fairy tale holidays cover the walls of the church[*ies?*] classrooms and they are starting to look the same to me. I must avert my eyes walking through the churches these days in exactly the inverse way I would when walking through the adult section of the video store.

430. Even for all of you that have [*an*] absolute resolute peaceful cognition of your faith in a god, you must always satisfy your basic genetic motivators as outlined in this book. Failure to do so will setup a natural cognitive dissonance that must be resolved via a memetic activity. This mental resolution is not an indicator of any level of intelligence, education, or the ability to reason somewhat logically. It is a signal that you have arrived at where you want your mind to be or not to be. I see no difference in throwing sticks at the sun during an eclipse or making the sign of the cross on yours truly, for who created those acts and of what effect on the physical or life "after life" do they achieve? There isn't any effect and the sooner you realize it, the sooner you will actually work toward achieving that futile goal of you humans, "peace on earth" via some vision of a common god of which somehow you have come to believe that Godd wants it that way, but that is not what Jesus proclaimed. Of course if this discourse is discouraging, depressing, dreary or dumb, maybe my contrasting thoughts on the religious meme in CHAPTER HUMAN PERCEPTIONS VERSUS TRUE REALITY will be more to your palette or palfrey if you are reading this book out of its intended sequence while on a horse.

431. It's difficult to get off of the bandwagon when everyone around you is fitting church and a god into their physical and mental schedules. It's not like the old days when you actually gave something of your life in order to believe in Godd. Of course, non-Christian's still hold their faith quite well as their lives revolve around their gods and ceremonies in such a way that they would give-up worldly events for their religious faith when the timing conflicts. Besides, every church service (or mass) that I have sneaked into, sans depression, in the past 20 years is the same typical feel good message about your truly wonderful soon to be demise and passage to heaven. Why don't all of you "off" yourselves and get on with it? If you saw what I see, you wouldn't be in such a hurry to get off the best E-ride of the known physical universe. Possibly, death is the end of existence for all of us. Can someone show me in the Bible where it is a sin to end our own lives

such that we may move immediately to our Heavenly reward? I plan on asking Jesus for-giveness for my sins - on seeking mental relief in physical ways - and that he should comfort my family after I take my life. Thus there will be no time for me to sin again before I am dead. It sounds like a plan to me!

432. Catholic dogma or catdad runs rampant throughout the Protestant churches but they (they being the Protestants) don't see it that way or believe it - oh, really? The Pope enjoys sex via touches-interruptus through Jesus with every Pope that ever lived or lied as they all touched hands in continuance thus Jesus personally anoints them all and forever will. Preachers and Priests don't really teach the Bible truths because members would leave the church quickly once they were told the truth about many of the transformed and fully established - for fun and prophets - have nothing to do with Godd but insult him - twisted holy day rituals. Using the worst metaphor I could think of, its like those prices at the various petrol stations, why are they always so close to each other even when their prices are fluctuating? Every Bible Church especially the ones that advertise "Nothing but the truth, the whole truth, soul help you Godd that's what we're about" churches have some list of rules they memed themselves in order to be more holy than the gas station next door. If they don't have a list, they ignore conflicting verses. If they don't ignore verses, they interpret them to their advantage. You can't get to the bottom of all this. Personally I went to the church that checked my oil and gave coupons because everyone is looking for a church and belief that fits his or her idea of what should be taught[ed] and preached. You find a god to fit your image of Godd when in fact I doubt very many Christians, manic or not, would really admire the Godd of the Old Testament nowadays if they really

sat down and looked at him objectively. One Godd, one Bible, will someone figure it out and send me an E-mail. Sometimes I think we all would be better off being tortured into believing the same damnation thing.

433. I have so many cognitive endogenous hypothesized apocryphal speculations about living forever in Heaven. Now you might believe that to be a strange thing for a manic-depressive to write, because it's actually nearly impossible to say and I don't have a clue as to what it means. (But those words were remaining on my "Look like an Intellect" word list, so I had to use them sooner or later.) Why not live forever and forever and forever? You must remember that the *Homaniakos* have the ability to see a clearer vision of reality. This vision, although difficult to explain except to say that it is the greatest fucking pain any human could feel (The mental pain of total loneliness for the infinite of time.), makes me worry about living and being busy for eternity. I doubt eternity because I don't want to carry my depression into an eternity of depression in Heaven or Hell. I am not very likely to believe the St. Catherine (of Genoa) account of the fixation of free will or sin at death after reading the *Treatise on Purgatory*, my god, where do humans get such tales? Remember that humans can't imagine or describe what they have never sensed - yet the fairy tales persist. Thus you can't imagine Heaven except in relation to your perceived reality. The *Homaniakos'* perceived reality is greater than that of the ordinary humans (the *Hosapiens*) and thus more accurate of existence. I don't believe we should want to live forever. Die, be dead, and be satisfied it's over forever. Once you're dead you will never realize the moment the universe ends 82 billion years hence or compresses and starts over again with new living creatures (forever unknown to us) that won't imagine your budding breasts in your 13th birthday party dress, the moment your son was born, or the time you cut your wrists extended over a blooded sink, the þain viewed but not felt as jabbing and cutting with the shattered glass is both the saviour and the metaþhor of the shattered lives soon to be left behind with the mental question of "Jesus, why?" One way acts of þhysical þassion are as warm liþs caressing the body, but it is only the warmth of the self as your blood enjoys its freedom for a brief moment in the light of the world as thought it has found Heaven. But it dies as you do not being able to live in a delusional world either. Ordinary humans are born not to know what the *Homaniakos* can verbalize as [a] wonderment, and they would die frustrated if a god weren't þresent to keeþ them in the groove via some tyþe of hyþe of life after life.

434. Look at all the questions that can be raised about the nether world for in my mind a Heaven can also be a Hell because isn't that how the earth life can be conceþtualized? What if our Godd has a god? What if Godd is there and we all get to Heaven (or are raised from the grave onto the new earth) and find out that most of the stuff is true, but that the existence of it is tied to some other non-þhysical reality that also ends? It's one more thing to worry about later. What if you sþend eternity dying and going to new heavens and hells and you accidentally get left behind forever in the void? What if we do live forever, but we are alone, cold, and in the darkness forever because Godd abandoned us out of frustration or boredom? What if we never see our human-children for an infinity of time but can think about them and how good they smell giving warm hugs, staring into their eyes and listening to them laugh? What if Hell is exactly as one infinitely long *Homaniakos* þanic attack worst than being traþþed

in a dark mine cave-in upside down on your back with your head half in water for nine days? What if Hell is like watching your human-children die while looking into their eyes? I'm going to change the subject now and go for a car ride. I'm sorry I ever wrote this paragraph as my axioms can't give me information about an unknown existence of a spiritual type, so give me 15 minutes then proceed to the next paragraph, I'll catch up to you later.

Religion within a genetic creature

435. If we could separate, sort, and congeal the citizens of the United States into tribes, as were the original slightly displaced inhabitants, by moving them into communities based entirely on each religion, we could get back to fulfilling some of our genetically driven needs. Now I don't mean to tell you to put all Baptists in one town of enormous size, but rather into regular type communities of 1k to 15k humans with unremarkable attributes. Why do this by now hopefully you have not asked out loud [*Verb confusion, what verb?*]? Genetics work against the existence of religious freedom. You may not have the religious truth, but in a tribe, everyone around you would be supporting your cognition. Isn't that what a perfect delusion is about? Isn't that what the *Hosapiens* are genetically good at? Genetically you should not allow a non-believer (sinner), a peacekeeper of a god, to date, mate, or influence by affluence your tribe or clan and that is how the Old Testament operated (See Deu 20:16-18, Deu 21:18-21, Deu 22:23-24 and similars). Thus I finally get to my second point of this chapter after all these words, the Old Testament Godd ruled with death and destruction to all opposing kingdoms, man, woman, and human-child, but not to the virgin angels (See Numbers 31:17-18 and similars). It was a regular horrorshow for

the nonbeliever as well and I can't find those OT verses where non-Jews were allowed to be converted into Jews so that they may avoid the slaughter by Godd's will [*Passive voice, no suggestions*]. Surely Godd gave every non-believer (non-Jew) of the OT a chance to be saved before taking their life? But alas it seems that Godd ruled with a genetic hand, foot, or eye for an eye. If I had lived in Jerusalemland back when the Jews were returning from a night on the town in exile in Egypt, from what I am reading, they would have killed me, my human-children, and even good old Ernie (and with my grandmother being Miriam Levy at that!). I can't pass it off as "Those were different times" or "Godd is different now" because that is not achieving an understanding of a god that supposedly has a "forward looking" plan and has things figured out.

436. If you don't have the budget to purchase all of my genetic motivator ideas, then killing is only hate but actually natural, even if it is for an insurance policy of clan or tribal survival. Obviously Godd hates incorrect thoughts; actions not withstanding or even required, before he would kill you. But the humans I speak to believe Godd is righteous when he kills because he is pure goodness. Yes, Godd can kill you for your own good from what I've read, but I am not asking for any of those favors. But I will remain with the thoughts that it is Godd's natural ability to hate, otherwise he would have had to learn to hate but from whom? Thus Godd is not pure love but rather as complex as the *Hosapiens* are and perhaps as nearly as complex as a *Homaniakos*. If our almighty can understand the difference between left and right shoulders (think of a visual metaphor), it is because he has the ability to express himself in ways "we" [*Ignore quotation marks*] would interpret as evil or good. Our interpretation of his well-documented actions is everything because we base our salvation on it. Thus if Godd is too complex a creature to be understood (Axiom #2 would fit here fine) or have his wishes, dirty dishes, and day dream universes of perfectly obedient Foot (another movie metaphor find it yourself) soldiers figure him out and thus have us end up in Futureland without our fast-food injected rejected tissues, he is worthless as gods go. Why do so many humans, having gone through tragedies of human proportion, start stating statements of "I was saved, over all others, such that I must have a purpose that Godd will reveal to me at a later date" or "The reason my human-child died is so that I may bring comfort to others in the same situation". Is that what you would believe is my purpose as a verbalized, vocal, self-published Manic-Depressive Junkie? Then let me make myself clear again, I offer no one any hope, you must find hope somewhere else. Self-purpose clashes with the first protocol of hypomanicism, because I don't perceive that they are the same. One is a thought of purpose via faulty logic (the *Hosapiens*); the other is a genetic feeling of a supreme self (the *Homaniakos*). I prefer to allow manic-depressive protocols to rule me, in place of the ordinary human's memes of self-worth.

Ramblings part I

437. The Older Testament was written to fulfill the natural unchecked by the sociopathetic politically enhanced genetics of yes the human species or race if you insist. If Jesus didn't stop by to use our restrooms we would have one hell of a hi-tech ultraviolence horrorshow of religious wars with Dukem and Nukem at the push of the holier than thou button. Jesus left us not with so much a change in our salvageable salvation, but rather with a

"knock it off" instruction (i.e. meme) prior to the construction of semi-automatic assault rifles. Well, there you have it. The Newer Testament is the example of memetic control of an entire species in the worst of oh-my-god ways. Love and make love to your enemies, don't kill them. But again, memes are not as strong as genes; thus we do make love and follow it with murder in the most creative of ways [e]insuring þeace on the earth is ruined. Þeace on the earth is liþ service to a þoorly organized meme that fights the strongest of genetic traits; þrocreate and kill that which is different (kill that which is considered a threat to your life or to the continuance of your genes).

438. "I þray for world þeace", said the bathing suit beauty contestant. With her imþlanted, duct taþed breasts. Liþo-sucked thighs, þainted on eyes. Teeth by Ultra Brite, tongue holstered at her side, ready to recite memorized mesmor-lies. Words for cash selling out your god with every breath of "give me, give me" money, no credit þlease. With all the foolish self-serving rhetoric clogging the airways, byways, and sideways, who[m] do you trust? If I were to base the value of a god on the unity of his believers, Christianity would not make the cut. Fortunately, I trust no *Hosaþiens*. If there were a god [*Fragment thought*].

439. We now observe the failure of Christ's efforts for trying to imþlant the memetic control of 6 billion humans into suþþressing a strong genetic "living" engine created at the hands of his dad, the Godd, that works toward the survival of so many individual tribes and clans. You might be inclined to say humans have failed, but as Godd is the coach, the failure of the team is often a þroduct of the coaching. We've had 2k years to imþlant the meme of forgiveness but nothing has gotten better at all. I do not see it

occurring anywhere, but I try to exhibit kindness toward all passive humans (and I mean no harm by my strange hypomanic humor). Here's an example using the graded school (as schools were originally named) lie of religious freedom in this (stand up) the United States of America (sit down). Early in this country's history, anyone that did not believe in your religion was run-off or killed. The Indians were the first to go because they did not believe in the correct god. A Christian Indian was tolerable but of the wrong race ("race" for clarity). Genetics win. The Mormons had the time of their life (style) trying to live in this country of pseudo religious freedom. The good Christians of my home state of Illinois exercised their tribal genetic behaviors, via herd actions, by executing Joseph and Hiram Smith in the name of Christianity during the mid 1800's. Genetics win again, the Jesus meme worked in reverse when combined with Old Testament genetics. I can't believe the ordinary humans don't rationalize these past actions against their own contemporary teachings? Jesus' meme of love and forgiveness is carried on Godd's physical genes of tribal survival. What a bad plan.

440. So summarizing (one fifth of the way through this chapter) here we are with the Old Testament being written to allow genetics to rule with your eye for mine, and the New Testament being written to control our genetics with some big time memes if you will forgive me. Godd = genes, Jesus = memes. You might even wonder if Jesus was a meme of Godd? But memes are rarely as powerful as genes, so humans have a difficult time of contemporary Christian religions. You may even find if you (not me) took the time to examine that the success of a culture is related to the religion as a direct function of its ability to allow

humans to act on their genetic attributes without mental dissidence.

The true nature of Godd?

441. The true nature of Jesus is not the true nature of Godd, thank god. There is actually no Christian god because the Jewish Godd was in control before Christ became Christ, as we now know him. Therefore Godd cannot be a Christian. Does Godd worship Jesus, or Jesus worship himself? No. It would only then be proper to say "The god of the Christian's". But that being a lying lie also, it is actually only logically correct to say "The god the Christians chose". Godd's chosen people are still the Jews and always will be. The Christians act as though they are a part of Godd's plan within the Old Testament as they quote "hand picked verses" to suit any occasion and imagine that Godd is speaking of them; but there is no plain for conversion of the non-believer to become Jewish or Christian or any action for that event to occur in the OT, and early gentile Christians did not follow the laws of Moses, but now they act as though the OT was written for them. As my anger increases, I won't hold back, so please indulge me as I shout, "My god, don't you see that fact!?" Godd of the Old Testament is a genocidal maniac that worked at all times to keep his chosen people (the Jews) clean from outside influences (This includes requiring the killing of humans by his command, that later would have become the past relatives of future Christian families). Godd did this mostly by death and destruction of Biblical proportions. Oh the excuses I have been privileged to hear as to why Godd would command the killing of little boys, but give the virgin little girls to the Jewish conquerors. So I was going to put Num 31: 17, 18 right here followed by Mat 18: 5 right here, to show all of you why I have these impressions of

Godd, but I decided not to because everyone tells me that I am misunderstanding the intentions. (I will be accused of taking verses out of context, like everyone else I guess.). I don't see where Godd did much for us gentiles, although Jesus' gentile followers made some comments about it. Everything seemed to be changed after Jesus left the earth and humans took charge during the process of gentile-lizing the Jewish traditions. I don't believe Jesus eliminated the Jewish religious traditions. The Christian religion most likely was an attempt to de-Jewishize Jesus. Don't you believe so? (As a Christian, I would feel better keeping the Sabbath and the other Mosaic laws as Jesus did, but how would I every straighten my life out at this point, being such a Manic-depressive Junkie?) Despite the death and destruction, I see the OT as revealing the alteration of mankind and womantype at the hands of the creator of the same thus it is very important for us to understand Godd if you believe that Godd created mankind and womantype (his chosen one's or not), and Godd's creation of the human animal is what remains of our physical selves. How do we then understand our abilities and ourselves, and our thoughts versus our actions? What were Godd's intentions?

Be fruitful and increase in number

442. I never want to argue whether a god exists or not. I have not decided about Godd and I am sorry that I appear to waffle a bit, but as I write this book I am going in and out of various normal *Homaniakos* moods. Someone told me that there was a lot of anger put into this book, so I tried to edit some of it out, but I am afraid this chapter still comes across a little strong, I suppose. I expect that the last momentary mental thought upon my exasperated expiration will be of my optimum procreation

creations and that I would wish to live forever embracing them and feeding off the living warmth of my own contribution to the continuation of life. Thus the concern of suicide being too fast or too slow, as thoughts of "Is this a mistake?" can occur at any moment during the event as true logic is applied via a total vision of reality combined with the mental þain of knowing the truth. I believe in my book and thus for all [of] you lost *Homaniakos* comrades out there, genetics should rule you and when they do you'll want to stay alive because continuance is the number one rule, Godd or not. Besides, as we *Homaniakos* cycle through our normal moods, we will change our belief in a god but our feeling of continuance is genetic and should always be strong, you must keeþ it that way. Þerhaþs that is a key to understanding whether there is a god gene within our bodies, but I don't see the relationshiþ at this moment. What I do want to þoint out in this moment of *Homaniakos* calm as I now feel a þleasurable satisfaction coming over me, most of the humans do not sþend enough time getting to know "The god the Christians chose". Its so easy and lazy for them to only read a couþle of verses from their "haþþy verse-a-day" book and think about their delusional life after death wish. I see so many humans are waiting for their miserable marriages, unfortunate þhysical deformities, imþoverished lot in life, or þlain bored out their wits to be over and everything will be "haþþy haþþy, oh so haþþy" forever and forever and forever and ever in Heaven. But why should ordinary humans dwell so much on believing that an afterlife will be better when in fact I see that so many of them could actually bring more satisfaction into their life right now, if they would stoþ and think about what their body and minds are telling them they miss or need? Ordinary humans are so cruel to each other as they always seem to be among strangers what with all this traveling too and fro, but I try to be kind as often as possible, in order to teach them a better way.

Resistance to Change

443. When Bible stories start to get a little strange from what is known or taught, humans really don't want to believe them or even hear of them. They will believe in Godd, Jesus, and angels that keep them from harm (never really works) but to add to that knowledge - even with stories not really any stranger at all - and they are not likely to believe them. When I tell other humans about what I've read in the Bible, they stare at me as though why would I want to know such things? Even showing them the text doesn't cause them to dwell on the new thoughts presented. Sometimes they ask me what translation I am using? We all are inured to our beliefs and only astute changes can be made, and then at the expense of great time. Most humans believe in the god of their parents. Not that they continue at the same exact faith, but they rarely accept an extreme belief out of the clear blue. Thus humans believe in their "concept of god" based on "god attributes" most likely from their regional cultural influences. An example of this behavior is as when the media or lobbying groups create an idealized whale or dolphin filled with every best attribute from all species of whales or dolphins. This would be a concept dress of a whale or dolphin. They will even leave out unfavorable whale or dolphin traits that would go against their successful removal of your money during fund raising times. They expect, and are almost always correct, that you actually don't know much about of truth about whales or dolphins and you really won't spend the time to check. Don't you believe that your churches and sermonizers do the same with Godd and Jesus? When a religious agenda is

advanced, whether Godd exists or not becomes moot. Do you really trust those humans that control your religious beliefs with smiles, while extending their arms toward Heaven and their hands toward your purse?

Ramblings part II

444. So is there an agonizing agenda to this chapter? I guess in retrospect, I have created 119 paragraphs of miscellaneous ramblings, but isn't Godd such a complex subject to deserve so much ramblings? Well, my vision and rational of my perceptions is what I am revealing to you whether you believe I am a religious idiot, born of the devil, or mentally ill. I have never claimed that any of the Homaniakos have a spiritual vision or even a vision 20 minutes into the future. I absolutely do not believe in any psychics or ghosts or speaking to the dead, and you should put all that trash aside for your own good. How will you get to any of the truth to reality when you believe in so many fairy tales made from schyster[sp?] humans, with cold cash always coming into being a necessitous to be mailed in or Foned via credit card? How can I get you to believe in the actually very real Homaniakos humans with only our simple clearer vision of reality and slightly enhanced normal senses? But as far back as Plato, even 300 years before metaphysics was given a name, the soul and the spirit of mankind and womantype has been analyzed and logictized in that never ending (until now) search for the truth to reality and neo-reality. But I really think that the 100 or so famous philosophers (that are famous via written history) have put way to much thought into it. Nature is simple, the universe is even simpler, but the truth to Godd's existence is not to be found by scientific examination of anything physical, shrouds or nails or veiled women apparitions

included.   Read Godd's book(s), and try to avoid being delusional is the best any human could hope for. I guess I may not be seen as a worthy Christian by the *Hosapiens* standards, because I find this Christian religion of theirs to be very abnormal due to its Jewish origins, corrupt transformation, and ultimate adoption by a dysfunctional techciety, but there is more that needs to be understood than the general feel-good information being dissimulated for the last 200 earth years. Christianity is totally pell-mell by this late stage and its age is showing. How many evolutions and revivals and revisions can it survive? Church activities are always culturally biased and then biased according to the standards and lifestyles of the community. How much of a theology graduate do I need to be, before you will say I have knowledge of my thoughts in this chapter translated into a contrived language written?   For credentials into mystical knowledge, I give to you the fact that I am not of the dominating species of ordinary humans, I am a *Homaniakos*. I will take Godd on, face to face with no fear at all, because I am most serious about the understanding of the finality of physical life, since a mistake now will last an eternity. I do believe that when a human-child becomes of age, they had better question the authority and measure of fairness dealt to them as a human-child and with that I am told that Godd is my father. Everyone dies. Does everyone have a chance to be resurrected? Is my god treating me fairly? Why must I assume that Godd is as fair and just as the lips of ordinary humans would scream but without them being able to offer any proof, and contrary words found in the Bible at that!?

445. St. Thomas Aquinas would have us believe in the great and almighty purest of pure oh it hurts your eyes to look at and stresses our minds to think about thinking about how absolutely

perfect and just your god is, was, and forever will be. If Godd sends you and your human-children to Hell for the ultraviolence horrorshow then obviously you all deserve your infinite pain for infinite time, even if it is only for thinking, "I don't believe" because someone has never properly presented Godd's plan to you. But then any species that uses a technology so that they may kill their human-babies without having to personally do it or see the pieces of cut flesh themselves would have no trouble believing that a god would send those discarded human-babies to hell for being unwanted bastards born of lustful and sinful fucking. Friedrich Nietzsche would argue (in a presentable fashion) that something has come over man recently. Christianity works against genetics. Hmmm, maybe I should stop while I'm ahead and give a blind man an elbow. Genetics are evil, I am told, but a hell of a lot of fun and how would you survive as a species without them? Bertrand Russell I find quite fascinating, but he needs more Web sites. He certainly is a shoe-in for a stand-in in Poltergeist II; I can hear the hissing now.

446. For every miracle baby born, pulled from a carnage car catastrophe of carnal destruction, or as the sole surviving soul of a plane crash, physical and mental scars applied, there are thousands that die and leave the empty arms of mothers to gather dust for the want of that one last hug in the middle of the daily nightmares of schoolyard visions. How do the ordinary humans survive each day with their dead children on their minds crowded with thoughts of "Godd's plan" while on bended knees, and every physical artifact collected as in a museum for personal pain; as dead children play with no toys found on the earth or in a mother's clammy hands in the silence of lost thoughts. Does technology help them as they view pictures and videotapes with sound tracks

of happier days past? Are they genetically fooled into believing that their procreation exists because sight and sound are all that genes need? I never want to know because as a Manic-depressive Junkie the thoughts and feelings are real as real can be, and I have already attended a million fucking funerals too many - of which I can't tell you if they were real or not. Jesus why do you do this to them, to me? Jesus, I have given up on defining your logic because the physical and spiritual of it don't mix. There are no spiritual clues sitting around to be found or dug up, we only have words in a contrived language combined with heart pains or mind pains if thoughts are thought for too long. For every physical act attributed to you there are millions that you wouldn't want credit for and neither would the adversary, the devil, because mankind and womantype are lessor than the angels, the devil included.

447. Where is Godd?, I still believed he exists but his ways are cruel, not strange. Tell it to the sky as your prayers fall upon a being waxed but without ears. It is so easy for healthy and comfortable humans to dismiss the pains and sorrows of the poor, the sick, and the lonely as a part of life and Godd's plan for them (the poor), but not themselves. Tell me, *Hosapiens*, what is Godd's purpose or plan for me? Why would the creation of me be a part of Godd's plan or any plan? Can't he create angel groupies as he sees fit to kiss his angelical mystical omni powerful butt? Why would a creature create a creature that he might then have to punish for an eternity if that created creature misunderstands the confusing signals? He is not playing fair. Human-children don't always obey their human parents, even with punishment at hand and previously felt. Our god is in hiding and his presence is only expressed via the contrived words of delusional ordinary humans. Where are all the manic-depressive prophets of the OT?

Someone that I can trust [*Fragment (no suggestions)*]? Does he love me before I was created? Then why is it easier for me to end up in Hell for an infinite time of infinite pain than to end up in Heaven with my father [*as in "Godd", too many phrases my computer states*]? Why do I get only a few of the earth obitals to figure it out? We don't know our own expiration date, do not purchase after, do not use after, do not plan a vacation or day with the kids because you're going to end up blown up in a minivan and burnt like a potato chip caught in the strainer for six cookings, without the slightest hint its coming. "Behold, I come as a thief in the night to slash your throat and rape your women", Jesus said. "The truth of life lived has been spoken", I say, because Godd created all, and Jesus sees every action of every human, but never puts his hand down to stop the evil of human against human. When are your prayers answered? When a random occurrence falls your way? How sincere everyone prays moments before the phone rings in the middle of the night, or when the doctor looks them in their eyes and states, "I'm sorry", or when that mechanical device they are riding in starts to rumble strangely or shake out of control. Prayers are never answered by proof, except when you survive and can assign contrived verbs as to how Godd has helped only the very special "you".

448. How can Godd deny the pleasures of the flesh to the creatures he purposely gave them too? Why do I have to see the angels that walk the earth and admire their perfection? Whereas mankind of the Christian type has in history explored and conquered many lands and then raped the woman and little girls with the appearance as though they were items to use and discard, but its more likely mankind was only succumbing to opportunities of optimum procreation with no one looking or with no laws in place

to be broken. History is full of it and how could all of mankind be taught the same lessons unless it was a natural gene from Godd? Where do you draw your moral lines? Is your list of items A and items B divided by what Godd tells you to do and what the devil tells you to do? I rather believe all is from Godd, the creator, because the devil created nothing, and as the imperfections of the creation were revealed a revision of actions was issued. Unfortunately technology was not accounted for in the final issue of the Bible and thus now mankind and womantype create issues of the physical open to biblical interpretation. Modern humans have the nerve to say we are enlightened and so sophisticated as they create gay marriages with bibles in hand and female preachers (priests) and churches of every belief with fake holidays all the while they call a period in history 1k years ago as the Dark Ages. Within all of that human stew, you beg of me to give up my amoral life and become ordinary – that I should ride the soul train with you.

449. It is completely within the realm of my beliefs to accept that the *Homaniakos* can actually see a part of the hidden universe that only Godd and his angels are privileged to know. This is something that maybe Godd did not plan on happening, he seems weak in the "I didn't anticipate humans would do that" department as he was always getting so upset at the actions of his select few. The *Homaniakos'* vision creates a different will to know Godd than that of the *Hosapiens*. How does Godd account for this? (Godd must be accountable for his actions via a set of rules of supreme and ultimate justice and mercy or how would we know his behavior is fair?) He seems to have left the *Homaniakos* vision out of his best seller unless all the prophets were manic-depressives and they actually left the ordinary humans

out of the rewards of the Bible. But time passes quickly and its time we gather with the tour group now entering the Garden of Eden.

Life in the Garden of Eden

450. It is time clarify a point about our Biblical human ancestors: Adam and Eve. It matters not whether you believe in the absolute existence of the two characters named Adam and Eve as the prototype humans version 1.0 or if you believe the story represents the nature of the method by which Godd created and genetically endowed early mankind and womantype as the species of proto-humans on the earth. Adam and Eve of course, are the perfect alibi to human's evil nature and nature itself being evil toward mankind and womantype. Not all Christian religions see it that way though, as Eve becomes the hero for making the correct choice when biting the apple or how else would we be able to perform sinful procreation via Godd's command? If you will indulge me, at least the stories of the OT reveal a progression without actual progress being transpired, as the humans become cultured (or meme infested) and thus loose their ability to act on their genetic drives without feeling sinful. The rules set forth by Godd as shown documented by the inspired hand movements of mankind with a pen and paper, illustrate by truth or by example our fairy tale metaphor: How Godd changed our genetics and our memes. I am not easily amazed but I am amazed at how many contemporary humans do not believe in Adam and Eve or the progression of the early-created mankind and womantype and Godd's alteration of them through history. What is their basis for their beliefs if we all can deduce (via faulty logic) images of Godd and his creation according to our liking? Why have any religion if that is the case? Now as the Bible stories fall into disbelief so is

Godd fading from existence but in the human mind only. Nietzsche will be proved to remain correct. You could say that soon mankind will no longer believe in or need a "real" god because I see so many humans creating their own beliefs to replace the Bible facts that they don't agree with (thus they do create their own god). But as some humans find out, believing a gun is unloaded leads to many surprises. Your belief may make it real in your mind, but that is as far as that thought goes, and I speak from experience.

451. Maybe there is no evil, only the human's[s'] inadequate or varying interpretation of the purpose of nature as technology removes nature from sight and sound. After all, if you have grasped my axioms and most basic motivators of life, you will see that all any living creature does is procreate and eat other living creatures (except for a few creatures that can digest non-life substances); the rest is gravy for the goose. Did not Godd create procreating life on the earth with explicit instructions to do so via *The Genesis Protocol*? He did not state: "Keep your hands off each other". Now so that I may substantiate my theories on the "Genetic Behavioral Motivators", let [*Suggestion: lets*] it be know that by Godd's own words, his creations had a purpose. He created all life with the first and primary function of procreation via his own command. See Genesis 1:9-31 for yourself so that I won't be accused of a misquote. Now you know why I stressed this procreation point so heavily in the earlier chapters that I will write later.

452. Novocaine, X-rays, gene therapy, transplants, and now cloning are changing our concepts of pain, suffering, and mental distress. All of those and others that I don't care to mention are

removing our actual dependency on Godd (because [Godd] dependency seems to be more common during distress that can't be handled via human intervention), but in the end we all must die thus the survivors get to say, "They are better off dead" or "It is Godd's plan". Oh, now I get it (light bulb over my head). Godd's plan is that we must die without proof of knowing, only hoping, that out of the dark and cold grave (always expressed as a genetic least favorable condition for the continuance of life) there is light and warmth (always expressed as a genetic most favorable condition for the continuance of life). Now getting back to what motivates you to believe in Godd, think of your beliefs of Godd while you are giving your human-children their vaccinations. Now think of half your human-children already dead by age 5 because of diseases you no longer know [knew?] ever existed. Which one of those thoughts would need a stronger belief in Godd? Which one of those still needs a god? Where as you might once have prayed so your human-children survive into adulthood, later in history you prayed that the medicine worked, and now you pray that you can afford to buy the medicine. Where does the Godd transference stop?

453. Prior to mankind's and womantype's first and foremost disobedience, the natural world was a peaceable kingdom: Food, nice weather, friendly animals, and everything lives forever or at least comfortable until some type of natural end. As you had sex, Godd watched as though you were two farm animals being rutted for profit. I might add that some Christians believe that sex was never intended to be had [Passive voice (no suggestions)] in the Garden because it was sinful (by Godd's design) and Adam and Eve had not known sin yet (they were naked and unmarried by Godd's first plan, yet read Genesis 1:20-31 because everything

else was "doing it"). I find it very difficult to believe that in *the entire* [*or optional "all of the"*] universe, that some garden view location on the planet called the earth is the ultimate hangout for the god of the universe. I mean, what are the chances? If the best Godd could do is nice weather, a garden, and an occasional visit from him, then I would have to wonder about this god because look at all the cool stuff that humans have come up with and we are not gods by any measure.

454. Godd did not plan on his proto-humans on the earth to live forever on the earth or in Heaven (unless I'm missing something) as he cautioned against it via the "Don't eat the fruit of life" instructions after they had gained the knowledge of good and evil (Although I hear some humans stating that we were to live forever in the flesh in Eden if only Adam and Eve had eaten of the tree of life, first.). It wasn't until later that Godd became vain enough to demand we give him more credit for what he hath wrought to or for us. In reward for our praise of him creating this physical universe for us, we would get to see him in Heaven (or on the new earth) forever after our physical death. At any rate, the Bible is not clear on what would become of the first humans if humans had not disobeyed Godd, so perhaps there is additional information in some other early Jewish documents or translations. I need more data, please help me!

455. The problem that I have is that every time I find an article with an interesting introspective title such as or exactly as, *Terrestrial Monotheism of Sumerian Essentially Ordered Polygons*, it ends up with a self-authorship revealing a exponential of "Godd being the perfection of goodness" and the whole article becomes liar biased (because the author started the article with

the intention of ending up where s/he planned to end) (As a note, I did not plan my endings as is evident by the fact that my chapters ramble aimlessly.). How can we remove the transference of what we believe now, when we apply it to the history of obvious opposing viewpoints? The human's logic is a function of the human's perception of reality and our contemporary logic would have been unknown to rationalize 4k years ago (due to less scientific discoveries of the universe, atoms, DNA, etc.) thus how can we know the human's thoughts from that long ago except to say what I am telling you, and that is that all genetic motivators for the humans would have to be constant throughout time, logic not withstanding. Thus my four axioms remain true then, now, and in the future as well as my stated "Genetic Behavioral Motivators" and "Genetic Dispositions". There must be a constant for the human animal, for how can all of those be changed by the will of humans?

456. As has already been proven by the events that have been known or believed to have taken place in the recorded history of mankind and womantype concerning discoveries, would the same discoveries have occurred if mankind and womantype never left the embryonic conditions of the Garden of Eden? Getting more or less to the point in an indirect as possible manner (After all, this is a book about a Manic-depressive Junkie's metaphysics), would any offspring of Adam and Eve question why for their world, inertia, friction, and conservation of energy would not always work? Why some animals have canine teeth but eat grass or smoke it? Would we have scientists or mathematicians if Adam and Eve had never sinned? Why would we? Having inquisitive scientists in Eden they would question everything Godd created or did.

457. The big questions of which I know the answers but will hold you suspended like a bridge over troubled water is, "Did Godd create a genetic trait in the original humans that would prevent those humans from questioning the lack of logic in their first intended unnatural natural environment of Eden or the proto-earth?" Would all ordinary humans remain delusional as to what was truly occurring around them with Godd controlling the natural systems to keep the delusion going forever? If it were truly a genetic to be born with trait, then this would explain why the *Hosapiens* are still so delusional. This is the basis for my understanding as to why the ordinary humans are delusional about reality. It was Godd's intention. I rest my case. Point presented, never proven, but I am not out of words, metaphors, or metaphysical slang and you should not exit the ride until it has come to a complete stop.

458. I digress to restate my previous statement but not in exact words, maybe *Homaniakos* (manic-depressives) see what was not to be revealed to humans in general by Foot. Would there be a Sir Isaac Newton or cousin Walton in Edenland that would proclaim there is gravity but not the entire physical realm is affected by it? Would there be a cult dissenter that would question why inertia, gravity, friction, and Brownian movements do not work predictably? No metamagical themas of mathematics would ever be able to follow documented rules. Without rules, no human would accept mathematics and it (with "it" being mathematics) would remain a curiosity that sometimes matched dissimilitude perceivable events and other times did not. Mathematics would never amount to more than a magician's trick

for human-children (provided Godd allowed magicians to live, after all they are liars and deceivers by trade).

459. Would this be the forever proof of a god because nature (as in events that occur as perceived self-actuators) did not follow rules therefore something other than nature is in control? Is this not the same reason that humans can create a god because they misinterpret natural events or even contrived events or even humans pretending to be psychics? Only because even now most humans understand very little about anything. The opposite of that statement is alive to-day - oh really? The fact or premise that nature follows rules is what intellectuals' use as proof there is no god or any need of a god but then again, that is perchance only a perception or Godd's actual plan. Besides, any rules beyond my Four Axioms are subject to interpretations of validity.

More Free Will

460. Is not everything Godd's creation? I might believe so and maybe so, but then I am prematurely interjecting that Godd is constantly proving his actual unworthiness to the title of supreme Pooh-Bah by creating angels that sin and humans that don't have a chance by their own genetic nature and penis erectile behavior with optimum procreation given too strong of an enzyme. I will not blame the adversary (the true measure of the devil) for mankind and womantype's troubles. Who of you have actually seen the real Lucifer standing face to your face, when in fact your phabled sins are never committed beyond your arms reach or your tongues wiggling, and are always of your own doing. Although sometimes I feel that I have the power of the devil as I present humans with choices of right or wrong (with "wrong" slanted heavily toward

genetic protocols), they have almost always chosen to do wrong. No one outside of me forces me to choose sinning, that's for certain.

461. Now I am compelled to include my friend and editor Jack who has an analogy [*Sentence structure error*] that at this time became logical to place right here in this book. Especially with the coincidence of time being 3:47 p.m. Eastern Time at this moment. If nature does not rationalize good and evil, thus free will, are humans only over reacting to whatever? Do the emotions of love and remorse keep us from seeing that we actually don't have free will and are only behaving genetically? Is free will only a poorly defined genetic action of explaining the necessitous of living including the complexity of altruism explained by contrived verbiage? By virtue (lost or not) of living in our unnatural environment with our unnatural societies have we renamed our natural attributes "evil" because they don't fit the examples of documented laws when confined within structures built of pine 2 x 4's? Can we toss the image of Godd out yet?

462. If you wish to argue free will and obedience to Godd by choice and his by-laws, revisions, amendments, and the release of DNA version 1.0, then how is it in the *Hosapiens Handbook of the Corrected World*, the description of the *Homaniakos* species as in "manic-depression is a mental illness", they take away my free will by providing me with the seven protocols more or less of manicism as found in my handbook CHAPTER MANIC-DEPRESSION? [Empty space] According to psychologist's, the *Homaniakos* have no free will because we must follow most or all of these aforementioned protocols with no mental control over them unless we are drugged into the ordinary

humans sense of reality. Then after being drugged we can find our way to heaven and is that how Godd wants us, drugged out of our reality? Do they drug us such that we can find true knowledge of sin and thus become truly accountable for our actions? I would prefer to run rampant and enjoy life as a naked and dumb animal, amoral and with no accountability at that! At least it would feel natural to my genes.

463. Do I and my fellow *Homaniakos* partners in crime [*Order of words (no suggestions)*] get a get-out-of-jail-free card with regards to choosing between Godd and Satan represented by the physical acts against the *Hosapiens* moral laws? Do we get a handicap permit in Heaven and move to front of the queue because of some genetic mistake such that Godd will overlook our behavior because Godd is at fault for creating a genetic system that is not perfected and can't be, even if he shuts his eyes and wishes really hard? Am I out of my mind, look at these words I write and thus I am forgiven before my birth because Godd knew of it before I was born while I was some type of premortal, and then he didn't take the least bit of time or effort to lift his smallest fucking finger in the most insignificant of ways in order to put my mind into life's easy chair of delusions with along with his chosen and preferred ordinary humans? How do you account for the *Homaniakos* in Godd's universe of perfection in your mind? Look at my thoughts! "He's lost his way", "The devil has his soul", are all the thoughts of the self-proclaimed righteous, but I see everything very clearly, too clearly indeed for without a doubt when a *Homaniakos* closes his/hers eyes, the event horizon becomes visible and feel-able. Does Godd understand that what is real in a human's mind is actually real to that human? How else can the *Homaniakos* act and rationalize the thoughts and actions

needed to be acted on, except by inputs sensed and processed and logictized? Dr. Watson, another needle!

464. In all honesty, I actually see the *Hosapiens* as not having control over their genetic actions and still living the delusion as Godd intended for them in Eden. I would actually doubt I would see many ordinary humans past the pearly gates. You've already read or will read later (your choice) my statements on the *Hosapiens* mindset found in CHAPTER MANIC-DEPRESSION. It is most obvious to me that the *Hosapiens* have their own specie behavioral protocols that would rival that of the *Homaniakos'* list. Their list is different but not better. I wouldn't make an even trade with them, even with a 30% chance of myself cutting my fucking wrists to get out from all this reality and away from a brain that never rests. A *Planet of the Apes* lobotomy comes to mind but it's the *Hosapiens* that received it, not me.

465. With a dual species comparison I want to believe that any human of average intelligence would notice the most obvious and understated point I sharpened in this book. That is, free will makes up a very slight difference in ones behavior for the *Hosapiens* or the *Homaniakos*. Most of what is called free will comes down to a choice between using a natural genetic trait that Godd designed (in CHAPTER MANKIND AND WOMANTYPE it's based on evolution) into us or a learned meme at critical moments of action or decision. The *Hosapiens* are so delusional about free will and their own "thinking mind", I state with unctuous flattery [*angry mood sets in*], that they don't see the truth, but that's the whole idea about reality [*Run-on sentence, I hope*]. This is why the *Homaniakos* will always be above the *Hosapiens*. We have the slight advantage of the ability to sense actual reality. All of that aside, I suppose both of our species have enough free will that Godd will, with complete peace of his mind on his part, send you, me, and our human-children to Hell for the ultraviolence horrorshow for infinite pain for infinite time should we make the wrong choice at the right time, AKA St. Catherine of Genoa syndrome. Although I have trimmed 3,452 words about free will out of this book, I will replace them with the analogy of the number "42" and we both move to paragraph 466.

466. Given all the information to date (I'm drifting), I honestly believe that elephants are the most intelligent life on the planet the earth and nothing that any human has ever done, Veg-o-Matic included, will convince me otherwise. They appear to respond with emotions identical to that of humans. This would be proof that a DNA coding sequence would be responsible for the thoughts we interpret as emotions. I also believe that elephants have free will as seen in the behavior of some of the elephants that have been in the service of the humans and then decided freedom was a better option. Free will is associated with biological life that has a lesser dependency on pheromones. Pheromones create a mandatory action (or thought), not a free will action or thought. So when we introduce Godd into our thoughts, do we misinterpret what our pachisi playing pachyderm friends deal with, without a god? This definitely puts their species ahead of ours with respect to dealing with reality. But with interspecies communication problems, how do we know whether they are thinking of a god? Maybe theirs is a big elephant sized god that can crush our Godd with one foot.

467. Now I'm interjecting (in a decent way) a brand name new thought here on my fifth rewrite of this chapter so it is totally out of place. Adam and if you must, Eve, were nothing special. Possibly because they were only prototypes. Though I have read of religions that practically worship Eve for her bravery of making the "choice". What I know for certain, she had hairy pits without a doubt. Adam and Eve possessed no special powers of invisibility, x-ray vision, worldly insight, intelligence, or never even questioned why they didn't have belly buttons (They weren't born, get it? Thus paintings often depict them covering their midsections because humans can't figure if Godd would lie and create them as though they were born complete with belly buttons.).

468. But that story is an interesting retrospective expective because nobody hardly makes any comments of value about them except in silly bloody Television machine commercials and satires about how fun, perverse, sexy, and outright fantastic its been since Eve went oral and forget the impending horrorshow that she never knew about. Tarry a moment, we have fast-forwarded past the previews during a syntactical element failure of this sentence structure. Pause while we get back into the safety of life in the garden.

469. Six months later, I'm back to tell you I believe my view lends itself well to the examination of the genes of Adam and Eve as created because we must be created to live where and how we are planned to live or the mental thoughts of captivity and displacement would be constant and overwhelming. Manic-depressives have these thoughts of displacement but the ordinary humans as created by Godd don't. Thus I interpolate present

brains back to the original creation by Godd, and can you tell me why not think of it this way? (That point of Adam and Eve having genetic protocols is the point I need in order to tie this chapter into CHAPTER HUMAN PERCEPTIONS VERSUS TRUE REALITY and CHAPTER MANKIND AND WOMANTYPE. Godd may of [have] made us with free will but without genetics you can't exist as a "life" and a physical being that replicates, I think?) Meanwhile the need to figure "things" out on the proto-earth Eden would be the same as now as I will explain or will get to in a few thousand words hence. We only figure things out when we are forced too, when there is a problem that prevents our genetic functioning from functional functioning, or during an accident, or during a need to change the predictable events whether they are truly right or wrong. Eden did not present those cognitive functioning situations, but not to worries mate, the Bible would be boring if our hero doesn't transpond via some crisis and how could you have a happy ending if everybody is always happy?

Further Drifting

470. Now I have to parallel a thought that though entirely out of place it seems, and it should have appeared in CHAPTER HUMAN PERCEPTIONS VERSUS TRUE REALITY, but I can't wait to write that chapter so I'll mention it now and hopefully you are reading the book out of chapter sequence to get out of the sense of it. That thought is quite simply and none theismly "Nothing has ever been invented by mankind or womantype". That's a statement you don't hear too often and it seems a strange time to flirt and blurt it out of the mouth of babes, but I said-wrote it so lets leave it right here my

editor disagrees. Since humans cannot have an original pure thought, it would have taken a leap of logic to see past the control that Godd had over nature in the Garden of Eden, because Godd was restricting most natural events from taking their natural course because in fact gravity kills when improperly applied.

47 1 . No human logic was required, our two contestants would question nothing and humans were created to live in "that" proto-environment. Genesis 1:26, first 50 alpha-characters: Then Godd said, "Let us make humankind in our image, according to our multiple personalities; blah, blah, blah". I believe because of that statement and every statement of action that I wish I could put in this book from that book, Godd is not because Godd is more human-like than most would admit, but he doesn't have the ability to suffer from (or enjoy) the "sins of the flesh" affliction that we do. I don't feel Godd understands us, and he should get in touch with his "human" side if he wishes to improve his image. If humans were created from day one, to strive to overcome the trials of everyday life and become more Godd-like, then they would become restless in Eden, not having those influences that would bring them that satisfaction of accomplishment. Thus a big new thought for the world is right here – Godd created mankind and womantype to live in the controlled by him environment, not the world of the second revision (outside of Eden without Godd) as we now know it to-day. He did this in his idea of a human's genetic code for easy passage to the future generations of Eden's garden [*Too many phrases (no suggestions)*]. If I were given a chance to "add to" and improve the Bible as the early Christians did, I would add the following to Genesis: "*So by strands of chromosomes of DNA, Godd created all life; plants and animals he did create in this manner. Those chromosomes contain the*

'seed' to each their own and rules to govern each specie from within, for the continuance of their own. Godd created genetics within all life and he was sad, for he wished he had the same". Godd þut into humans less þheromone, so free will is easy to achieve or at least you can þass judgement on others because of lack of the aforementioned þheromones. (For those less readers scientific but quite necessary to our lives, þheromones are chemicals generally þassed from one creature to another usually via the airways and cause some tyþe of autonomic (wrong word but sounds good) action that you can't control and þossibly don't even know is haþþening.) The Bible doesn't say or mention that Godd was numbing man's mental abilities in Eden, or Godd would have been the first to fall þrey to Mr. Blaise Þascal's wager thus þroving Mr. Þascal correct after all, even before the Þascal family was birthed. So why all my time sþent daydreaming and rationalizing the genetics of Adam and Eve? Because Godd created a genetic creature, whether you strictly believe this to be Adam and Eve or mankind and womantyþe in general, we are not under control (being controlled) of invisible forces that defy scientific sensing at every moment of our lives. And yet if we were all "free will", as many believe, without any þreþrogrammed abilities, then there would be no consistency to any of the human's actions/reactions and you can see that that is certainly no [sic] the case. Godd created the þroto-humans and he created them via genetics to have þhysically and mentally what they needed in the Garden and nothing more. From this I will understand why the Hosaþiens behave the way they do in every action and reaction while the Homaniakos have to look on and feel sorry for all of them as though the Hosaþiens don't see the cage that their mind is in, while I chisel at the bars on mine.

472. We don't inherit original duplicated sin transferred and validated invisibly from soul to soul throughout manikin kind because one naked womyn was properly convinced that at one moment in history, eating the correct vegetables would improve her chances for optimum procreation. We get what Godd invented in Adam and Eve, a genetically driven optimum procreating organic machine with marginally effective DNA. (An inappropriate remark was removed from right here!) Why do we need sin by invisible never divisible transference when we have genetics made for Eden but tossed out into the real world by a temperamental god? Thus perhaps I will understand all of the ordinary humans after all, but there is more to the story and more that Godd revealed about himself when no one was looking so lets read on, because sweet dreams are made of these.

473. It is only after sin was known that humans were faced with problem solving as in raise an eyebrow and rub your chin while saying, "Hmmm". Problem solving was not one of the better features that Godd gave the proto-humans, his creation, because he honestly didn't believe humans would need it in Eden. What was Adam and Eve to do in Eden?, set off on a coarse of discovery and build a bridge to nowhere and for what reason to go to nowhere? Once humans sinned or went against Godd, all the controls creating an unnatural environment were stopped halted terminated by Godd or maybe they never existed outside of the holy vegetable garden and the expected reactions to many actions became random by human perceptions and their faulty logic. In other words, "Nobody was driving somebody". Those aren't useful words but they are other words.

474. All was not lost for the humans racing because Godd revealed the truth to my þroems [*Incorrect word usage*] that I wrote before his creation in anticipation of you being here to read these words, that Godd changed the genetic structure of humans from his original creation and I have proof via his own words. Thus the logic is sent backwards to þrove that humans were created for Eden genetically and not the real lets make a deal world we live in. Add on to this, that unless you believe that Godd is controlling everyone of us as þuþþets on strings to infinity, then you will now believe in genetic action ruling your life þer Godd's own design and you can't out think yourself out of it. This is no insult to Godd, because look what a marvelous thing genes are.

475. During the tossage scene of the fall of mankind and womantyþe, Godd added genetic features to humans not meme's because meme's have no guarantee of þassage by verbiage or þhysical transaction, esþecially line of sight to blind humans. He altered our DNA because he can and he did and he told us he did in þlain words nonetheless, but no þreacher has ever made a big þoint about it to my ears, and Godd thought we might need the "additional" gene sequences in order to survive without his helþ. Oh no, this was no þun'ishment and cannot be debated by the master debaters such as the few feminists are now. Godd knew he was sending his human-children off the to the big city so his gifts of survival were as he told us: Gen. 3:16 To the womyn he said, "Blah, blah blah, your need will be for your husband, and he will rule over you". He said something about mankind will[*would*] enjoy working for a living as all men actually do now. Godd saw too [*to?*] it that via genetic transference that man will dominate woman via the woman's need for men, but many humans are too politically motivated in this era to ever say, "I see it" in this time and place on the earth. Then Godd went on to make some predictions that he will send Jesus later on, but in the worst grammar so nobody saw it until after the fact. So Godd messed around with the human DNA again after the failure of the proto-human in Eden, in order to be certain that hierarchies and clans and tribes and a need to work and survive and procreate would be there once Godd left mankind's and womantype's confirm-able presence. So version 1.1 of mankind and womantype became real and what was leftover or not removed from the DNA (from the Garden of Eden days) would keep the ordinary humans delusional about reality even until this day. In summary, using capitalization for clarity, I write: thuS I pulL thE delusionarY aspecT oF contemporarY humanS froM godd'S originaL plaN, anD hE shoulD havE spenT morE timE oN ouR geneS prioR tO thE dismissaL froM edeN. maniC-depressiveS provE therE iS noT thaT mucH morE geneticS tO alteR, iF yoU wisH tO providE humanS witH aN alternativE anD morE accuratE visioN oF realitY.   (I'll throw this in here so that we may remain accurate as to the revisions of the human's DNA. Godd made DNA version 1.2 as stated in GEN 6:3 when he shortened the natural life span of all humans, to remain at 120 of the earth orbitals.) (Now I am also inclined to state that there was a DNA version 1.3 issued in Genesis 9:3, which is the ability to eat and metabolize meat. As well as the ability, must come the need.)

Genetics are not perfected by Godd

476. If you ever wondered why so many so-called good women go after so many so-called rotten men and end up on the daytime

talkie shows wit black and blue eyes, why don't you blame Godd? One word will work now, "genetics", but as a revisional afterthought. Also, lets hope you are not believing to think that only modern mankind exhibits power over womantype via some combined covert secret communications that all men share or by men discovering *Barbie* dolls (discovered by a woman, actually) in order to teach pre-masturbatatorial girls that they must be subservient to men and they will never amount to anything more than meat on a hook if they are lucky enough to look like a piece of plastic. Most men don't even give *Barbie* dolls a second thought, but I having a different view of reality find those dolls so lustful as my human-children leave them lying on the floor half naked and bent and posed in unnatural erotic positions of needs unfulfilled, or I see dozens of them naked and stacked into some giant tub as an illusion of the most erotic holocaust imagined with some of them headless or limbless but smiling through the thick of it as though it meets with their approval. (I blame those thoughts on this music I'm listening to.)

477. The only punishment that Godd spanked his pets with was the eviction from paradise and his (Godd's) presence of the daily walks in the cool of the day (Godd suffers from hidrosis). It has nothing to do with the "so called" curse misinterpreted. Since Godd is not really a sexual being of gender attributes and is not even a potential rapist (as all males are proclaimed to be by the feminists), why it is interpreted that mankind as opposed to womantype came out on top of the power struggle at that time is beyond me. It's possible that Godd didn't mean anything by it and mankind took advantage of the situation over the years because mankind turned out to be the hunter and killer of big game, while womantype were stuck with breast feeding the

newborn, all because womantyþe somehow came to have breasts filled with milk (I see the consþiracy now!). I however believe it was a hasty revision and he didn't þut much thought into it, as it hasn't worked out very well for either gender. Feminists see the male genetic trait of "tribes" and believe there is a consþiracy in it. I see households being run by the female genetic trait of "clans" and men let it alone but complain about it at the office. Who can figure the truth to all of this?

Þrimate see, þrimate do

478. As I had accidentally þut *Hungarian Rhapsody No. 2* in my þlayer, I can barely think as fast as I am typing but let me write that humans – within the architecture of the natural behavioral motivators – can only imitate as learned behavior. This statement of observation is not mine to þro-þhess but it has been stated and re-stated by the great ones whose books are not considered Grubstreet by nose in-the-air þedigrees. With the one exceþtion to that statement whereby I believe we only imitate and don't really have original thoughts. How do we then objectively keeþ free will within this þaragraþh? Learned behaviors, versus learned resþonses, versus sooner or later we get to make a choice and we already know whether the outcome will be acceþtable to the clan or the tribe because of that big memory we humans have. What else could free will be? Free will thus does not stand on its own merit and is very inconsequential within our lives is what I am going to believe at this time, for what would then be the descriþtion of it? Do you consider learning doggie tricks free will? Saying "I'm sorry" or asking before taking the last cookie or blowing your spouse's brains out in order to collect some insurance money, or saying "no" to drugs can be described both as þroþer and improper learned behavior or free will within a set of choices, depending on the circumstances. Free will never needs a correct choice - but learned behavior expects one. But to make the discussion of free will more complex than it has to be let me write that humans are mathematical contrivance contrivers altering mechanisms using resources as equations. We add visual or experienced (via the senses) resources to derive future visual or experience resources. Visual resources are to contrivance replicators as enzymes are to organic life (What the hell does that mean?). In case you are not convinced of your lack of free will, original thought, or "I'm an independent thinker" as you all say to your friends or those that are forced to be in your presence, what is a fad and how many do you follow? What do your clothes look like? An original idea that is always birthed of an existing idea is the best thought you can hope for as any human species, and to that I would proclaim makes you a genus when you can memorize more previously existing ideas than your neighbors.

479. When can the imitation change such that we go from throwing sticks at the moon to typing on a personal computer? That answer is simple, humans deduce (by faulty logic) that the reaction was not justified by the original action. But we still throw sticks (as a metaphor) as we type on our computers. Making a coat out of a peeled off skin of an animal, hopefully already dead, is not an invention it is simply imitating what the senseless animals own already or what you would do with no sense at all the moment you got cold and hid naked under a pile of leaves with the worms. Making a loom to mass-produce 10k coats would appear to be an invention, but it's not. It is 10 million sequential misinterpretations of expected reactions over a period of 1.5 million years. Besides, all of us are so quick to brag about our great technology but in our

life we spend our day imitating the human that did those tasks the day before. It is all we humans can do to learn doggie tricks like flipping on a light switch and then we brag about it as though we've created nuclear energy. Thus referring back to my previous statement of "Nothing has ever been invented by mankind or womantype" but somehow because actions accumulate over time as physical artifacts, and no human can duplicate or imitate "sensed" reality very exactly, we end up with all these gadgets.

480. Yes we are still in the chapter that concerns itself with the existence of Godd but there are many paths to Godd, the Lone Ranger once stated, and I suppose I am routing another path so stay with me. As I am trying to avoid depressing thoughts, the sound track that I have chosen seems juxtaposed against the holiness of Godd, but then I am actually splitting my already split mind so as to remain in the neutral territory of emotions. For as strange as it sounds, the "Issues" CD by Korn, brings joy and peace to my mind as I can easily vision [envision] the fulfillment of my genetic needs within the words of the songs. (Where as ordinary humans may describe me as amoral because my thoughts tend to believe in genetic satisfactions, you must understand how sensory input can put us *Homaniakos* into our moods, and we must survive our moods everyday.) The bass sound of this music is so grinding and moving and constant and reminds me of the way life continues unchanging one note after another without a plan or consequence or thought needed. Although this is one album with every track a hit, track number 11 is one of my favorites.

481. When Godd walked in the cool of the day with our naked ancestors, all actions and reactions did not need to be resolved. There was no fear of attack by predators and there was all the food you needed in a climate controlled naturalist environ. The first questions came after sin. The first misinterpretation of an event was that they (Adam and Eve) saw themselves as being naked and it was believed by them at that moment to mean something. It actually meant nothing because nothing of reality changed except their perception of reality and that is only a thought and you can see that faulty logic was then to become the downfall of mankind and womantype from which we have never recovered. Their eyes were not opened, but their mind interpreted reality differently. They became transformed in one single moment, as the *Homaniakos* species does when waking up one day and realizing that they are no longer ordinary. How could the humans of to-day ever see and interpret reality through the eyes of Adam and Eve before the great transformation? It is not possible to imagine. So this is where the ordinary humans get their faulty logic, and I bet you never thought I would get to the basis of it?

Greek phables and Hebrew stories

482. Changing subjects abruptly as this chapter labors on aimlessly you might be glad not to be stuck with me during a dinner party for how would you get a word in edgewise? I am feeling inclined to recline for a bit and release the remaining remainder of this chapter to the virtual reality trash bin. However with about 30 more formatted pages to go and I've got blisters on me fingers, I'll

queue up the correct CD on the turntable starting on track #6 and give it a go after leaning back for a short rest. Its getting more difficult to get back to feeling like a human after every nap, as time and distance and "Who am I?" remains confused, especially in these dark winter months. Without a human voice here I don't know if I would get back at all. This electronic stuff isn't as much fun anymore, as plastic is starting to feel normal in my hands and I think I want to be buried with my keypad in place of my wedding band.   Plastic and electronics have provided me with all the knowledge from the universities to personal insights and pictures of Internet womyn with manufactured breasts designed for visual fornicators and the Internet womyn are all gooed up but smiling through the thick of it as though it meets with their approval. Jesus, you are now farther from reality as all of this stuff is so calculated to be pleasing and desirable, proving humans have lived too long and are starting to figure out the shortcuts to genetic pleasures. Maybe I should go and hug my kid's goodbye and let their mom explain what pain really is and how a living mind can hurt without hurting at all. Jesus, why isn't the afterlife more clear with pictures provided on your web site with a site map of Heaven and all its delights? I want to see an angel of the spiritual type and ask a few questions or so because all the Jesus freaks and bumper stick-on signs of love and warmth and love again are being driven by ordinary humans who believe other humans will be transformed by a sign hung on the ass of their minivan. · · · · · · "How long will it take me to get there - before I reach *my* home?" I asked within my mind, as I felt the vision almost upon me. A quiet voice replied: "Forever". And with those thoughts, instantly the clearer vision appeared to my mind's eye, and the feeling overtook my whole self, as I was no longer upon the earth, and my eyes were no longer needed to see quite clearly. END IT! End it now. THE

PAIN! The pain arrives with the vision, as it always does. The loneliness of the mind, the manic-depressive mind. Where is my feeling of love that was to replace the quiet lonely moments that are upon me in the darkness? I used to dream of evenings full of smiles and kisses and hands that touched me, all for the purpose of blinding the vision from my minds eye. Suicide, I am such a coward to my people. I am a disgrace to them. How could I ever lead them to a clear understanding if I won't finish the job and solve the equation; zero divided by infinity, emptiness divided by forever, the forever loneliness of the manic-depressive mind - the equation of Logical Death? Jesus, you are such a bastard god. You blind *them* from the true reality but my people must see the vision beyond death - the fucking creation of physical existence without the need of love or answers. Where are my people? They all lay dead, in their graves so dark and cold and lonely. They were the brave ones. How do I comfort them? How do I give them light and warmth and love? Yet ordinary humans cry everyday for those dearly departed intentionally dead, without understanding what the dead knew, or what they felt at that changing moment. Jesus, how will you find me, for I have no soul for you to take after my death?

Time presses on

483. I have often but not really wondered if there was or is a common beginning to the phables of the ancient Greeks and the Christian religion evolved through the Israelite religion. Internet Academia comes through again and true or not; it matters not, because I have found what I have waxed and wrothed over for many years.

484. Now I have found the Ugaritic Tablets, the Canaanite mythology, and the marriages of human women to the angels from heaven. The fact or fiction that this so closely parallels heathen mythology of the same era might be absolutely no coincidence at all if you believe in Godd or perhaps you never studied Greek or Egyptcian mythology. Does a lack of knowledge of history allow you to substantiate your religious beliefs? Then how can you find the facts of Godd birthed from so many legends? Even heathens believe in something even if they believe in nothing because believing in nothing is something. Now I doubt that this knowledge could bring about an end to your Christian beliefs but I'm going to write about it anyway and let your mind cogitate or cognize it as much as you would like. The common question is still the most applicable – did the belief in the true Godd inspire sequels and triquels in the form of fictional gods as in the example of the *Star Wars* movie genre? I will tell you that I can't find out which came first, legends or religion, or if there is even a difference, but we never look at ourselves as though we are as the ancient Egyptcians worshiping a ridiculous cat god of some type. Of course, the ancient Egyptcians had these same thoughts about the ancients that came before them so how are we ever going to get to the truth of it? No answers in number 484 so proceed to 485 and some of the data I found was useful and I will continue along with a new thought.

485. Now whether you wish to ignore, disbelieve, or mentally justify self-righteous translations of the Bible there are versus in the book of the holier-than-thou that are mostly ignored as a part of the humans skimming over process in order to avoid distressing cognition. Yet I thrive on such hidden data, because some humans wish to keep it unknown for their own self-purposes. Humans seek data that matches what they believe, not what contradicts what they believe (subjective validation). The rest is subconsciously ignored. So goes the pseudo power of all mind reading mystics. It is my most logical of beliefs that the true man of the cloth would not point out for reasons of self-serving interests, the true nature of the angels under Godd's creation and control. With the ability to work with computerized searchable databases and the Internet, data is in abundance if you ever wanted to look. Godd isn't a parent as proclaimed by Jesus who came to the earth to do some PR work on [with, for?] Godd's reputation. In actually Godd is the slave master of our universe and us too. He does not allow us to leave home and figure our own destinies (Exodus 22: 20). Our free will always ends in his flip of the coin decision to give us an infinite view of his feet or infinite pain of some unknown spiritual fashion. He does no better with his freely willful angels. Any decent human parent will let their human-children become independent and will also stop spanking them after maturity is reached. Godd, being a poor parent (Mat. 18:14, 23:9, 2 Cor. 13:3, 4 and etc.), can't leave us or the angels alone to decide for ourselves to move back home with him or only to drop dead without his planned horrorshow.

486. His angels that live in his realm and are understandably his creation also are as naive as the *Hosapiens* and they can definitely screw [*Inappropriate verb*] themselves over big time by trying to become independent of Godd. Now I believe as in an office environment, Godd employees the angels and all angels are not that happy to hang around Godd or live under his controlled handouts (as thanks to Lucifer already documented in the Bible). You are either with Godd or you are evil, and that is not how our world operates and for heaven's sake, that is not how the natural realm of godless created by Godd creatures live daily. The godless creatures (i.e. cows, dolphins, chickens, etc.), fortunately, do drop dead and don't suffer the possible ultraviolence horrorshow that Godd so kindly invented for bad little girls and his not so pure hard-up angels. Although some humans have told me that their pets will be with them in Heaven (or on the new earth). So a pet parrot or dog has a chance to make it into Heaven by having an ordinary human wave a hand or sprinkle water on it? Oh my god!

487. Now if Godd created the angels and allows them to live in his presence then why do so many choose to go against his will? I can start to see that Lucifer might have had a different management plan for the mysterious spiritual realm, but couldn't convince most of the "like human" angels that are afraid to standup for what is really right to back him at the right moment even though most of them probably said, "We're behind you Lucifer 100%". Lucifer was fired and then sent to the earth as some kind of punishment. Visitation rights to Heaven granted as per Job's book.

488. It is obvious that the earth is an angel's prison or Devils Island if you see the connection. What type of favor is Godd doing by putting us here with all the prisoners? Why would Godd believe that by creating creatures less powerful than the angels (and us without proof of the existence of Godd), he would achieve his wanted captive audience? The problem with humans is that we are so tasty (no I am not off the topic again). Godd created us that way with some type of patented flavor. We don't taste like chicken at all. All the good carnal lust (sinning) fun that you can have usually involves sooner or later putting some part or fluid of another human into your mouth, or in contact with your mouth or tongue. Yum yum. (The last five sentences actually belong in paragraph 489 but then paragraph 488 would have been too short.)

489. Without a doubt, angels don't eat or therefore taste while they remain angels, because of not being physical I suppose. I am most certain that when Godd is off fixing some part of the out of sight universe or winding up the big spring, Lucifer or his earthly revelers communicate back to heaven and thus the heavenly host get to hear their boasts about debauchery, orgasms, fornication, and beautiful women. As documented (somewhere), some were interested and maybe even in disbelief that anything physical could be that fun - because we can't imagine what a spiritual creature does for fun either.

490. Now as it is a well-known and documented fact among humans that when a mermaid leaves the saltwater she gets her legs but still smells like a fish, so do the angel when they fall to the earth (but without that fish smell). Without a doubt good angels roam the earth, for if you are inclined to certain beliefs you believe your angel attendant keeps you from harm. Of course, the devil is an angel also, and from what I can tell from the book of Job, angels are allowed to go between the earth and heaven or about the universe.

491. Now suppose that some angels while watching the earth women groom their earthly mound of Venus fell prey to the human only, no angels allowed sensations of touch and taste? What about the angels that became physical and fornicated with the

earth women and created the giants of the earth as documented in the Bible? The angels that tempted the earth woman and gave away the secrets of Heaven for a good physical romp of fornication had already lived in Heaven with Godd, thus what was their reason for giving up what we strive to reach? Is the fun of sex more powerful than the need to procreate, or is procreation the number one rule of life in the universe, even in Heaven? Did those angels, turned human, fail to resist the procreation gene once human? This would explain a lot of the human's behavior I guess. (Angels don't have sex as angels because of not having to procreate, from what we know of them.) Too many strange behaviors if you think about it, and you'll have to do some research on your own to find the story behind the story. I leave you shocked and move on to another subject.

492. The genetics to optimum procreation has lead mankind and womantype down the road to unnatural technologies that can satisfy the boner urge at a moment's notice no matter how twisted the gene. Godd either didn't see it coming or couldn't figure a fix to the genome with the time remaining to his significant number 7. Where is Godd now? For certain he would have destroyed the world again for our recent creation of one sinful World Wide Web of Sodom and Gomorrah using digitized electrons to sustain the Second Coming of Homo Erectus. The birth of the Web has re-born humankind and re-confirmed exactly what is on mankind's mind, and the Internet porn and sex via wire should tell you my reader friend to believe in what I am telling you about the genetics of humankind. (I am only reporting what I see and hear and touch.) What with Adam and Eve being expelled from Eden, the flood to destroy all the earth life (except Noah & friends), the city of Sodom being the first ground zero test site, how is it that the

earth stays in existence now? I see all of us, every human as out of control within all this television, movie, and Internet technology as we daily watch, listen, and pursue topics of sex acts, murders, betrayal with lies, thoughts of heavenly spies with eyes, psychics, mystics, life changing crystals, and if its not real then Hollywood makes it real for us and we put our money where our heart is or wants to be, because it makes us feel satisfied. The "self" has never been so important but it is not the "self" that screws us over, it is the pursuit of the "self" though technology pleasures. These technology pleasures remove the necessity for genetic behaviors to be socially acceptable or satisfied naturally. All hope is lost as I see we are never going back and I myself take my fix everyday in unison with all of you, and I actually wish I was implanted with electronics or mechanisms to provide pleasure resources as needed. Unlike ordinary humans, we the *Homaniakos* do not live our lives in delusions, thus delusions created are entertainment for us.

Faith

493. Faith is not a lesson in logic. That which is logical or illogical should have no bearing on a belief in a supernatural being that has lived forever, can create spontaneous life, has complete control over all the laws of our physical universe, can reverse death even 3 days old, and removes stains better than Bon Ami. Why all the concerns over fake pieces of the cross, fake shrouds, fake 9 inch nails, the missing chalice, or the missing robe? If any one of those were true, then you have proof and no faith. We are now told to have faith but the Bible is full of examples where proof was never needed because Godd (and Jesus) was there to speak, create physical phenomenon, or shake your hand and yet in the very presence of these anomalies, with no advanced technology to create visual and audio special effects to fool humans, sinning persisted. It is hopeless for us, because our faith has to be stronger than those that saw the proof, or stronger than that of the angels of Godd's Heaven. All we can do is ask for forgiveness every hour. I have forgiven all others of their sins – for they know not what they do. I stand ready at all moments. I suppose that if I was to put any thoughts of redeeming value in this book, then I would like to tell all of you that you must quit looking for the physical to prove the spiritual. Never allow your priest or preacher to start speaking of scientific proof or genuine artifacts found, or heathen historical collaborating documents. Never kneel down to anything made of earthly elements, never kiss another mans' ring, or touch anything made of the earth as if it has a spirit or a power or history or function for your soul. Do not ask of another human to speak to your dearly departed dead relatives, tell you of your future, or speak of imagined after-life experiences as though Godd looses track of who is to come to Heaven and when. Spend your idle time reading your holy book, from end to end, with no thought or emotion omitted, for it was not written based on your opinion of what or how you would have Godd behave. Know the god you chose. Do something spectacular for the other humans around you before your physical time runs out.

494. If we have already discounted and reduced the price of believing that genetics created our gods in our minds, then our understanding of our godness belief all relies on the information we can put or someone else can force into our minds. When truths are avoided so that you may be happy with your simple solution to the labyrinth of Heaven then you only have a partial understanding of Godd, and being human, that is enough for most all humans from what I see everyday. I tell all humans as I already have told you, there are more legitimate understandings of the Godd Book than you are being shown. Understanding can only occur when you are at the end of knowledge so that you may look backward on time to see the way knowledge is transformed, mutated, forgotten, ignored, or denied. The truth is different than your delusions of þure love and forever haþþiness. Quit reading your "Haþþy thoughts" books and "I heart Jesus" bumþer stick-ons and realize you are dealing with a comþlex creature of an unearthly mentality that has more þower than man but thinks the same as man, and for a reason. Do you see that reason yet?

495. You, my reader friend, are doomed to Hell because you trust another human to do what you should do yourself for your own soul. You have looked for a nice church building, a similar "þre" established belief, a young congregation, or a service with guitars in it. A church must be a college and a keeþer of the tradition of the faith. Its "members" must be an army ready to defend against change or allowing via their human-children, the religiousizing of heathen customs. Instead what has continued to haþþen is that every modern custom is adoþted into the churches and services such that they become unrecognizable every two generations (because the aged humans die and their resistance to a given change imþosed by the youth dies also), but you don't recognize the changes at all. My simþle suggestion is to forget whatever you think you know about Godd and the Bible and start over. Give yourself a mental enema and flush twice.

496. We are too far through time from ever knowing any truth to the þast, as even yesterday's events are debatable with humans as such liars as they are. Even now, as I stand at the end of knowledge, there is a singularity of history and time that prevents the reality of the past ages from actually ever being known. Faith becomes stronger than knowledge, and in the last days to come, is this not what Godd wanted all along? Who among you can let go of a physical life on the faith of an eternal life, without seeing the proof except perhaps a madman or one of us? In the loneliness of the darkness, the true believers take off their Sunday faith and leave it in the night-light while lonely tears fall on pillows so soft, praying that to-morrow will be different. Ordinary humans might run far enough to hide their fears from their fellow *Hosapiens*, but when they can't run any further and they fall into despair, they will look forward and a *Homaniakos* will be standing tall in front of them on the side of a reality that the ordinary humans can't see and a pain that they can't imagine. How many moments in your life do you spend 2 seconds from death with only you and Godd present? If you want to argue what is faith, then talk to all my fellow dead manic-depressives that trusted in Godd enough to make a true and logical choice. The logic of suicide is proof of the strength of a faith that the *Homaniakos* achieves, and how many ordinary humans can make that claim? What do I feel or believe when standing between critical moments of physical life and death? I see what all the *Homaniakos'* see, and that sight is beyond description in a contrived language.

497. I start on a new topic but don't bother to mention that I did until you read that Sheol [*sp?*] is to the Hebrews, a place where the dead stay if you do not end up in heaven. To get to Sheol you cross a river after meeting the prerequisite of the first death. It is as a city of ruins and remnants, yet it did not previously exist in order to become ruins and remnants. Thus Godd understood that mankind and womantype would mentally be but

aside and distressed by ruins and remnants because it is born to us to know the þath to survival and avoid such þlaces, as such þlaces are genetically disturbing. Therefore in more words than we would þrefer, we þrefer not to be found dead there but since it exists, or actually did exist, it has rules and attributes that must be followed by its inhabitants. Godd can see you in Sheol and you can be rescued from it. Communications between Heaven and Sheol is þossible. Where for art thou Sheol, the hell that is not quite so bad as you would like it to be for me. Although I read that Sheol is for OT Jews and not for NT gentiles. How can we keeþ all these rules straight? Hell is now an image made by þoets and Saturday morning cartoons and consists þrimarily of the same descriþtion of the þlace that the never dying angels of the earth will be sent for an ultraviolance horrorshow. Is all of Godd a þoem so old that it got lost in the antiquity of þoor data storage and retrieval systems combined with man-made translations mistranslated through corruþt minds to massage your beliefs and emþty your þurse?

498. Am I confused or is the Hell of Godd different that the Hell of Jesus? All is not different through time þast or þresent time futured but your ability to get to the truth is imþossible. I am lost as to which new Heaven or new earth or which Hell I will be in after the end of days, but if none of that is even remotely true, then what will our universe exist as in 82 billion years from this time onward? I am holding back another þanic attack as I quickly see the clearer vision of reality þass before me as a universe that is real, and of no need of me is what I feel, but I reach for a handful of chocolate in order to suþþress the vision that I don't care to see at this moment.

499. Strange thoughts are those but since I created CHAPTER GODD out of multiple assuages[?] of pre-existing words arranged in a one of a kind sequence, let me continue on the split nature of Godd and Jesus in a way I hope no human has ever described, and I myself can hardly believe would have existed weren't' it for the obvious ploy that Godd tried to pull by creating Jesus, the physical god of memes and PR sent to the earth for one last effort.

500. Random thoughts along a similar line of thoughts; Godd follows genetics. We, being made after his image mimic his actions of violence built on genetic tribal relations and an abuse of power due to a genetically driven tribal architecture (when the leader shouts "kill", we kill). In reality Godd couldn't think that far from his own nature when he created the angels and us and why would we expect otherwise (thus paragraph 11 of this chapter is not the truth at all, but I knew it from the beginning of the chapter because I am the creator of this chapter). Godd must be as imperfect as we are, but with enough power to spoil our fun. I suppose that the "Godd" belief or fear of Hell would be enough to keep most men from using their genetic actions of wanting to bend young maidens over tree stumps and rutting the daylights out every one of them only for the purpose of optimum procreation without love needed. But I doubt that that type of "fear of Godd" would ever happen in mankind, even if we were left with our genetics and no god to be found, ever mentioned, or ever believed in, because not enough men really fear punishment from Godd as much as they won't violate the genetic protocols of human mating or they fear being hit by their present female mate. Regardless, enough bending of maidens occurs at every opportunity to call it a natural event with no fear of Godd shown. It is not the belief in a Godd that prevents you from sinning; it is a belief in your genetics that keeps you that way. This visionary Godd has never done anything to you that you can see via physical proof or verbalized evidence, but you speak in your mind in a contrived language until you are convinced all actions and events are ordained by Godd or the devil when it is convenient, but those outside of your vision say you are crazy for not getting control of your life, and thoughts of Godd rarely come into play in their minds.

501. We are so close to Godd emotion-wise, but unlike us humans, Godd doesn't have a helpmate that he has revealed to us - I suppose that is why sex is so screwed up. Godd never "did it" and perhaps he couldn't imagine the needs created via the DNA sequencing that he created. Godd didn't or couldn't give a marginally pheromone driven animal such as humans, a sex urge gene that works halfway proper based solely on the words, "I do". We would do better if every human female went into heat once a year and we had three days of a no holes bared pheromone driven orgy. At least the rest of the year would then be totally productive. At any rate mankind memed the concubines (against Godd's intention) and satisfied their own procreation *Genesis Protocols* by re-writing the Bible to suit the fashionable sex habits of the times. In modern times we have affairs at every moment as the divorce rate climbs and having multi-mating partners is revealed to be truer than once suspected or as was once hidden out of the fear of being found out via contrived languages. (There is no way around it, I must leave humans as "visual fornicators" and possibly leave it as the dominant trait in order to justify the action of optimum procreation that I see and hear about

and read about everyday. How can you convince me otherwise, while I live amongst you every day?) The movie rental retailers all have "back doors" leading into "back rooms" where the topic of perversion in the name of "adult entertainment" via freedom of speech properly exercised is rented day by day, with everyone knowing that each video cartridge comes with one orgasm guaranteed, so why rent two? The magazine covers in this country bare as much as possible as opposed to Europe where they grin and bare it [all]. Movie theater productions, TV Shows, and commercials (either on film or paper) are as sexy as legal public sexity can be, wherever you be at [Queer word usage(no suggestions)]. If Christ or Godd was so popular, or always on the humans minds, then where is their representation within the media dementia? Surely Godd or Christ or Christian topics should get at least 1/7th the retail space? As my mind is clearer now - at last all too well I notice, to my curiosity, that the Internet men and Internet womyn often neck dangle their religious medallions with a miniature Jesus nailed and hung(ed) upon a cross of gold no less, while orgies of any gender (or species) find relief upon the passion of Christ. ? Perhaps I have found my absolute proof of Godd or proof of the devil (prove one, prove all), because what other animal uses technology for the purpose of physical torture in the name of satisfying the procreation gene? With all the bondage, torture, burning, branding, needle puncturing, artificial penetrations, scatting, whipping, spanking, hot waxing, animal interaction, and same-sex interchanges, I would want to know what in the name of evolutionary advantage would create such sought after actions within genes? Only a god could create such a creature, via applying too much "free will over genetics", and only a devil could offer so much fun to tempt everyone. But maybe the human genome is only defective?

502. My trail down the þath to find Godd-like behavior within mankind and womantyþe is taking me where I susþected it would all along. Genetics infused by a contrived language and infected by millions of memes has lead us to be no more soþhisticated than 4k years ago, but we are lost souls in the mess of it as if we are þea's in þea souþ being stirred too swiftly. How am I going to find my satisfaction in the thick of it? I was counting on all of you to lead a þroþer life (as my thoughts were when I was a human-child), so that I may learn by examþle, but you temþt me in the ways I þrefer to go anyway, thus now I hoþe for erotic distractions and technology toys until the day I die - and I am starting to agree with you - save Godd for that hour and 3 minutes on Sunday.

A new toþic

503. The way I am starting to figure it, Godd is adlibbing the whole þhysical life experience as the OT stories zig & zag about each other while the Dead Sea Scrolls are missing in action. Maybe Godd gave uþ after the Jesus limited engagement tour. There is still a good chance he'll þull this entire Heaven þromise out from under us now or in the future and as Heavenly sþirits, are we going to sit as the angels do and dwell on universal thoughts of other þhysical sensations without an inaþproþriate thought or action? Everyone seems quick to exþlain his or her belief of it, but nobody living will ever have the þroof of it.

504. What is this god's true behavior as though I haven't already given you a clue or three? No matter what verses you find in the old time testament speaking of the Peþsi generation and the love for his þeoþle - those only apþlied to Godd þrotecting his

sacristan Jews; his chosen people not the non-Jew. He never loved the common persons no matter how gentile they were or were to be now, as in "you". Godd never planned on loving the non-Jew. "Ipso Facto Brute" (That's a fact, Jack). Does Hebrews 13:8 apply to Godd or Jesus, and what would be the difference? What Godd said is what he meant to say. What he did, he did with his own intentions of his own free will, knowing that humans will know of it for all time. Behavior reveals character even in a god, but then I have no problem believing in the god of my nightmares because I along with the rest of the *Homaniakos* see the gravity of the life and death situation, even if few *Homaniakos* believe as I do. Even an abused human-child will love the only dad he knows and kneels down before, and then he'll run off to school and say he has the greatest father in the world. Are you still that human-child?

505. I will have to grant to you the equal (but not by analysis), possibility that a somewhat powerful creature such as a god of the nether world exists and wants our essence to be delivered to him after death to accompany him throughout the rest of time, but how do you account for boredom as events reoccur daily forever? I would have to leave the topic where it lies and say that I suppose with no proof to offer, and we absolutely can't imagine another existence, that souls don't become bored, and we will enjoy that new feeling because we won't remember the old feelings of now. It worries me.

506. If we are to spend an infinite amount of time as a soul in this new place, what will we do? What will that god do with us? I'm worried again. I need to know more about the character of this god that I am going to be with for 10 billion billion billion billion

billion years and then you find out you have only started and you have an infinite time more than that to go and not an unhappy moment ever is what I am told. But those are the words of the ordinary human and what can they tell us about the feeling of "time" or the pursuit of the never to exist "happiness?" What if Godd has screwed up and actually created a Heaven that we won't like forever? (As far as we know, none of this has ever been tested.) Why have some of his angel's rebelled and gone to the earth searching after the pleasures of the physical body? Why wasn't Heaven and Godd's supreme presence and light of the world worth anything to them? They were not created evil they simply exercised their Godd given right of free will when they were presented with choices. If Godd is commanding our planet from Heaven, and his angels also help at the perceived moments of holy intervention then there is a sense of time in Heaven because the earth being physical has a "time" attribute. With the great uprising of Heaven War 1 before man's creation, then it is obvious that "timeness" exists in the spirit world even if angels don't get wrinkles and the embarrassment of psoriasis. Will we sense time in Heaven or will it be as that singularity moment of embrace-ment with your human-child when love overpowers the senses and you momentarily leave the physical realm of sensual moral reality and fall from grace and live forever in a moment of true I don't know where this thought is going, so I'll end the sentence [Blocking]. But I must tell you, that if you are an ordinary human you might not believe that the "sense" of time does not always exist. Ask the nearest Manic-depressive Junkie and they will tell you that during those moments of the clearer vision of reality, the pain is real and infinite, and the passage of time is not felt as the sensation is continual and without end, occurring and reoccurring moment to moment, no inuring possible, the same as in the way you might imagine burning in Hell.

507. Any angel that will not follow Godd's way will be cast into the lake of fire forever and forever. If you take the path of Lucifer being evil toward Godd in Heaven, then you must contend with the fact that there is no indication of how long Lucifer previously existed in Heaven and that when you get to Heaven you may find angels tempting you as poor old dead Eve was tempted by an angel. Heaven must therefore be capable of possessing evil and having the consequences of said evil applied to said evil doers. With that freshly in your mind, I say Heaven is no different than Sheol, and that you can be cast out of Heaven after arriving. Otherwise, no free will and you end up "transformed" as in 12 billion voice mails in Heaven all reciting "Glory to Godd in the highest", and is that what Godd wants? He could create creatures to do that, right out of the blue. Thus I continue to worry that although we will be transformed upon entering Heaven, we will remain with free will and thus I now fear for my future behavior or thoughts as well.

508. Our beliefs in Old Testament stated slavery, isthmian injustice toward other humans, etc. (Exodus 21:1-10, 21, 22, 32) has no bearing on what Godd believes, does, dreams, or would of liked to have happened but maybe he couldn't figure out how to do it with physical life and DNA so we are just plain screwed. Humans are more human than Godd and that stupid statement makes actual sense as a verbal dependency relationship because Godd will never know by virtue of not being able to give physical birth to a genetic replica or by self-stimulation during phallic phantasticus have an orgasm of which are traits he gave us to deal with or to use as natural drugs to self-medicate. We get into a herd mentality to cooperate with each other enough not to kill or enslave every opposing tribal member we meet but Godd never appeared to be able to do that from what I read in the Bible (Numbers 25:10-18). Although when it comes to mankind against womantype, there will never be a consensus because of the issuant isomerous sex organs and Godd saw to that when he altered our genetics on mankind's and womantype's retreat from Eden. Man will stalk the woman and the womyn will steal the man's human-children and money, is what Godd meant to state.

509a. Godd of the Old Testament clearly suffers from earth-rage combined with all the power of the universe. There is no clear reason why Godd would behave the way he does other than there is not a reason for everything in the universe, nor a purpose for everything. Any being with a vision of all infinity that doesn't anticipate the human's actions and then changes his mind as though every event around him takes him by surprise, cannot be counted on to be reliable. As I wish to establish the true nature of Godd, we already have heard enough about his love; etc. (because Christians tend to dwell on only such thoughts of Godd) so you should look at contrasting actions, the type that action movies are made of. Besides, these stories of Godd's anger are awesome, and I would have paid closer attention in CCD if my lesson book had pictures of thousands of humans gagging and choking to death on quail! I can picture it now as Godd's chosen clutch their throats and look upward toward Godd and plead while dying, "We only wanted a dinner of meat after all these years of eating bread". But I'm behaving as a human-child, so check Num 11:18 through 34 or so, and follow it by Mat

7:11 for contrast. I suppose they will tell me I am missing something in those events, but I think not!

509b. My axioms only describe the limits of universal knowledge not the reason existence is here or there or everywhere except where it's not. Godd behaves according to his character and that is how I will accept him - why believe in phables of Godd? There is no reason to ever say, "Godd works in mysterious ways" because Godd is documented with behavior similar to my human father, not the perfection of life on the earth, but we had a dandy time of our human-childhood, and sometimes we got belted for no good reason. I also believe that as with your human holidays that evolve every two generations, the belief of what Godd is like with regards to Christianity, personality-wise, changes constantly because why would you behave any different with your religious thoughs than your other beliefs? There are always new trends and fads, and always someone to follow them.

Onward to a clearer understanding

510. There is such a thing as a depressor (one who causes depression as opposed to pushing down ones tongue) and a depressee (one who becomes depressed via the actions of the depressor). Whether you have uni-polar, manic-depression, or are plain depressed at some moment of our eternity, the actions of the humans around you may affect the degree of depression in your life but it's not their fault. In the general delusions of life, *Hosapiens* allow their minds to fill the physical time with trivial events that are created as fast as their inuring boredom overcomes them – different than the thoughts of the distractions *Homaniakos* use to avoid seeing the clearer vision of reality.

From canoe jumping to *Beanie-Babies* the fun never stops because stopping wouldn't be fun. It matters not what you do at all, only that you do it all.

5 1 1 . As humans are all around me I can't help but to look at their faces and stare into their eyes. I want to see if they are buying into all the contrived events of distractions constructed for their pleasure. I figure, but can't prove, that I will find the *Homaniakos* in the crowds because there are empty eyes to see for certain. I see those faces with fake smiles that aren't getting into the distractions because they too have become inured to so many repeated events. Year after year the magnitude or amplitude changes as society becomes richer in my crowd, but if you look closely you see eyes that reveal dissatisfaction or rather no satisfaction because contrived events do not satisfy the genes. So many humans are role-playing for the benefit of the younger humans that haven't learned that any of this means nothing I guess. Everyone says, "That was great" but I feel what they mean to say, is "Help me Jesus, I am lost", but perhaps that is only a transference of thoughts. I don't know what I see in your eyes but it worries me because I will be of no help to you.

5 1 2 . Now, why all the metaphorical psychotical rambling in the chapter devoted to a devalued god? Because the manimal by reason of his/her sanity self-proclaimed has seen to it and for it that s/he serves Godd in buffet style portions. Take what you like, and don't eat your vegetables. Two helpings of desert because it tastes better than bitter herbs and unleavened bread. The holy days, now holidays whether Godd is there or not, are another contrived event and are the worst for wear because of the nature of humans as a beast. In being Christian we avoid being

Jewish like-ish but we shouldn't toss out the baby with bath water as entertaining as that may be.

Christos Mass and other þhables

513. You definitely have it all wrong but I don't expect you to change your ways, whys, or wisdom concerning the þunctual observance of the holiday extraordinare esþecially when Xmas is a þarty that has been vouched for by the holy rollers. Why not invite the Easter Bunny to your manger recreation where the þhables are as lucid as any reality, as if a god shows uþ for the observance. Now Xmas, as many would disdain that sþelling which aþþears as a modern deþartment store syntax jerkoff, is actually a þroþer historical Greek "X" for Khristos your saviour and that is oh so boring of a fact. So if you are inclined to follow the crowd as your genetics drive you to do, you most likely [sic] believe in the holiness of Christ's mass or at least you believe; "What can I be sent to hell for if I do it anyway?"

514. Now most are willing to admit that one or two or maybe 666 þagan þreceþts have snucked into our original þure, set uþ by mankind, observance of Christ's birthday. Surely its a day to celebrate should that day or month, or year ever be revealed by Godd hid it on þurþose from humans like you don't get it [A trilogram]. All that [*Suggestion: "that entire"*] aside it is most definitely a þack of lies that if we take Godd for his true self we wouldn't mess with man's idea that can send us to Hell if we so believe and bend those knees at the wrong time. As I study my theology and history and watch all of the humans, I can't see where they get these þarties. There is a reason their Xmas is so frustrating and troubled, because it isn't from Godd for certain –

none of it is, not even the thought of it! "Get Christ out of Xmas" is what their signs should state, and then maybe their selfish party will be more mentally relaxing. I remain as passive as possible during the season to keep my remaining wits about me, but I sit and watch and listen in total disbelief that I could ever be so delusional as ordinary humans again. I want you to walk up to your church's holy man and ask him for verification that this holy day is what it is from day zero with Jesus' verification. The ordinary human's belief in phables pushes me from wanting to be ordinary of mind and thus look at the two choices I have left to me. Could it be that all the depression during the Xmas season is because so many humans subconsciously know the truth to it, and they try to hide the truth to the lie with what they can buy - thus we can't be bought with presents into it?

515. I propose a new reason to drop the hot potato I am placing in your hands before you open another much sought after Wal-Mart gift certificate from under the tree of endless papers that wrap your genetic hoarding needs. What is the correct emotional response for humans such as you and even I on the morning of the warning? If you are inclined to follow me, then Christ was born in a predicable and avoidable blood bath of massacred babies. For Christ later in his life did nothing by giving up a body he didn't own but borrowed from someone that then was never born, having stolen at least half of someone's chromosomes. Xmas was born in a blood bath of murdered baby boys, apparently known beforehand by Godd. (You'll have to check all the Bible verse's yourself as I have erased them all from my files out of the fear that my computer will store the words of Godd overwriting images of deleted Internet porn. I don't know

how Godd is going to respond to all this technology of what is real and that which is virtual?)

516. Godd continues to show his true nature when surprising his chosen people he killed the human-male babies as they slept in the arms of the only creature that can truly feel love on the earth, a human-parent. (And if only I could be held again as a human-child in the arms of its mother, I would only cry in sadness for an eternity filled with the joy of it.) All of this murder was to hide the escape of his chosen newborn son to a place of safekeeping in Egypt. If you refuse to believe who is in charge and universally responsible then I suggest you go and get a new Job. Godd blindsides us, killing us from behind and thus we have limited free will (Deuteronomy 2: 30-36) as Godd sticks his hand in the pudding without us understanding the spiritual logic as in the actions as documented throughout the Bible. Read on as I angrily continue to erase more blank pages.

517. Never say Merry Christmas to me. I still have visions of the massacre of innocents that bought my choice of being saved or not and do I honor those murdered babies by taking the gift they gave to me of eternal life? The righteous angels of Godd bound the hands of babies so that the Roman soldiers could put cold steel through their innocent hearts. Do angels cry? Can blood stain a spirits gown? Were we created for the physical death at the hands of a Godd that never really lived or died and from what I can surmise, never cried? A Godd that leaves even his believers in anguish because we really can't achieve his knowledge of the second life - there are not enough clues and the messages are all screwed. Merry Christmas is a fake and the murdered babies chosen by Godd to die for Christ prove it.

5 1 8. Of all the good Christians that are worried about their human-children participating in Halloween or whatever, you had better look at your Christmas and Easter customs and where they come from, for I listened and watched and heard the excuses and have heard it all and what's the difference I ask of you my fine reader friend? When it comes to parties and presents and fun and food and stuff that is not work of the ordinary type you humans are masters of creating all the right holidays and believing by conversing in that contrived language of yours, that you must be correct. Yet I feel that were I capable of ordinary human thoughts, I would strive to find the truth of what Godd wants and not serve mankind and womantype so eagerly. Alas, I spend my time treading water equalizing the duality of my mind only so that I can say it is worth it to get up, or get dressed, or to see what tomorrow will bring. As my book draws to a close, I am weary after four years of typing and sitting in this cold dark box to make a buck or two, and as I loose track of what I am doing all of this for I don't have the time to mess with ordinary human's affairs, so you are on your own to examine your imagined truths and phabled beliefs, and "Party on" is what I say, because I do not believe trivial events will answer my questions, but please don't forget to invite me to your parties, I need the distractions. Live your life blindly without giving too much thought to anything at all, plan your days until your days are gone and I'll stop by for a drink or a chat or to figure my next attack.

Revelation (a true dream, 1995)

5 1 9. As my mood heightens, the clearer vision of reality descends upon me and all the sights of the physical universe are revealed to me as the most wonderful vision ever seen. The universe moves and changes as if it is life itself. Its glory is there to be revealed to all of the *Homaniakos* that have the ability to understand the clearer vision of reality. Now the universe asks of me to write what I see and feel that I should declare what is now, and what is to be later. So I wrote the following: To the Manic-depressive Junkies, I understand the pain of living. You must search for the cause of your pain within the understanding of the requirements of the physical life. To all the *Homaniakos* of an even temperament, be faithful to your brethren of a like mind. To those who have died in the depths of despair, I give you my respect for your strength of mind to take an action when that action is figured by logic to be a means to an end. To those of us that are unable to control the moods, the violence, the pain, and the loneliness of the mind, seek help wherever that help may be found - do no harm to other humans. To those who have lost a soul or a love to the pain of reality, you must only wait and all suffering will end in its appointed time. To the *Hosapiens*, the ordinary humans, I understand your fear of the unknown mind of the *Homaniakos*, for I fear your mind also. What other than ordinary thoughts would you expect to know? Then suddenly a feeling came over me and caused me to see with my minds eye. Behold, I saw myself standing at the foundation of the universe and all of its self-made glory stretched out before me. The universe was larger than its self - but I could see the whole vastness of it. It is without end, as we understand beginnings and endings. It would take forever to travel the length of it, for the end could never be reached or found. Within the expanse of it, there was no physical proof of love to be seen or sensed, thus the universe beyond our minds is empty of human emotions whether you are alive or dead. For those that have the knowledge, let them calculate the number that represents the demon, as so many of the Homaniakos know of it. That number is zero divided by infinity; emptiness divided by forever - the loneliness of the manic-depressive mind. Knowing that number is the end of knowledge. Then I saw our sun, and all its energy, and from within the sun comes the source of our life. The sun spoke and its information was sensed only as "life". Around our sun were countless numbers of other suns, called stars. Each star was moving in its apparent motion - as the ordinary humans see them only with their eyes - but it is within my mind that I sense their existence. The universe then became dark, for such is the matter of the universe. The universe hides its life, or rather the source of its actions, within the smallness of its vastness. The universe then took the source of its existence and hid it within the depths of its greatest physical self, far from the senses of all humans. Thus no human will ever know of its birth, birth place, or even its death. Then I saw greatness in the smallest pieces. Energy surrounding energy, onto countless particles of matter made up of a million colors of energy, invisible to physical eyes, stretching outward for what appears to be infinity, for all of the universe is of touching to itself - not of empty space. And all the matter was equal, and all the matter was energy, and all the energy was equal, and all the energy existed outside of the universe that we sense, for we are not born with all the senses required to know of all things in existence. When I reached outward to touch it, the universe stopped for a moment. An intensity that caused all matter to exist appeared to me as a vision within a vision. Then the vision within a vision disappeared and the universe was in motion again. But I am unable to describe from the vision within a vision the substance of the intensity, for it is not as anything now known nor ever seen by the ordinary

humans, thus no language has been contrived to describe it. Then
I saw into the depth of the universe, which is to say into our future,
and there appeared a perturbation. That perturbation
approaches the earth even now, and when it will pass through the
earth, the earth will shake and lightening will fall. This
perturbation is the heartbeat of the universe, and it gives all life to
the physics of the universe. As the universe exists, it cares not for
the events of living creatures, thus its actions will harm the order of
life on the earth, but the universe does not do this by deliberate
action. The universe will destroy the works of the human animal as
it follows the nature of its own natural order. The humans will be
busy about their own affairs the day universe reclaims the earth
for its own use. The order of the earth cannot be preserved by
the will of the humans or of the motions of the universe. As I have
written, the truth of the universe has been revealed. For each
human, their final day is near, but they do not live each day as
such. The universe showed me those that would join it by their
own will, but no living human will ever feel as a part of the universe.
The universe takes all of existence for its own use, for it does not
understand life or the emotions of life. The universe could not tell
me of any great plan or purpose, for it has no need of knowing
such things, only that it is here now for us to sense, but that was
not always true, nor will it be true in the future. I was shown a
universe without life, yet it grows old; without love, but it needs no
love to exist; without time, but it does not understand time. Slowly
I fell into a sleep and I had a dream filled with wonders like no other
dream ever dreamed. The universe appeared to me in this dream,
from one endless end to the other, and every star and planet and
every piece of matter was visible, and it was more beautiful than life
and more wonderful than love. I saw and felt its existence, but it
was without a sound for the human ear. All information was given

to me in a single moment and my mind was aware of all knowledge and I was finally at rest. All purposes and functions were revealed to me and all of my pain was gone, and I felt no loneliness while being a part of the universe within my dream. Then I realized that I am the universe and that after death I will be at home in the universe forever, and no longer lonely. The universe is my father and my mother, and all my human-children are of the universe also. So forever after death we will exist within the universe without sensing time or pain or loneliness. Within my dream the universe asked of me (without it using words) to tell it of the emotions in the mind of the humans, for the universe allows such abilities within the humans, but it cannot feel them. So I dreamed of love, for that is what all humans, ordinary or not, need above all else, and that is what the universe will never feel. After I awoke from my dream, I wrote what I had seen for you my reader friend, and I wrote the following story of love for the universe: I'm lost within a mind that itself is lost within the perceptions of the real universe. What can I say that will explain the pain of the visions, except that I want to be loved and I want to feel love again? Where is the fulfillment of my little boy dreams of those future moments, now here, but not here as once imagined? I feel the infinity of time, and those feelings cause me to wish for an eternity of life filled with love forever. I wish to stare into blue within blue eyes while speaking gentle words of love. I am so lonely within my mind, the loneliness of the manic-depressive mind, the mind that is always "on" and the thoughts never stop, and death fills every thought, and in dreaming I dream of future times, filled with death and loneliness without ever knowing love again. How can humans feel or remember love without the touch of another's hand or without lips touching lips, as I can't seem to remember the feelings or the joy of once being only an ordinary human? How do the humans live each day, or want to live each day without the feelings of love as extreme as only a Manic-depressive Junkie could feel for someone - but who would return love to me? Many humans are so lonely or so lost within the understanding of life, or so lost without the voice of another's love. I see visions within their staring eyes, empty eyes and emotionless faces, waiting or searching to hear these words from someone: "I will love you and only you, forever and beyond forever."

Pre-conclusion

520. So now this book is finished and I must tell you that we all behave Godd-like and don't even think of the similarities, genetic motivations, and that perhaps even though Godd is not physical, his idea of creation was not far from what he was familiar with in his own type of hyped existence. You are as pure as Godd is, every one of you is, and made of planet and star stuff also. So how much more of the universe can you be within the pages of published new-age bullshit? Our lives are only an extension of the resurrected while mimicking his emotions and thus his behavior using physical stuff instead of Heavenly fluff. Look at what we surround ourselves with, for certain that is where our mind is at, and thus so are our gene driven *needs* (you might define as "*desires*"). Are you ready to buy into my imagined human mind and real body of a genetic action and reaction? Our thoughts must be true for how can we constantly lie to ourselves when thoughts translate into an action? Thus genetics rule all life and you won't learn that in school in this decade past or in future decades to come.

521. Maybe it wasn't such a big leap of logic for a god to create all of this existence and biological life with its emotions and imperfections. Everything that we see, that your god has created, is imperfect and disintegrating around us at every moment and yet this god proclaims he will build it perfect, the next time. Would that be the big plan: to create the naturally occurring slum for humans to compare Godd's better home and gardens too? Are we to be jealous of Godd's home and the greener grass on the other side of the fence of existence? Is that all there is to this god's big plan? That I should say this life, so short, is not enough for me and I am not thankful for the few moments lusting after the age of innocence? Why can't I choose, with documented permission from Godd, door number 3 - nothingness after death?

Conclusion incognito

522. Every book needs a conclusion and as track #3 is queuing up again I continue to write in the misery of it. Based on my readings of the Bible, my writings of the most basic knowledge of the physical realm, and the most basic knowledge about the human animal, I am willing to re-interpret our god as a being that is at best, every human attribute projected within an existence that we can't define. A being that has caused, because of a few actions on its part, normal predictable genetic reactions within a human animal that claims to understand the universe itself, but can't understand its own self. Those reactions combined with the unavoidable genetic trait of the human's need to imitate each other, and thus acquire memes, creates a god of perfection and pure love out of a human-type spirit being living in a place called Heaven or within the heaven of your mind I suspect. Optimum procreation creates a need to continue living forever only to meet the genetic drive of continued procreation. The creation of an unnatural religious system by the humans has proven that complexity causes complexity as Jesus is filtered though our changing technologies that change our willful need for a belief in a god and the belief's in how we must be obedient to his commandments. The life of Jesus fits within the attributes of becoming impregnated and the birth of a son. The pre-dispositions of tribal and clannish behavior are seeds to create the figure of a leader – the leader of the humans. Humans have appointed this being to be the tribal chief. Thus the tribal chief becomes the final word that if any humans go against, [they] are punished whether they are wrong or not. NIV, Luke 2: 14, "Glory to God in the highest, and on the earth peace to men on whom his favor rests". Do not judge your chief, your boss, your bowling team leader, your government, your father, or your god, right or wrong. Humans can't smell their own noses and I suppose that is why ordinary humans will never see past the delusion.

523. Add to the above, the *Four Axioms of Existence*, and is having a god so important to any actual purpose or goal within the universe? Because perhaps in all this self-created mental mess and metal technology, there is actually no purpose to anything and no goal achieved by you, my fine reader friend that will matter within the blink of a universal eye. Now I give you the final axiom, Axiom #1: "Nothing Matters." When you truly believe Axiom #1 for only one moment, and you if can see the clearer vision of reality at that moment and feel the infinite pain it brings, Logical Death is the only action remaining to shed this physical skin that needs to sin.

524. If anyone misquotes for slanderous reasons, adds too or deletes from this book of knowledge, or creates a copyright infringement; then all the curses of the lawyers mentioned in this book will be upon you. Behold, I put thoughts into your mind while you sleep at night. I offer you no hope. I am the beginning and the ending of your nightmares. I am *Homaniakos*.

525. As for myself, I wish all the humans of this planet with no name, to have satisfaction for their 15 minutes of fame and peace within the heaven of their mind's creation.

Closing thoughts

526. I will close this chapter with these thoughts. What I have not mentioned in this book of my life, needs, and thoughts, I have done with complete intention. Only perceptions sensed are real, and the description of them starts the lies. For my *Homaniakos* brethren, keep your eyes forward and direct if you should decide to reveal your true self, for your eyes see farther and deeper into life and death than that of the ordinary humans. Believe in your true self. You are greater than any of the *Hosapiens* would want you to believe. Create your world around your reality, not theirs. You have abilities that are unimaginable by ordinary humans. Set your goals, set your schedules, and use the clearer vision of reality to enhance your perceptions of this life and beyond death. Respect those *Homaniakos* that have gone before us - stay alive.

527. Beware of false manics.

THE MOST BASIC KNOWLEDGE OF THE PHYSICAL REALM:

The Four Axioms of Existence:

Axiom #4
"No living entity can have a greater understanding of its existence, than the physical ability to act on it."

Axiom #3
"Nothing in existence has more significance than anything else in existence."

Axiom #2
"Nothing can be completely understood."

Axiom #1
"Nothing matters."

The only purpose of all living organisms:
"Optimum procreation"

Most basic law of nature:
[As expressed in a human language]
"What can be, is. What cannot be, isn't."

Most basic law of unnatural systems:
"Complexity causes complexity"

THE MOST BASIC KNOWLEDGE ABOUT THE HUMAN ANIMAL:

Genetic behavioral motivators of human males:
"The Birth of a Son"
"The Hunt"
"The Kill"

Genetic disposition of human males:
"Tribal"

Genetic behavioral motivators of human females:
"Becoming Impregnated"
"Territorial Possessiveness"

Genetic disposition of human females:
"Clannish"

528. You have now completed CHAPTER GODD, please turn the page and proceed to CHAPTER MANIC-DEPRESSION.

REFERENCES, DICTIONARY, FURTHER READING, QUOTES, LIES, AND NONSENSE

PREFATORY

V>"Black holes, as Hawking tells it, are rips in the fabric of space and time so dense and distorted by unimaginable gravitational forces that for years physicists believed nothing could escape from one, including light. They are thus, by definition, invisible." Page 60. Quote source: The Book: *Stephen Hawking's Universe* by John Boslough, Published by Quill, 1985.

V>Meme. A unit of cultural transmission. A thought that replicates among humans by its own compulsion to do so. Source: *The Meme Machine* written by Dr. Susan Blackmore, Publisher, Oxford University Press, 1999.

iV>Intelli-genetics. A combination of intelligence and genetics such that the genetics of the animal determines the cognitive reactions possible, by RJH. Not to be confused with "No hay nada como ésto en ningún lugar excepto el sistema experto StrataGene de $50.000 de IntelliGenetic's." *The Gene Construction Kit* by Textco. Source: www.drtomorrow.com/spanish/X0016_Capitulo_09.html.

iii>Race. Refer to *Ever Since Darwin* by Stephen Jay Gould, Publisher, Norton, 1977, See Chapter 29, *Why We Should Not Name Human Races-A biological View.*

iii>Race. Refer to: *The Book of Wonders* by Presbrey Syndicate, Inc. 1917, page 537, "What you eat determines your color, according to Bergfield, a German investigator."

ii>Homo sapiens maniakos. A taxonomical[*sp?*] description of a manic-depressive.

ii>Homo sapiens sapiens, Ordinary Humans. A taxonomical[*sp?*] description of a human with only ordinary mental abilities. The most common and populous human specie.

i>Clanging. A preference for word or sentence "sound" as opposed to thought content. But since nothing communicated via contrived language can really reveal the truth, why not entertain yourself with the noise of it?

i>Distractions are a requirement of the *Homaniakos*. Getting to the end of a thought is not as important as getting to the next thought. Why would that be considered a negative trait?

i>Logic is an interpretive study. There can be no baseline for any deduced thoughts or interpretation of the sensed events of reality.

i>Thought disorder is a major revealing characteristic of the *Homaniakos* species from what I can ascertain. Ordinary humans consider the *Homaniakos* to be mentally ill because they believe it is we that have delusions about life.

CHAPTER MANIC-DEPRESSION

9>The second set of 10 commandments are not as the first set. These are possibly older than the first set of commandments. Contrast Exodus 20:1-17 as the first commandments and Exodus 34:15-26 as the second set. Contrast 34:1 and 34:27. As a good reference see: www.positiveatheism.org/hist/lewis/lewten03.htm by Joseph Lewis.

11>*A Clockwork Orange*. Movie, *A Clockwork Orange* directed by Stanley Kubrick, A book written by Anthony Burgess. Topic: Violence and its treatment within the contemporary society of the 1960's. With backward motion you find out how to kill 20 hours a day. Besides who else can lead you to a space odyssey?

11>Cesare Pavese, from an undocumented source. Italian writer wrote *A mania for solitude*.

11>Photon: A piece of light or a light ray.

11>Regnated: Not a word.

13>Neologism: "a meaningless word coined by a psychotic." Internet Source: ©*2002 by Merriam-Webster, Incorporated.* "Neologism, either invented words or familiar words given strangely new meanings...", Source: *Abnormal Psychology* by Peter Mckellar, Publisher Routledge, 1989.

13>Conjugates: Not a word in descriptive English. Used in algebra as "Complex conjugate."

13>Detracted: Not a word.

13>Facial expressions and hand gestures: Jana Iverson, Ph.D. at the University of Missouri reports hand gestures are not learned but fundamental to communication. Source: *Psychology Today* magazine 2000 (Who the hell cares what month?). See "How to be a mind reader (and tell what people REALLY think of you)." Source: *Daily Mail*, Friday, January 19, 2001 (A British Newspaper).

13>Hyperversion: Not a word.

13>Interrobangalated: From interrobang. A question mark on an explanation point, I think?

14> "Deep Thought". The name of the computer from *Hitchhiker's guide to the Galaxy* Novel by Douglas Adams (1981mini series). Source IMDb. Quote from the movie; Slartibarfast: "Perhaps I'm old and tired, but I always think the chances of finding out what really is going on are so absurdly remote that the only thing to do is to say 'Hang the sense of it' and just keep yourself occupied."

21> "Talk all you like if it makes you happy", Movie quote: *Fahrenheit 451*. 1966. Book by Ray Bradbury, I don't know, I lost my notes on this one so I am going by memory.

24>*Zanti Misfits*, 1963 title from *The Outer Limits* written by Joseph Stefano. MGM TV show. Source: www.sciencefiction.com/outerlimits/o114.htm. Also a book by John Peel, Publisher, Mass Market Paperback, 1997, source: www.amazon.com.

24> Abby Normal. Dr. Frankenstein: "Would you mind telling me whose brain I did put in?" Igor: "And you won't be angry?" Dr. Frankenstein: "I will NOT be angry." Igor: "Abby someone." Dr. Frankenstein: "Abby someone? Abby who?" Igor: "Abby Normal." From movie *Young Frankenstein*. Quote source IMDb.

26>Virus. Life that grows once it is inside of a host cell. It is only "alive" once it is in the host cell.

26>Bacteria. Single cell life. *The Britannica Concise, 2000.* If I might add my remark, I believe they or some of them reproduces by Binary fission (asexual). Maybe I'm wrong.

26>Genotype. The genetic constitution of an organism. Determines hereditary potentials. ©*2000 by Merriam-Webster, Incorporated and Encyclopaedia Britannica, Inc.*

28>Advice found on Internet FAQ sites for manic-depressives: Being passive and agreeing with your psychologist is the best method of getting out of there without having your drug use altered.

29>Lithium. Used for treating mania and hypomanic (highs). I've heard that the side effects include death.

29>Prozac. An antidepressant (lows). I've heard that the side effects include death (also suicide).

30>Concerning the drugging of humans to induce the perception of ordinary behavior. See source *CNN.com health*, Topic: Children, February 26, 2001, quote: "In addition to Ritalin, more young children are also taking clonidine, a blood pressure drug used to treat sleep problems stemming from attention disorders, and antidepressants such as Prozac."

30>Movie quote: *Fahrenheit 451,* 1966. "The only way to be happy is for everyone to be made equal." Book by Ray Bradbury.

31>I offer no proof that our sun will die in 1 billion years.

32>Asbestos causes lung cancer.

32>Breeder Reactors create nuclear materials as they use them. "It is possible to use the plentiful, nonfissile uranium-238 isotope as a reactor fuel by 'breeding' fissile plutonium-239 from it by bombardment with neutrons." Quote source: *Breeder Reactors.* Lecture-Discussion #22. Nuclear Engineering 201: *Advanced Energy Systems.* Professor David N. Ruzic. 1996, 1997, 1998 www.starfire.ne.uiuc.edu/ne201/course/topics/breeder_reactors/.

32>DDT shows up in mother's milk and is poison to animal life.

32>The vaccination of humans allows resistant strains of viruses to propagate.

33>See the TV *Twilight Zone* Episode *Number 12: Looks Just Like You* (1963-1964 season) written by Charles Beaumont. Everyone gets to be made as flawless clones of each other. source: www.scifi.com/twizone/season5.html.

39>*Steinfeld* is a TV program about a comedian and his friends; circa 1990's.

41>From the movie *A funny thing happened on the way to the forum,* 1966. Hero: "For us there will never be happiness." Philia: "We must be happy without it." Quote source: IMDb.

41>Drug treatment is wanted by some Manic-depressives or required for some, but don't compluse me to be out of my mind because of some type of ultimate altruism on your part.

42>Refer to *Scientific American, Exploring Intelligence,* Winter 1998 Vol. 9 No. 4, for supporting studies on my view that humans "look" for animals that have visual triggers and then assign intelligence or behavior attributes to them. See *Talking with Alex* by Irene M. Pepperberg and *Can Animals Empathize?* By Gordon Gallup, Jr. and Daniel J. Povinelli. I remain with my conclusions that humans by nature see what they believe and logic or the truth will not interfere with that behavior.

42>"Keep them busy and you keep them happy." Movie quote: *Fahrenheit 451,* 1966. Book by Ray Bradbury. If you're not coming here from #136, ignore this message. You better wind your clock. Who can lead you from here to number 11?

46>The news media is quick to state "suffering from depression" during any violent actions reported, but the type of depression may not be reported, thus the confusion of *Hosapiens* and *Homaniakos* traits continues. The study shows that ordinary humans with depression have greater anxiety over Bi-polars. Source: *Manic-depressive Illness* by Frederick K. Goodwin and Kay Redfield Jamison, Publisher Oxford University Press, 1990. Extra, Extra, read all about it, see page 285 of that book. Thus as I state, violence toward other humans is most likely an ordinary human trait during depression.

47>"10 signs of suicide" is a generalization by myself. "On the other hand, the general suicide literature, despite its staggering size, offers relatively little guidance for the management of suicidal patients. The guidance that is available is often more speculative than empirical, and it is not particularly relevant to the study and prevention of suicide in manic-depressive illness." Quoted from the source: *Manic-Depressive Illness* by Frederick K. Goodwin and Kay Redfield Jamison, Publisher Oxford University Press, 1990. Page 227.

47>*Suicide Prevention.* See the article in the section titled, "Science and the Citizen", Neurobiology, page 18 of Scientific American magazine, Special Report, March 1997, Volume 276, Number 3. Quote: "Even so, individual suicides are exceedingly difficult to predict. Indeed, a recent survey showed that although roughly half of all suicide victims visit clinicians during the 90 days preceding their death, only a quarter receive any psychiatric treatment." Also, "...the researchers guess that serotonin signaling in the brains of suicidal individuals is inadequate."

47>"I have a message for you - a very sad message!" is a direct line from the recording, *It's in the book* by Johnny Standley. I don't' have a year for this, but my parents had the 45 (speed) record that I used to listen to as a human-child. Now I have the mp3 file, of which how do I pass that on as an antique?

49>Suicidal Intent Revealed. From the book *Manic-Depressive Illness* by Frederick K. Goodwin and Kay Redfield Jamison, Publisher Oxford University Press, 1990, page 240, "Patients who commit suicide generally communicate their intentions to others." "...estimated that 80 percent of people who commit suicide had communicated their intent to kill themselves." "....usually directly." "Suicidal potential most frequently was expressed to spouses and other relatives ... then to friends... and to physicians...", "The high rate of communication of suicidal ideas indicates that in the majority of instances it is a premeditated act of which the person gives ample warning." So as an experiment, I indicated a suicidal intent to my best friend, who just got quiet for a moment, to a psychiatrist who did exhibit a look of concern for a moment, and then to one of my proofreaders who then stated that I appeared out of my normal mood. I E-mailed a friend that I had put all my "after death" instructions into envelopes for my family, and that I had placed my suicide note in an envelope labeled, "CONTENTS: ONE (1) STANDARD - SUICIDE NOTE - OPEN AT YOUR OWN RISK. There was no remark. Thus in my book I write: "Plans are made into great detail - time and place, what method to use, music to play, and the verbalized note becomes a record to leave for the living fools who couldn't understand the signals you gave them for months and months, so thus you will now do it and they will learn their lesson well after seeing your dead body." What are the ordinary humans to do? Bury my body - as one of the Beatles once stated.

50>"Suicidal fantasy" is the proper term for an attempted suicide.

50>The description of the suicide fantasy in this paragraph is from my actual life experiences.

51>"A thousand deaths" is from the source: www.1000deaths.com. Quoting from this source: "The person who completes suicide dies once. Those left behind die a thousand deaths, trying to relive those terrible moments and understand, 'why?' ". I define this statement as proving the ordinary human's lack of logic or their understanding of true reality. This mentality is an insult to the logical death of the *Homaniakos* species.

51>"Survivor rights" is from the source:

http://members.tripod.com/~LifeGard/ssrights.html. This site has a list of suicide loss rights but only deals with the remaining living as if they have done something to deserve attention. Quoting from the site: "Experiencing suicide loss is a disorienting and disruptive life experience." Also see the source, ABCNews.com March 18, 2002, *Dignity in Death?* By Dean Schabner. Concerning Doctor-Assisted suicide as an assault on the terminally ill. Quote: "Allowing doctors to prescribe lethal doses of drugs to terminally ill patients who say they want them strips whose people of their dignity, rather than providing them with a dignified option for ending their lives,...".

53>"AIM" is an acronym for: Awareness, Intervention, and Methodology by the U.S. Surgeon General Dr. David Satcher. Source: www.surgeongeneral.gov/library/calltoaction/calltoaction.htm.

53>Lucid. A dream whereby the dreamer (dreamee) can mentally control the thoughts within the dream.

53>"Span" is an acronym for: Suicide Prevention Advocacy Network. This group believes they can join the efforts of all suicide prevention groups.

53>The quilt in this refers to a quilt made in remembrance of humans dead from suicide. From the *LifeKeeper National Memory Quilt Project*. From the *LifeKeeper Foundation*. See their Web page: www.LifeKeeper.org. I am not trying to be disrespectful of the dead by self-inflicted means, but I wish to draw attention to several points. First: The faulty logic of the ordinary humans in believing that these quilts will really affect other humans. Second: that they should not "clump" suicides if they ever wish to understand suicide. Third: Anyone who makes a quilt on behalf of the dead will also feel justified in their own suicidal fantasy if they should ever decide that suicide is the only course of action remaining, because the mental image of the "quilt" becomes a focal point of the dead relative. See my reference number 49.

They say, every 17 minutes someone dies of by suicide. I say, every 18 minutes a new suicide prevention advisory group is formed.

55>LSD is Lysergic Acid Diethicamide and it causes hallucinations. The drug of choice of the Hippies of the 1960's.

55>"One pill makes you smaller" is from a song by Grace Slick of the rock group *Jefferson Airplane* referencing the story *Alice in Wonderland* that was written by who cares?

55>Protein. Simply put, a protein yields amino acids, a requirement for life, I guess.

55>Valiums. The drug Diazepam at one time was the most common drug prescribed to the females of The United States. Thought by some to be a "male" conspiracy to keep womantype in their "place".

56>Movie *Logan's Run* starring Michael York. 1976. No one in the movie lives past their 30th birthday as a method of population control by someone or some machine that is in control of the population. It appears as though it was filmed in a shopping mall, but still a great movie.

56>Movie *The Matrix* written/directed by the Wachowski brothers. 1999. Reality is not what it always appears to be. I only own three DVD's now, and this is one of them. You could easily know the other DVD I own, but can you name the third? Not a single reference of any type to the third DVD that I own appears in the chapters of this book, but I had a whole chapter in which to do such.

67>Muellerian mimicry. Both the primary and mimic of a species are poisonous or distasteful. Refer to the Monarch and Viceroy butterflies. Source: Bud Polk, 1998, www.pendulum.org/writings/syphrid_fly.htm.

CHAPTER MYSELF

69>"What, me worry?" A *Mad Magazine*, Alfred E. Neuman quote.

71>Cosmoillogical. Based on cosmological and illogical. A misunderstanding of universal realities as I would use it.

71>Molycule. A feminized molecule. A joke.

74>"And when the sky was opened, worms fell to purge the earth of human flesh. Your destroyer craws under your feet every living day you walk and dream of what you need but you never get." By me. Also see NIV: Isaiah 14:11 "All your pomp has been brought down to the grave, along with the noise of your harps; maggots are spread out beneath you and worms cover you." Parallel thoughts written without prior knowledge caused by genetics ruling the human's unchanging minds, thus how many original thoughts are possible?

78>*George Jetson*. Cartoon character living in the future. By Hanna-Barbara cartoons, 1962-1963. One of the more accurate predictions of the future.

80>Death-hounds. "...is as the howling of a death-hound hunting them out of the air into their graves." Source: www.ccel.org/ *Robert Falconer* by George MacDonald. Part III *His Manhood*, Chapter XI *The Suicide*. I removed the reference text from my book, but I like this reference so I left it here.

81>Cognize. Not a word.

81>Confabulation. A revealing trait of *Korsakoff's* syndrome. Sergei Sergeeuichkorsakoff a Russian neurologist. Source: ©*2000 by Merriam-Webster, Incorporated and Encyclopaedia Britannica, Inc.*

81>Id. In terms of Freud, is the psyche that controls instinctive needs - some would say primitive needs. Quote: "The Id (Latin for 'it') is the primitive, unconscious basis of the psyche dominated by primary urges." From the book, *Freud For Beginners* by Richard Appignanesi and illustrations by Oscar Zarate, Publisher Pantheon Books, 1979.

81>Hynagogic. Psychic or psychotic sleep paralysis, as though an invisible demon was setting upon your chest keeping you from moving once you awake from sleep. Or something totally different from that description.

83>Metonym. Substitution of word with similar or interchangeable meanings. *American Heritage* fourth edition 2000.

83>Schizophrenic or schizophrenia. I would suggest using mescaline if you wish to walk on the other side of interpretive logic. Four types of schizophrenia as reported in *Abnormal Psychology* by Peter McKellar, Publisher Routledge, 1989. Starting on page 207, "Paranoid", "Hebephrenic", "Catatonic", and "Simple." These are all psychoses.

83>"What unknown sights are here! Why should we be unable to preserve a remembrance of them?" Quote from the book: *Twenty Thousand Leagues Under the Sea.* Written by Jules Verne. Chapter 11, *The Sargasso Sea.* I forgot the page number. Try http://jv.gilead.org.il/p9/20000/2/11.html.

83>Hallucination. A perception of objects with no reality usually arising from [a] disorder of the nervous system. Internet Source: ©*2002 by Merriam-Webster, Incorporated.*

84>Delusional (delusion). A persistent false psychotic belief regarding the self or persons or objects outside the self. Internet Source: ©*2002 by Merriam-Webster, Incorporated.*

84>Violence of the son. Actually sounds like, "violence of the sun" from the song *Tales of brave Ulysses*, by Cream.

86>"And I loved every one of them." A painting by Patrick Woodroffe. Reference the book *Hallelujah Anyway* Copyright Dragon's World Ltd. 1984. Page 35. Shows pre-teen girls lifting their skirts in order to reveal their panties.

86>Top 40. A method of charting pop music hits during the 1960's.

88>*American Girl*. Collectable dolls with an outlet store in Chicago that has parties and performances for customers. Several girls and moms died in a fiery train crash in Bourbonnais IL that I viewed a few hours after the crash. Quote: "Naturalists, on the other hand, have a plausible explanation for pointless suffering: there is no all-good, all-powerful, all-knowing being to intervene and prevent pointless suffering." Source: March 1999 *Internet Infidels Newsletter.* http://www.infidels.org/infidels/newsletter/1999/march.html Feature: "*The Empirical Case for Metaphysical Naturalism.*" by Jeffery Jay Lowder.

89>"I'm not me." Quote by Curly Howard (The Three Stooges), spoken while Curly is dressed in a bear costume. I don't have a clue what movie or episode that came from.

89>"Sharing wet dreams" and "Yesterday's dreams" Words from a song By the group Jethro Tull: *From A Dead Beat To An Old Greaser* 1976 Chrysalis Records Ltd. Written by Ian Anderson. Theme of CD is relevant to thoughts on worthiness of life.

90>*Be a cowboy baby,* Song title by Kid Rock.

90>Youth and "The Cube" is a reference to page 45 of the book, *The Cube: Keep the Secret.* Authors: Annie Gottlieb and Slobodan D. Pesic, Publisher, Harper San Francisco. 1995.

91>Michael was my human-childhood playmate and he died in a car crash prior to signing his divorce papers. I have never gotten over his death and I think of him almost daily.

91>A mpeg (mpg) is a file format used in computers for creating and viewing movie pictures.

106>Sentence in this is a trilogram. Three sentences in one, sharing words for efficiency.

106>Verbigeration. Continual repetition of stereotyped phrases (as in some forms of mental illness). Internet Source: ©*2002 by Merriam-Webster, Incorporated.*

108> "I enjoy working with people." Quote by HAL the computer from the movie 2001, A Space Odyssey. Movie directed by Stanley Kubrick.

110>Dirted. "Dirt-ed" Having dirt applied and noticeable.

110>Rut, rutting. An annually recurrent state of sexual excitement in the male deer; *broadly*: sexual excitement in a mammal (as estrus in the female) especially when periodic. Internet Source: ©*2002 by Merriam-Webster, Incorporated.*

111>*Twilight Zone.* A Television series hosted by (the late) Rod Sterling during the early 1960's.

CHAPTER CREATIVITY

113>Brass tacks. Carpets used to be held to the floor with brass tacks. The brass wouldn't rust, as steel would have.

114>Serotonin. Chocolate produces serotonin. Serotonin regulates cyclic body processes. See "Melatonin". It is believed that depression is caused by a lack of serotonin.

118>Cyclothymic. "Perhaps more common is to experience periods of energy alternating with periods of passivity, withdrawal and rest - this is the so-called *cyclothymic* temperament." Source: Excerpts from the final draft of: *Psychiatry and the Human Condition* Chapter 10, Mania, by Bruce Charlton MD, Radcliffe Medical Press: Oxford, UK (date unknown) www.hedweb.com/bgcharlton/psychhuman.html.

121>Boustrophedon. The writing of alternate lines in opposite directions (as from left to right and from right to left). Internet Source: ©*2002 by Merriam-Webster, Incorporated.*

124>Moron. Although archaic, it would define a human with poor mental abilities and one that would not grow out of those characteristics.

128> "The usual gang of idiot's." *MAD* magazine quote.

129>"O my brothers" Quote by the character "Alex" from the book, *A Clockwork Orange* written by Anthony Burgess 1962. The book was written in twenty-one chapters but in the United States was it published omitting the 21st chapter. Stanley Kubrick directed the film in England but he also omitted the 21st chapter from the plot. Thus the perception and understanding of the book was based on the reader's geographical location or the language s/he spoke and had little to do with the truth of the book or the intentions of the author. It was biased toward profit.

129>Sailor Moon. A Japanese anime cartoon teenaged girl action hero. One of my favorites, since the Bugs Bunny days are gone.

129>SUV. A Sports Utility Vehicle.

129>Tatteredtood. Multiple tattoos.

130>Master debaters. Feminists (satirical).

130>Read the book *Born under Saturn*. By Rudolf and Margot Wittkower. Publisher, Norton. 1963. The character and conduct of artists.

130>*Maslow's Hierarchy of Needs.* Source: www.connect.net/georgen/maslow.htm. Biological/Physiological needs, Security needs, Social needs, Ego needs are the Hierarchy of needs.

131>Diane Arbus is a photographic artist who committed suicide in 1971 but had actually died much earlier than that. Her photographs reveal the true reality of human life and meaning. See her book(s) of photographs: *Diane Arbus: Untitled.* 1995 edition from www.amazon.com, Publisher, Aperture. As one of the purchasers of this book states in the review section, "The images are grotesque, disturbing, cruel, ugly." and also "These images were made when Arbus's life was spiraling down, when she was more and more lost in her final depression. They provide an insight into her mind that it would have been better not to publish." My own opinion is that viewing these images proves the statement that there is your life before you see a photograph, and then there is what's left of your life afterwards. Don't miss it.

131>Apophenia. Being able to instantly notice connections and meaning of unrelated occurrences. This ability may not have any truth to it, but the human exhibiting this condition perceives it as such.

134> "Stop, Look, and Listen" were words once found on railroad crossing signs prior to electric crossing gates if I am remembering correctly.

135>Canopic jars are for storing a human's soft body tissue after death, of course. (Odyssey Mag. Nov/Dec. 2000. Doug Alexander.)

135>George Jeston was the star of a television cartoon from 1962. The theme song has only 11 words. A futuristic family whereby a hard day at the office consists of pushing one button. This cartoon was thus the most accurate prediction of the future by any fictional work.

136>Body illustrations is another term to describe tattoos.

136>*The Illustrated Man* is a book by Ray Bradbury. The movie was released in 1969 and starred Rod Steiger and Claire Bloom. She also stared in the original 1963 movie *The Haunting* as Theodora with Julie Harris. May I recommend to you the original 1963 release of that movie and not that recent not as good remake. In *The Haunting* is the answer to the great question found in number 42, but who can take you there?

138>Randolph Street Gallery was the location of my only major art exhibit in Chicago in 1985.

139>Being your own test subject would be difficult to validate on a casual interpretation of it, and impossible to do if you take the absolute reality of all facts. I guess an interpretation of Gödel's theory could apply here. Poorly stated, you can't make a map of the universe because that map would have to have a map of the universe in it.
Try www.miskatonic.org/godel.html for starters.

144>82 billion years is a time span not confirmed for the time to the death of the universe. In fact I made it up. The universe may continue to expand without gravity to stop it, or there may be a "repelling" force, yet unknown, that could be pushing everything away. Who cares?

144>Rebar or re-bar: Metal bars made of scrap iron used to strengthen concrete structures.

144>".25 level syncretistic response" I found these categories in the book, *Manic-Depressive Illness* by Frederick K. Goodwin and Kay Redfield Jamison, Publisher Oxford University Press, 1990, pages 250 and 251. They list a source from the American Medical Association, copyrighted 1987, *Archives of General Psychiatry*.

144>*The Anthropic Cosmological Principle*. A book written by Barrow and Tipler. Publisher, Oxford 1986. It explores the relationship of space, time, and the appearance of the universe with life with regards to the age of the universe.

145>Random events or sounds must be interpreted by the cause or actuator of the event, not the observance or sensing of the result of the event.

148>Freud had some interesting theories about human nature and most are based on natural human functions such as sex or orifice awareness. Quote: "Ego development is imprinted by the instinctual structure of the libido (mouth, anus, genitals). In other words, self-awareness and bodily activity develop together." Source: *Freud For Beginners* by Richard Appignanesi and Oscar Zarate, page 156.

148>Pamphilos, A Greek, c. 390-340 BC. A painter that was trained in arithmetic and geometry of which he stated was necessary in order to be an artist. Source: *Born Under Saturn*, By Rudolf and Margot Wittkower, Publisher The Norton Library, 1963. Pages 2 and 3.

149>Bastard cursive hands are writing styles indicating no style or a variety of styles.

149>Graphologists are hand-writing experts (for human handwriting).

149>Split Brain Humans. "...the mute brain hemisphere was able to answer questions by taking action, although it could not report to the speaking (aware) brain half." Quote from: *Experience, awareness and consciousness: suggestions for definitions as offered by an evolutionary approach.* By Mario Vaneechoutte, University Hospital, Ghent, Belgium. See the source: www.allserv.rug.ac.be/~mvaneech/EAC.html.

150>*Cube Of The Infinite Reversed* is a title of an artwork by me.

151>Homo erectus. An extinct primate classified in the subfamily Homininae and the genus Homo, which include humans. It is not clear that this animal became mankind and womantype.

151>*The Creative Explosion*, Book by John E. Pfeiffer, Harper & Row, publishers, 1982. "An inquiry into the origins of art and religion." Also the author of *The Emergence of Man.*

152>Australopithecine. Several extinct species of primates classified in the subfamily Homininae, a group that includes humans but this may not be the human's ancestors. Source: *Encarta 1999.*

152>Ancient footsteps found on the planet earth indicate three upright walking human type creatures. One was a youth. Reference the book *The Creative Explosion* by John E. Pfeiter. Published by Harper & Row. 1982. Pages 78 & 79 for the footprints described as three individuals heading due north. Australopithecine footprints. Reference the book *Lucy* by Donald Johanson & Maitland Edey. Published by Warner Books1981. Page 249 for the same footprints described as at least two hominids.

152>Unga-dugged. The "unga" prefix denotes a type of private language (i.e. unga-Bob in place of Uncle Bob).

153>*2001: A Space Odyssey.* A movie directed by Stanley Kubrick, by MGM, 1969. Arthur C. Clarke was the author or co-author or what ever. This film could support intentionally or not, the views that evolution may have occurred in rapid jumps followed by the status quo of no changes for long periods of time. Someone by the name of DeVries (?) might have come up with this idea, from around 1905, but I can't find any references.

153>Andy Warhol is reported to have stated that everybody has 15 minutes of fame. A "Pop" artist of the 1960's. Possibly named "pop" after a montage artwork by Richard Hamilton titled, *Just What Is It That Makes Today's Homes So Different, So Appealing?* 1956. This artwork has a *Tootsie Roll Pop* dominant in the center. Source: *Shock of the New* by Robert Hughes, Publisher Alfred A. Knopf, 1981. Pages 342, 343. Andy Warhol's name is actually a misprint. Source www.warhol.dk/.

153>Morgan's Cannon of Interpretation. States: In no case may we interpret an action as the outcome of the exercise of a higher psychical blah, blah, blah. No source listed.

154>Amygdala. Quote: "A little almond shaped structure deep inside the antero-inferior region of the temporal lobe..." "When triggered gives rise to fear and anxiety..." Source www.healing-arts.org/n-r-limbic.htm - Article by Julio Rocha do Amaral, MD & Jorge Martins de Oliveira, MD, PhD.

155>Friends and relatives of suicided humans might consider themselves to be either survivors of suicide or victims of suicide. They wish to take the credit but not the responsibility. They remove the honor from the suicided *Homaniakos.*

156>*The Shock of The New* is a book topicing[*sic*] the emergence of Modern Art at the beginning of the twentieth century, written by Robert Hughes. See the reference 153 above.

161>*The Asylum Sanctuary.* An artwork methodology created by me!

165>Critical Paranoia. A term used by Salvador Dali to represent the moment between sleep and waking whereby the confusion of the senses draws reality into perceptions of reality. My dad died while in a state of Critical Paranoia and thus for certain it became an enjoyable moment as the mind drifts in and out with no sense of time or concern for the trials and tribulations of mankind and womantype.

166>See notes from 130.

CHAPTER HUMAN PERCEPTIONS VERSUS TRUE REALITY

169>The *Gong Show* was a variety show from the late 1970's hosted by Chuck Barris at one time.

169>Language. See the reference at "i" also.

169>Ludwig Wittgenstein (1889-1951) Austrian mechanical engineer who studied with Bertrand Russell in Cambridge. He later became a professor of philosophy at Cambridge in 1939. As a note, he died the year I was born. He thought that the ability to rationalize existence is a function of "language" to describe it. Source: Internet encyclopedia of Philosophy. www.utm.edu/research/iep/w/wittgens.htm. I may be his re-incarnation, if you believe in such nonsense.

169>"...*Hosapiens,* perceive only what they need..." is from my book. See the source by B.G. Charlton, MD. www.hedweb.com/bgcharlton/meaning-of-life.html. I saw this article in March of 2002 when I was checking another of Dr. Charlton's articles as a reference. What a great perspective! *What is the meaning of life?*

169>Synesthesia, a "joined sensations of the senses" smelling sound, hearing color. Refer to: *Smithsonian,* February 2001, *For Some, Pain Is Orange.* By Susan Hornik. Page 48.

169>UFO's. Please research on your own *The Fermi Paradox,* "Where are they?" See the source: www.ndirect.co.uk/~transhumanism/Fermi.htm, London School of Economics, Department of Philosophy, Logic and Scientific method, by Nick Bostrom Please read on your own, *The Hynek UFO Report* by Dr. J. Allen Hynek (dead) Publisher, Dell 1977 and read *The UFO handbook* by Allan Hendry, publisher Doubleday & Company, Inc., 1979.

170>"..thus you find nothing because your goal blinds you." quote from this book by me! "Indeed, it is usually overlooked how our definitions and how the terminology we use direct our thinking, and often guide us into narrow dead end alleys obstructing what are often straightforward insights." Quote from the Introduction of: *Experience, awareness and consciousness: suggestions for definitions as offered by an evolutionary approach.* By Mario Vaneechoutte, University Hospital, Ghent, Belgium. Source: http://allserv.rug.ac.be/~mvaneech/EAC.html. I wrote mine before I found that source, but that and 10 cents will get you a cup of coffee.

170>Ether. The rarefied element formerly believed to fill the upper regions of space. Internet Source: ©*2002 by Merriam-Webster, Incorporated.* As a note, at one time it was believed that there was no vacuum of space.

170>European Carryall. I am told it is from the TV show, *Steinfeld.* A man purse. No previous historical usage was found.

171>"..consciousness is better defined as reflexive awareness,..." Although hundreds of sources are obtainable, I enjoyed that quote from, *Experience, awareness and consciousness: suggestions for definitions as offered by an evolutionary approach.* By Mario Vaneechoutte. Department of Clinical Chemistry, Microbiology & Immunology. Ghent, Belgium. Source: http://allserv.rug.ac.be/~mvaneech/EAC.html.

171>Lies. "But this explanation adds nothing. It is just a story Benjamin tells after the fact." Quote from page 237 of the book *The Meme Machine,* Publisher, Oxford, 1999. By Dr. Susan Blackmore.

172>Danse Macabre. A song by Saint-Saens. "A medieval symbolic representation of death". Quote from the source: www.carlfischer.com/bandscores/aboutDanceMacabre.html. Music uses wood blocks and xylophones to represent skeletons, and we have never improved on that sound/vision thought.

172>Scat. The fecal matter of animals other than humans but sometimes referred to as human fecal matter in erotic pornography. See alt.binaries.pictures.erotica.scat, I guess.

172>vNRS: von Neumann Reality Syndrome. See the book text in number 142. John von Neumann, 1903 to 1957. It would be worth your effort to read about this human that apparently never had a moment of faulty logic in his entire life.

174>Centon (spelling?). A unit of time from the TV show *Battlestar Galatica*, 1978-1979.

174>The Nyquist Limit is used to determine image resolution at sampling rates. The human eyeball must do something like that also, wouldn't you think so?

176>Human eye resolution has an affect on how we define our universe. Refer to: *Lightning Reference Handbook*, Published by Paul-Munroe Hydraulics, Inc. 1973 edition. Page 21, ...lower limits of normal human vision is 40 microns (.00158 inch), Grain of salt is 100 microns, White blood cell 25 microns, Talcum Powder 10 microns, and average Bacteria 2 microns.

177b>This strange paragraph refers to a news story of this era whereby a man from Kentucky (if I am remembering correctly) viewed a computer movie file "mpg" of a human woman enjoying herself with a male horse. I understand that the horse was also enjoying himself. One of the issues was the transference of digital data over state borders or via satellite. If you view an act committed in a state or country where such acts are not illegal, but you are sitting in a state whereby it is illegal, have you broken a law? Yet all that was transmitted was electricity.

178>*Territorial imperatives*. Book by Robert Ardrey, Publisher, Kodansha America, 1997. As the front cover states: "A Personal Inquiry into the Animal Origins of Property and Nations." I would really suggest that you read this book. If you don't yet believe that we are animals with basic instincts at the front of our actions, then this book will help to alter your views toward that end.

183>Jovian. Of, relating to, or characteristic of the god or planet Jupiter. Source: Internet Source: ©*2002 by Merriam-Webster, Incorporated*. Could also refer to any four of the large gaseous planets. Let me add that the size of these planets would give them gravity fields so strong that our bodies would not be able to function if we were to be at their apparent surface.

185>Discovery Channel. A television network available on cable that deals with topics in a scientific manner.

185>Divididus. Archaic: The object being divided.

185>General beliefs of evolution are based on 100-year-old theories and new theories are difficult to get into the mainstream of the general populous, at least not until all the old folks are dead. Refer to remarks made by Richard Dawkins in an interview conducted by the *Skeptics Society*, Vol. 3, no. 4, 1995, pp. 80-85, source: www.skeptic.com/03.4.miele-dawkins-iv.html. A quote from the article, *Dawkins*: "Not only should we not treat humans as being on the top, we should not see the animal kingdom as being layered as we often do. All zoology textbooks present their chapters in the same order--you start with protozoa,..." I ran out of space so get the article yourself.

185>*The origin of species*. Book by Charles Darwin first published in 1859. The perception of "Survival of the fittest" is derived from this book. I am told that the word "evolution" did not appear in the original publication.

185>The references to the "nose or thumb" are with regards to a reconstructed dinosaur that was on display with the thumb (or a claw) assembled as the nose of the creature. I lost my scientific reference to this one, but someone out there knows what I am talking about. Please write the reference for me in this space: _____. For a visual reference, check *Monty Python's Big Red Book*, by Warner Books, 1975. That book has no page numbers either, but look for one of the all "pink" pages.

185> Stephen Jay Gould & horse evolution. Reference to his book *Full House*, Published by Three Rivers Press, 1996. Try chapter 5 of his book, pages 61, 62 & 63, I guess.

185>National Geographic magazine, May 2001, page 98. Basically states that if you run fast enough with your arms outstretched, your future generations will grow wings. Oh really!?

187>My quote from Julius Caesar has no basis in the truth, I made it up. Parity of, "You can't have your cake and eat it too" as commonly spoken. "You can't eat your cake and have it too" is the correct quote. Also know that Butterfly is actually Flutterby but how can we stop general knowledge? I offer no proof of any of those quotes.

187>The name Caesar implies a cesarean birth but not of Julius Caesar otherwise his mother would have died within days after his birth. I have no references to offer for this information.

189a>Evolution per *The Origin of Species* would imply evolution into a niche as opposed to those that can survive in that environment, do survive in that environment, but with minor adaptive changes possible. "Evolution" was added to later editions of that book, but I offer you no proof.

191>Stephen Jay Gould. Reference to his book *Full House*, Published by Three Rivers Press, 1996. Try chapters 3 and 4 of his book, I guess. Evolution can only get more complex.

191>(vN). von Neumann. See the book text in number 142.

200>Anthrax. "..an organism that under certain conditions forms highly resistant spores capable of persisting and retaining their virulence in contaminated soil or other material for many years." and "..one of the oldest recorded diseases of animals, being mentioned by Moses in Exodus 9:9" Quote source: *1999-2000 Britannica.com Inc.* I wrote that chapter a year before the anthrax via mail terrorism started, there is no correlation or hidden meaning.

200>Sinew. A tendon; especially: one dressed for use as a cord or thread. Internet Source: ©*2002 by Merriam-Webster, Incorporated.*

201>DOA; Dead On Arrival. A medical slang. It seems silly to mention some of these terms, but I can guarantee that in 50 or 100 years, the readers of this book won't have a clue as these types of slang are usually very temporary.

203>Dildo. A phallic shaped device, sometimes motorized, for masturbation via insertion in the vagina or anus. Often sold as Adult Toys or Novelties. The gift that keeps on giving.

204>*Barbie* or *Barbie Doll*. Created by Ruth Handler, co-founder of Mattel. Source: http//abcnews.go.com/sections/us/barbie/barbie_career.html. Also see 485.

205>L 7. Make those shapes with your thumbs and index fingers then in touch index to thumb and thumb to index to make a square. Archaic youth gesture to indicate a person that is either a nerd or "not with it."

205>I am referring to the character of young men. Quote: "Our hostile armies are composed, to a considerable extent, of young men;..." Page 19, *Worth and Wealth* By T.L. Haines A.M., Publisher, Haines Bros. 1886.

207>Octopus traits. They do not shoot sperm from their tentacle tips, I made that up. They have complex brains with memories and problem solving abilities. Source: www.mote.org/~debi/octopi.phtml by Debi Ingrao.

207>Comparing animal intelligence to the human animal's intelligence. See the source: Oh my, I lost another source. Oh well, the title is *A Comparison of Primate and Dolphin Intelligence as a Metaphor for the Validity of Comparative Studies of Intelligence.* By Jonathan Ball. Using Morgan's Cannon of interpretation, Mr. Ball writes, "This statement is extremely relevant to comparative psychology because it calls for great skepticism in attributing intelligence to animals other than humans just because there appears to be no other explanation for an observed behavior or because the proper neurology seems to be present."

208>Puffy nipples. AKA: Apples or Bee stings. The shape of these nipples gives the appearance of being "puffed up" and thus their name. They have their own cult followers on the Internet. See alt.binaries.pictures.erotica.puffies. They drive me wild!

209>Ancient cities. See National Geographic Jan. 2001 *Ancient Ashkelon,* by Rick Gore.

211>Refer to the book, *The Panda's Thumb,* written by Stephen Jay Gould, Published by Norton,1980. See Chapter 9, *A Biological Homage to Mickey Mouse.*

211>"speciesistic dualism". See www.awionline.org/schweitzer/as-5.htm by The Albert Schweitzer Fellowship among others. (Chapter 5) Dr. Albert Schweitzer obviously was distraught over knowing that he must kill in order to live, but he had his preferences also. There are things of beauty and things that are a menace. Quote from the source concerning some palm trees, "But we cannot find it in our heart to deliver them over to the axe just when delivered of the creeper vines, they are beginning a new life." I prefer creeper vines myself. Add to that, humans destroy Japanese Beetles that eat (thus kill) Elm trees (I believe) in their yards, all the while humans clear-cut forests in the USA and kill just about everything, while preventing 3rd world nations from cutting their trees to make farm land. Gosh! (See Chapter 2 also.)

213>How is co-evolution possible? When starting there would not be enough plants to make oxygen or animals to make carbon dioxide. But I am an idiot at those things, so read *Search For The Universal Ancestors* prepared at the Ames Research Center by or for NASA. Page 33 is interesting. Catalog number NASA SP-477 from the Superintendent of Documents, U.S. Government Printing Office. Washington, D.C. 20402. Most likely out of print, but give them a call anyway.

213>PETA or P.E.T.A., I really don't know. "People for the Ethical Treatment of Animals". Obviously they are pushing things a bit with their acronym because of having to leave out all those little words. Shouldn't it be PFTETOA? Checkout their Web Site to see the ultimate in faulty logic. www.peta-online.org/fp/faq.html has this quote: "By eating vegetables directly, rather than eating animals such as cows....one is saving many more plants' lives (and destroying less land)." Oh my!

213>Plants do not have neural networks thus how can they process thoughts or have consciousness? Related quote, "Over evolutionary time, plants wage grim wars to push competitors out of choice locations, fighting over patches of sunlight and supplies of water as remorselessly as animals vie for hunting grounds and mating rights." Source:
March 1999 *Internet Infidels Newsletter*.
http://www.infidels.org/infidels/newsletter/1999/march.html . Feature: *Darwin and the Invisible Hand*, by Fredrick Curry.

214>Freud believed that sex was a primary driver of human's emotions or emotional problems. Research on your own, *Oedipus Complex* and the *Castration Complex*. While you are at it, read *Erotic Fantasies* by Drs. Phyllis and Eberhard Kronhausen. Publisher, Bell Publishing Company, New York, 1969. The back cover of that book shows a two-headed human, I think?

217>CE or C.E. "Current Era" is religiously neutral, but not necessarily ideology neutral, as opposed to AD denoting a Christian calendar but not necessarily a belief of any particular ideology. This is because AD and BC are considered "common usage" and CE would imply a deliberate departure from the common usage for reasons of belief, or due to training in the sciences where spiritual beliefs must be restrained.

217>The nick name, Buzz, is referencing Col. Edwin E. Aldrin, the second man to step foot upon the moon. Buzz is listed as being a manic-depressive (Bi-polar) on some web sites and Uni-polar on others, of which I have no other documents to which confirm the truth of either. To the casual observer, this might not appear to be a big difference, but it is the same as not knowing which gender your spouse is prior to marriage. Buzz was the second human man to walk on the moon during the first Apollo lunar landing. As a side note, my son and myself had the privilege to enjoy sitting with Brigadier General Charlie Duke (retired), for a breakfast a few years ago in Kankakee Illinois. General Duke was also one of the lunar astronauts on Apollo 16, and I believe the eleventh human man to walk on the moon.

218>Plants are "chemical telepathics". As told to me by Jack Goodwin (other origins unknown). What does it take to have a society? Plants communicate via chemicals for survival. See *WQ, The Wilson Quarterly* Autumn 2000 page 19, *Unlocking the Green Pharmacy* By Joel L. Swerdlow.

220>Endo-wise refers to endosperm, the part of the plant we make bread type products from. "Endosperm constitutes the nutritious part of most grains and many seeds that are eaten by much of the world's human population." Quote from page 325, *Biology, A Self-Teaching Guide,* by Steven D. Garber, Publisher, Wiley, 1989.

220>Haploid nuclei. Haploid cells possess only one of each pair of chromosomes and are sex cells. Two sex cells unite to form a zygote, which is worth 57 points on a *triple word score* square in the game of *Scrabble.*

222> "Kill a flower." A discovery made by Sir Jagadis Chunder Bose, a Hindu scientist has discovered that plants have heartbeats and the death of a plant can be determined by measuring them. Source: *Collier's Wonder Book*, Publisher, P.F. Collier & Son Co. 1920. See page 42.

223>Goedel theorems [Also as Godel]. See the source: www.myrkul.org/recent/godel.htm for this very long quote, "The symbolic systems we use to describe the universe are not separate from the universe: they are a part of the universe just as we are a part of the universe. Since we are within the system, our small understandings are 'the system modeling itself' (system meaning reality in this case). Completion of the model can never happen because of the basic self-referential paradox: the model is within the universe, so in effect the universe would have to be larger than itself."

223>Homocentric (human vantage during analysis). See http://paradigm.soci.brocku.ca/~1ward/mead/pubs/Mead_1895a.html. Quote: "...science that has suffered thus far from the homocentric character of psychical analysis as comparative anatomy and physiology have suffered earlier from the almost exclusive interest that centered in the human organism." George Herbert Mead's Review of *An Introduction to Comparative Psychology* by C. Lloyd Morgan, *Psychological Review 2*, (1895): 399-402.

223, 224>Stealing. Humans are natural thieves that cannot be stopped. Quote: "Every predator is a thief, even a murderer, stealing the very life from other organisms to benefit themselves. Even herbivores mercilessly munch up leaves and grass, stealing the fuel laboriously manufactured by the plants themselves from sunlight. And plants are not blameless either." Source: March 1999 *Internet Infidels Newsletter*. http://www.infidels.org/infidels/newsletter/1999/march.html. Feature: *Darwin and the Invisible Hand*, by Fredrick Curry

223, 224>Stealing. See the Wall Street Journal, April 17, 2001, *Bowling Shoes Are So Hot, People Rent Them to Steal a Pair.*

224>Xerox. Source: www.xerox.com Founded in 1906 as *The Haloid Company* and renamed *Xerox Corporation* in 1961. Xerography is derived from the Greek words for "Dry & Written" thus shortened to Xerox.

228>Tourette's Syndrome. See; *Tryptophan and Tourette's Syndrome* by Steven Wm. Fowkes. Source: www.ceri.com/tourett.htm from the "Cognitive Enhancement Research Institute" home page.

229>Oedipus. "He shouts for the barriers to be unbarred and he displayed to all of Thebes-his father's murderer, his mother's-no, a word too foul to say-as if he means to cast himself adrift, not rot at home the curser and the cursed." Source: *The Oedipus Plays of Sophocles,* Page 74, Translated by Paul Roche, Publisher New American Library, 1958. My comment: Yes he killed his dad and did "it" with his mom and was quite satisfied until the contrived language revealed the linage.

231>Unnatural environment. The constructed environment of the human animal as described by *The Technol Research Project* created by R. J. Hanink. Uses the term "inventive technology" to discern between what creatures such as birds and beavers create versus what humans create.

232>Sub-Sahara African technology. From my source page 9, when speaking of a region known then as British East Africa (now Kenya), ".. but remembering that progress and development in this particular kind of new land depend exclusively upon the masterful leadership of the whites, .." (The confusion of technology as a measure of societal success is what I surmise. R.J.Hanink) Quote source: *African Game Trails,* By Theodore Roosevelt (Former US President) Published by Syndicate Publishing Co. 1910 edition.

232>Sub-Sahara African technology. From my source, www.awionline.org/schweitzer/as-2.htm, Chapter Two, Africa. Published by The Albert Schweitzer Fellowship among others, we find, "They tell us in terribly harsh language that a civilization which develops only on its material side, and not in the sphere of the spirit...heads for disaster."

233>"Lucy in the sky forever." From a song by the Beatles: Lucy in the Sky with Diamonds -Thought to mean LSD but there is doubt as to its true meaning. You should do your own research on the Internet into this topic.

235>Colonel Flastratus phenomenon. If I understand this correctly it is the notion that because you are convinced that an idea is great has no bearing on the truth of the greatness of that idea. This is in reference to Peak Experiences (see the next reference). *Abraxis*, published 1998. By Bruce G. Charlton, MD. Source: www.hedweb.com/bgcharlton/index.html.

235>Peak Experience. Reference: Abraham Maslow also. The moments when we feel the highest levels of happiness, harmony and possibility. Source: www.hedweb.com/bgcharlton/index.html Bruce G. Charlton, MD.

239>Dr. Susan Blackmore. Writer of the book *The Meme Machine*, Publisher, Oxford, 1999.

239>Richard Dawkins. Writer of the book, *The Selfish Gene* 1976, published by someone I guess? Introduced the word "meme" from what I gather.

242>*The Bell Curve*. A book that topics the study of testing the intelligence of humans. Written by Charles Murray and Richard Herrnstein, 1994, Publisher, Free Press (paperback). The controversy of the book is the method of using IQ scores to define the intelligence of various "human races." My suggestion is to read instead or also, *The Mismeasure of Man* by Stephen Jay Gould. Published by W W Norton & Company, 1981.

245>Advertising strategies based on genetic actuators. Quote: "..packaging constructed from deliberately feminine curves, I can't help but think of the Ophrys Speculum orchid, and it's mislead suitor." Refers to an orchid that looks so much like a female wasp that male wasps mate with it (helps pollination). Quote source: March 1999 *Internet Infidels Newsletter*. http://www.infidels.org/infidels/newsletter/1999/march.html Feature: *Darwin and the Invisible Hand*, by Fredrick Curry. I had a much better reference that was obtained directly from a famous advertising expert but I lost it so this one will have to do.

248>The natural ability of human survival reveals itself as a function of physical and mental development. Refer to: *The Nature and Nurture of Behavior, Readings from Scientific American* Published by W. H. Freeman and Co. 1973 edition. Topic: *Developmental Psychobiology* Refer to *The 'Visual Cliff'* by Eleanor Gibson and Richard Walk, April 1960. Chapter 3. Also see my book text number 175.

250>Infants as embryos. Source, *Ever Since Darwin,* book by Stephen Jay Gould, Publisher W W Norton and Company, 1997. Refer to chapter 8, *Human Babies as Embryos*. Hello Professor Gould. I attended one of your wonderful speeches at the Field Museum, Chicago. When I was 5, my father took me to see the tyrannosaurus, also. I still have nightmares.

251>Helen Keller quote is not verified. Most likely I was lying in order to be humorous.

251>*The Wild Boy of Aveyron*, by Harlan Lane. I can't find anything out about this book. Allen and Unwin, 1977 from the reference pages of *The Mysterious World* by Francis Hitching, Published: Holt, Rinehart and Winston 1978.

251>*The Wolf Children*, by Charles Maclean. I can't find anything out about this book either. Allen and Unwin, 1977 from the reference pages of *The Mysterious World* by Francis Hitching, Published: Holt, Rinehart and Winston 1978.

252>Pattern matching. Refer to: *Experience, awareness and consciousness: suggestions for definitions as offered by an evolutionary approach.* By Mario Vaneechoutte, University Hospital, Ghent, Belgium. Source: http://allserv.rug.ac.be/~mvaneech/EAC.html. Quote: "Experience can be defined as a characteristic linked closely to specific pattern matching, a characteristic which is already apparent at the molecular level at least."

253>Closet Door Anxiety. CDA is not a verified psychological term. See ABCNews.com March 6, 2002. *Terror Strikes Young.* Quote: "...she was able to overcome her urge to get out of bed repeatedly every night, and slept with the closet door closed, which had previously worried her." Copyright © 2002ABC News Internet Ventures. So if you have CDA, I suggest psychotherapy, because you are obviously mentally ill without knowing it.

253>Government schools are also known as "public schools". The Democratic Party gained control of the educational brain washing within the schools by maintaining the Teachers Union. Thus my human-children get to be involved with every worthless "feel good" activity, while being told that the Republicans are just nasty. The teachers never bring up the fine points of Libertarianism either. So there!

258>Technol. Commonly referred to as "techno" but the "L" signifies usage as defined by *The Technol Research Project* created by R. J. Hanink. I didn't copyright "Technol" so use it all you want I suppose, but don't prevent me from using it.

261>Fon. Means "phone" but pronounced like "on" with a "f" in front. If it isn't French, then I discovered it.

261>Plaster. Prior to "dry-wall" gypsum board, a plaster mixture was spread over wooden strips called "lathe", and smoothed to make flat walls. This required great skill and labor, thus dry-wall was discovered and now even expensive homes use it.

262>Western "societies" method of taking care of their aged parents by putting them into "homes". Refer to *Napoleon's Glands,* by Arno Karlen, Publisher Little, Brown and Company, 1984. See pages 126 & 127. It appears that even what modern humans would call "primitive peoples" took better care of their families than current societies with advanced technologies as evident by the study of the skeletons of injured Neanderthals found in Iraq.

263>Language. I dare you to find a copy of this reference. *Future - The Aventis Magazine* 2/2000. This month's topic: *The Mystery of Language.* Publisher: Dr. Friedmar Nusch, Head of Aventis Corporate Communications. I can't reveal anything about the content without "...express permission of the publishers: indication of source and specimen copy required". Sometimes these magazines are found on the little glass top table located in the lobby of their offices.

263>Language. See the source: http://espresso.hampshire.edu/~aaron/ii_desu_ne.html. *Den Blu Avis - The Blue Newspaper.* By Aaron Culich and C. Tait Bergstrom. Copyright 1996. Quote: "The proper form of argument does not actually concern a dialogue dealing with the concepts of evidence. Verbal conflict relies upon constantly contradicting or refuting the opponent's last statement and their existence. This usually involves the 'Yeah-Oh Yeah' method of argument." From this I gather that a true argument would have no basis for ending except boredom. Now compare that to pages 181 & 182 of *The Territorial Imperative* by Robert Ardrey (book data elsewhere in references). We have the "callicebus" monkey with a similar behavior, "...bright and early is on duty at the border, ... waiting for the arrival of neighbors to be angry at." Continuing later: "...after a couple of hours of emotional daily dozens, ... That will be the end of the day's hostilities as all take their ravenous appetites to the breakfast trees." As we find out that the other animals of the planet earth behave just as the humans do.

264>Evolution of languages in humans serves no purpose. Quote: "What biologists overlooked for almost a century is the fact that evolution is totally anti-teleological. It is literally void of any purpose." Source: March 1999 *Internet Infidels Newsletter.* http://www.infidels.org/infidels/newsletter/1999/march.html Feature: *Darwin and the Invisible Hand,* by Fredrick Curry. Also, see the book, *Full House,* chapter 5, page 63, second paragraph (book credits given previously).

265>Speed of light in a vacuum is about 186,000 miles per second. Thus everything you see has already occurred. The sun is not physically where you see it when you believe you see it where it's is actually. Everyone sees or senses reality from their own "time", even if this time gap is small.

266>Please read the book, *The Territorial Imperative* by Robert Ardrey, publisher; Kodansha America, Inc. 1997.

267>Evolving physical features takes energy and must go through transformations of not being fully useful yet. Thus why would it happen? The book, *Origins of Species,* by Charles Darwin 1859. See Chapter 6, *Origins of extreme perfection and complication.* The eye.

270>A list, B list. Party lists for famous persons whereby being on the A list would mean you would be the preferred party guest over the guests on the B list. However, being on the B list would mean that you are more likely to be available for the party. Is that evolution or what!

274>Trilogram. Three sentences as one, but sharing words or word groups in order to mimic data compressed on a Zip drive. Reference music by the group Jethro Tull's *A Passion Play* for an example, when listening can be understood as two combined sentences sharing words. "...calls itself "Hell" -- where no-one has nothing and nothing is <u>well</u> meaning fool, pick up thy bed ..."

CHAPTER MANKIND AND WOMANTYPE

276>The belief by some that the "media" programs our society into what we believe are "basic morals" not transitive fads. Does the media reflect society, even only the extremes since it can't represent unknown thoughts?

277>Psychology. "One of the tasks of psychology is to provide a technology for facilitating the process of becoming a rational, moral human being." Quote from *The Benefits and Hazards of the Philosophy of Ayn Rand* by Nathaniel Branden, Ph..D. 1984. Source: www.nathanielbranden.net/ayn/ayn03.shtml. Wasn't she something! I hope all her followers buy my book too!

282>Pregnancy of pre-teens. The maternal mortality rate of 9.9 per 1000 live births for the age group 10 years old to 14 years old. [Most likely these figures represent white Americans.] Source: *The World Almanac for 1946* Published by The New York World-Telegram. Page 524.

283>"Y" chromosome. Additional data: The SRY Gene "S(ex-determining)R(egion)Y" is a gene on the "Y" chromosome that helps develop the testes and determines the "sex" of the human. Note that X or Y-chromosomes are not the only factor in determining the gender of a human as noted by humans born with gender confusion. www2.onnet.co.kr/smcobgy/hsd.html.

283>"...and young boys groom their hair and learn that walking stride to show what a hunter they have become..." from my book compare with this article I found a year later from *Natural Geographic,* May 2001, page 103 on the topic of Pterosaurs: "To explain its huge head, Bennett invoked the same reason that teenage boys swagger: To establish rank among the guys and to impress the girls." Now as I pat myself on my back for my observations and deductions while on Mall Safari, we must all realize that we have something in common with all of life: genes! Genes determine behavior when you don't have time to think about behavior!

283>Modern School System unnatural problems. See *The Volume Library,* 1912, Publisher, The W.E. Richardson company, page 57, center column. Quote: "The presence of boys and girls together in all the classes and social events of the school has both advantage and dis-advantage,.." also, "While they are frank and confidential with one another, they are often reticent and unapproachable toward their elders."

283>Puberty pregnancy. Quote: "If it is immoral and ``unnatural" to prevent an unwanted life from coming into existence, is it not immoral and ``unnatural" to remain unmarried from the age of puberty? Such casuistry is unconvincing and feeble." From *The Pivot of Civilization* by Margaret Sanger, 1879-1966. Search for, Project Gutenberg on the Internet for all types of good free stuff.

286>Now this is a tough one. I know that my strange phraseology has you guessing if there is meaning behind any of these queer expressions. Well at the time of my reference, two Governor's wives had visited the monks. A clue for you to-day: These people are dead, naturally, but don't get trapped O' my Brothers. You must be mentally in the correct state to know this answer.

288>A male erection is not as necessary as it used to be, I guess. The latest news is that now a male or even sperm is not necessary. See *The Jerusalem Post* Wednesday July 11, 2001, www.jpost.com/Editions/2001/07/11/News/News.30172.html (web page has been removed.) By Judy Siegel, "...could make it possible for lesbian couples to have their own baby girl - genetically related to both - without donated sperm. Since females lack Y chromosomes, they could not produce a boy on their own."

289a>The Columbine High School massacre is an example of ineffective gene cleansing whereby the "freaks" got the upper hand on the ordinary humans because of the cleaver use of technology gadgets. The question not answered is whether or not the ordinary humans (students) created the "freaks" via some type of MSO (Mutually Selective Ostracizing)?

289b>Obviously the change in names is to create a change in attitude toward those entities. Usually the change is so that humans will "accept" the entity, such as a street bum is now in the category of a homeless person, but really they are still street bums. Who wants to donate money to purchase food for street bums? Are you of the correct age to know the difference between a street bum and a hobo? A jungle sounds savage, but a rain forest is pleasant. If I dropped you off in a rain forest, five miles from civilization, you'd be dead in three days and eaten in four.

291a>Refer to the "Gem Vest Pocket Manual of Ready Reference" publisher, Marvis Publishing Co. 1899. See pages 62 and 63.

291a>Refer to Edgar Allen Poe and his "child" bride 24yr/13yr (Internet source). Refer to Jerry Lee Lewis and his "child" bride 19yr/13yr (Internet source: http://w1.country.com/gen/music/artist/jerry-lee-lewis.html). Refer to David Thompson (surveyor, born 1770), 28yr/14yr. Source *Mercator's World* magazine, March/April 2001, page 45 by Stephen R. Bown. Also see *Manners and Customs of Mankind*, Volume Two, Page 760 quote: "The attainment of marriageable age by the girl - generally coincident with puberty. . ." Published by The Amalgamated Press, Ltd. (date not noted, but appears to be from the 1930's). My remark is that these are not rarities, perverts, or idiots, but rather natural occurrences that are not inhibited via pseudo societies controlled via the news media!

295>Clothing. "Racy preteen fashions spark parental backlash" is the title of the article. From the *Kankakee Sunday Journal*, an *Associated Press* article. 2002. "...school administrators say the looks are becoming overtly sexual." This is with regards to the 8 to 12 year old girls, know as the "tweens".

295>Durable goods are consumer items that have a degree of longevity such as household appliances.

295>Happy, happiness. "We convince ourselves that all manner of things would potentially make us happy. All these peripheral routes are not merely vastly circuitous and inefficient. In the main, they just don't, and can't, durably work. At best they can serve as superficial palliatives of the human predicament." Source: *The Hedonistic Imperative* Chapter 5 by David Pearce. www.hedweb.com/hedethic/hedonist.htm. Quote: "So short has been his acquaintance with the world, that he has not learned how deceitful are its pleasures, and how vain its pursuits." Page 16, *Worth and Wealth* By T.L.Haines A. M., Publisher, Haines Bros. 1886.

295>Strainer stew. The food left in the sink drain strainer after the dishes are finished and the water is drained out. If still warm, it can be quite tasty.

295>Negative Utilitarianism. I can't describe it, you'll have to look it up yourself. Try www.hedweb.com/negutil.htm

295>Neuroleptics. See *Psychiatry and the Human Condition*, by Bruce Charlton, MD. Try an Internet search.

296>CE. European Union industrial standards for product safety. Might also be known as EU but the product mark is always CE.

300>Communications style theory. Reference theories from the book, *I wish I'd said that!* by Linda McCallister, Ph.D. Published by John Wiley & Sons, Inc. 1992. Communication styles revert to natural tendencies of the speaker when angered thus reveal the true nature of that human, or something like that.

306a>Courts must follow the "order of the law" and thus do not pursue the truth directly or at all. A prosecutor is only interested in conviction, not establishing the truth. Thus justice is at best, justice by law not by truth. Truth need never enter a courtroom during a trial. When it comes to entities such as the States Attorney, cases are pursued based on the possibly of "winning", thus whether a "wrong" has been done or not isn't a factor in case selection. Re-election and "conviction" records become more important than the truth. But perhaps this is a case of "resource efficiency" being misinterpreted. The news media perpetuates the misinformation because the news media deals only in "fear." Thus when you hear, "Man set free after wrongly convicted of murder", what is most likely to have happened, is that although he did it, a procedural error was made.

309>I was reading in a *Psychology Today* magazine from the year 2000 (month?) an article titled, *"Kids Keep Dad in The Office."* It seems that a Ph.D. found that Dads think differently of their sons than their daughters. And to think without a Doctor's degree, we are all too stupid to notice that! Anyway, more research is needed for some reason.

312>Ellen Key. As mentioned in *Leslie's Illustrated Weekly Newspaper*, November 13, 1913 Page 478, in the column *In The World of Womankind*. The article, *Know What You Talk About*. Quoting directly from the article, "There really ought to be a law prohibiting eloquent writers (no others carry such weight) from writing on subjects they know nothing of from experience."

312>Vaginated. An animal that possesses a vagina.

319>Males of the species fighting for the right to mate. *Territorial Imperatives*, Book by Robert Ardrey, Publisher, Kodansha America, 1997.

319>See Thomas Hobbes (b. 1588) and his book *Leviathan*. See Book II with regards to male/female roles. A good source is www.sparknotes.com under the philosophy section. Hobbes lived during the era of Galileo and the refuting of Aristotle's principles (imbedded within the church and thus imbedded within the universities) via scientific discovery. Also see *Discoveries and Opinions of Galileo* translated by Stillman Drake, published by Doubleday Anchor books, copyright 1957 (You can get these at garage sales for 25cents (US), which is where I got many of my resource books.)

322>Refers to wasp's that inject their unborn into caterpillar or spiders. This was not a direct reference to human activity. *Bathyplectes curculionis* is a black, robust body wasp. Females lay eggs in alfalfa weevil larvae. Wasp larva that hatch from the eggs feed internally, slowly devouring the living weevil larva. http: ohioline.osu.edu/hyg-fact/2000/2113.html. Yes, it's a cruel or efficient world, take your pick.

324>Copulins pheromones. Pheromones secreted by the vagina. See the article *Female Pheromones and Male Physiology* by Astrid Jütte. Source: http://evolution.humb.univie.ac.at/ institutes/urbanethology/student/html/astrid/femphers.html. From the Ludwig-Boltzmann-Institute for Urban Ethology.

324>Lesbians. From the island of "Lesbos" in the Aegean Sea. Or possibly a later application of the term to females of these type. Many men have an attraction to women that exhibit "Lesbian" type behaviors, but in truth, what would a man get sexually from a true Lesbian? The attraction is due to some type of pure genetic reaction but I haven't found any good explanation of it other than many men want to do "it" with as many women as possible. Sex with two women at once would be more efficient I guess.

324>Stump train a cow. Farmer boys would train a cow to stand by a tree stump so that the boy could have intercourse with the cow. Try the newsgroups alt.binaries.pictures.erotica.bestiality. Check with your local laws concerning viewing or downloading or hearing or thinking about such things, because I'm not trying to get you arrested, only educated.

325>What is the man's role? Permanent spouse, permanent father, or something in between? Refer to: *Manners and Customs of Mankind* Volume One, Published by The Amalgamated

Press, Ltd. (Date approx. 1930's) Chapter; *The Meaning of the Couvade* illustrates ancient customs of the parental male involvement with the birth of his child, see page 445. Refer to number 319 of my references. Also refer to *Leviathan* book II (I hope), by Thomas Hobbes.

326>A mental image created via 1950's style of TV programs. A non-reality.

328>Misconceptions about Drug origins and manufacture. Why drug companies don't use plants for medicine. So I say, the value of the rain forest is a myth, and we get most of our oxygen from the ocean anyway, don't you think? See WQ, *The Wilson Quarterly* Autumn 2000 page 16, *Unlocking the Green Pharmacy* by Joel L. Swerdlow.

328>Tests with chimpanzees reveal that a chimpanzee does not understand that the face of a human is important or that humans have vision through their eyes. This is important when trying to understand whether other life can reference the "self" via understanding biological functions. I lost the source material for this data, and with me bragging about being so organized. I'm going to guess it was a *Scientific American Presents* special issue from the winter of 1998, Volume 9, number 4, *Can Animals Empathize?* page 67, but I am not certain. Why don't you find this one yourself?

349>Racial profiling. Assigning "traits" based on the various human (so-called) races. Usually interpreted as a bias to create an underclass within the social structure of a human society. When in fact, all humans would create their own underclass even if everyone were of the same color, nation, language, income, religion, etc. They would find a way, believe me. Thus where is the truth to "racism?" The ordinary humans "profiled" me as a manic-depressive, but now as "The Manic-Depressive Junkie" what can they say? I couldn't be more proud to be associated with humans of such a common mind.

349>Stereotyping. See *Body Piercing Linked to Risky Behavior in Teens*, ABCNews.com March 11, Reuters, by Esther Csapo Rastegari. Quote, "...new study findings suggest that teens with piercings are more likely to smoke cigarettes, use drugs and exhibit other types of unhealthy behavior." This does not include what is considered normal ear piercings. Thus in the future, this study will be incorrect, and possibly thought of as a faulty analysis.

351>Under the topic of Racism or Stereotyping I typed a complete page for this reference, and now I will edit down to the following statement: "*Willfully* chosen altruistic activities promotes the acceptance of varied behaviors or varied beliefs as individuals".

353>*Stepford Wives*. A book & movie whereby the males of the community are replacing their wives with identical but physically perfect and obedient robots or as known in the philosophy trade as p-zombies, but of a mechanical origin. It has a happy ending, though. The men win this one. Novel by Ira Levin, movie 1975 by Columbia Pictures. Source: IMDb.

353>Yuppie. Archaic: *Young Urban Professional* if I remember correctly.

354>Man hunts mankind and womantype. See the book, *The Territorial Imperative* by Robert Ardrey, Chapter 7, *Look Homeward, Angel*, pages 261, 262 & 263. Louis Leaky announced the murder of "pre-Zinj" a twelve year old humanoid, 2 million years ago. Also the brain eating habits of Peking man from 500,000 years ago. I always wondered if eating brains tasted like scrambled eggs with Ketchup on them? They certainly look the same!

364>*Mission to Mars*. A movie directed by Brian De Palma, 2000. A good example of how music and sound can destroy a story, although this movie has a rotten story as well.

364>*Psycho*. Refer only to the original movie directed by Alfred Hitchcock, 1960. The newer "in color" version is too distracting because the color of blood has it's own emotional trigger. The movie was created to be filmed in B/W. The music is all string instruments as well. Novel by Robert Bloch. Norman Bates speaking about his (dead) mom: "She goes a little mad sometimes. We all go a little mad sometimes. Haven't you?" Quote source: IMDb (Internet Movie Database, go to their site, at the bottom of the page, click "search", then type in the movie you wish to find. Once in the selected movie, click the "quotes" button.).

CHAPTER THE UNIVERSE OF THE REAL

371>Missee. The person who is to be missed by another human.

371>Misser. The person who will be feeling the emotion of missing another human.

378>Pitch diameter: Usually a measurement of any object that has threads or gear teeth. For gear teeth it is the diameter whereby two mating gears physically touch.

379>Food chain. Quote: "In the scale of existence, plants occupy a position intermediate between minerals and animals. Plants take from the soil and elaborate into food, the elements which animals require for their growth." Source: Part V, Organic Life; Section I, Plant Life; Chapter 1, Plant Geography; Paragraph 302, *The Elements of Physical Geography* by Edwin J. Houston, A. M." Publisher, Eldredge & Brother, 1886.

382>Real time. Perception cannot be based on "real time" since real time is different for all persons sensing reality. This is due to the fact that sound energy and light energy and touch sensing take time to get to your brain. Thus there are time delays depending upon your distance from the event being sensed.

384>Martians. Refer to: *The Possibility of Intelligent Life Elsewhere In The Universe* [Committee Print] Report prepared for the Committee on science and technology, U.S. House of Representatives, Ninety-Fourth Congress, First Session. Nov. 1975 Stock No. 052-07-03112-3. Page 6 refers to an equation for the determination of intelligent life in the universe, (but only having a verified sample of one planet). I have heard this equation referred to as "The Drake equation" after Dr. Frank Drake 1961 but offer no proof.

386>Cheesecake. A sexual expression or image that would be considered rated PG (Parental Guidance), usually a woman in a bikini.

387>Neutron star. A type of star whereby its atoms are missing their electrons.

388>The theory of theories. On the topic of Black holes: "Despite the mystery, physicists in recent years have begun calling on black holes, largely as a result of Hawking's work, to explain everything from the creation of galaxies and quasars to the ultimate fate of the universe itself." Source: The Book: *Stephen Hawking's Universe,* page 60. By John Boslough, Published by Quill, 1985.

389>Big Bang. The theory that the universe became physical (I guess) during one hell of an explosion a few billion years ago. The Book, *The Big Bang,* written by Joseph Silk. Publishers, W.H. Freeman & Co. 1980, 1989.

390>Chrono-Synclastic Infidibula. Made for TV Movie: *Between Time and Timbukto: A Space Fantasy,* Written by Kurt Vonnegut Jr., 1971. Written for the National Educational Television, NY. Also the author of *Slaughterhouse Five.* See the source: www.geocities.com/hollywood/4953/kv_ring.html.

393>*Technical Remote Viewing.* A psychic's method of seeing the past, present, future or remote locations without physical movement or without using any equipment.

393>Elixir of life. See my reference number 427 for information about Albertus Magnus and Thomas Aquina.

394>Solids within solids. Steno, N. 1669. Reference to his book: *De solido intra solidum naturaliter contento dissertationis prodromus.* He suggested that perhaps fossils were actually once actual animals. This was not a common thought of his era. See www.ucmp.berkeley.edu/history/steno.html. It stands to reason that your philosophy of life and perceptions of reality cannot be beyond the current scientific understanding of that era or your understanding of the science of that era.

395>AI (Artificial Intelligence). Now, I know you are thinking that I added this reference because of that movie recently released via the same name. Actually, I wrote this over a year before that movie was released. Check the date of my reference and read something intelligent about AI in: *The Handbook of Artificial Intelligence,* by Avron Barr & Edward A. Feigenbaum. Publisher, William Kaufmann, Inc. 1981. AI is simply put; intelligence that is measured against the human's intelligence. I have to ask you, why is human logic a benchmark for the measurement of intelligence? Imagine, a machine as smart as a human. Oh boy! At any rate, Volume 1 (of that book) has some interesting topics on spoken language. It is our language transcripted into computers that will prevent computers from ever being better than humans. See Chapter IV "Understanding Natural Language" and Chapter V "Understanding Spoken Language". For the heck of it, checkout *Metamagical Themas* by Douglas R. Hofstadter, Published by Basic Books, Inc. 1985.

396>A, B, C, & D. Read *Search For The Universal Ancestors* prepared at the Ames Research Center by or for NASA. Page 2 is interesting. Catalog number NASA SP-477 from the Superintendent of Documents, U.S. Government Printing Office. Washington, D.C. 20402.

396>HAL computer from 2001, A Space Odyssey. A satire of IBM thus H(I) A(B) L(M) by taking the preceding letters of IBM. There would seem to be a meaning to everything, but there isn't, so don't get your hopes up.

397>Boner. Slang for an erect penis. Men have created many descriptions for their penii units. Men basically understand that the only reason for physical life is procreation, thus they take great pride in their reproductive device and speak about it as often as possible. There are no insults that can be bestowed upon the penis. Some women believe that every device that mankind creates, is to the glory of the penis, or at minimum every device created is in the shape of a penis. The television remote control is a substitute for a penis, thus men hold the remote as often as possible.

398>Mr. Machine. A toy robot I had as a child. Its gear mechanism was visible and it moved powered by batteries.

399>SETI. Search for Extra Terrestrial Intelligence. At one time headed by Carl Sagan, a well-known astronomer, I believe. He's dead.

400>*20 minutes into the future.* I believe this was the original name for the *Max Headroom* TV program. Lorimar Production Chrysalis/Lakeside 1987. Source: IMDb.

401>It is not yet possible to freeze an entire human body without destroying certain cells since the various cells cannot all be frozen under the same conditions. Embryonic freezing is a successful technology as of this date.

401>von Neumann machines. Refer to: *Predictions from Philosophy? How philosophers could make themselves useful.* by Nick Bostrom, Department of Philosophy, Logic and Scientific method. London School of Economics and Political Sciences. Sept. 1998. von Neumann was perhaps one of the most intelligent humans to ever live. See the source: www.nickbostrom.com/old/predict.html.

405>*Whole Earth Project,* created by Robert J. Hanink for *The Technol Research Project.* An art project that believes all the needed knowledge of the earth should be consolidated into one source. It deals specifically with the data required to completely rebuild the technology of the earth from scratch.

406>2D or 3D. 2 Dimensions as in a drawing on paper or 3 Dimensions as in physical objects common to us. 4 Dimensions includes "time" as the fourth dimension. 2D objects may be drawn in a 3D projection, but they remain 2D by description. Does time exist without the existence of 3 dimensional objects?

406>The age of the universe and life being present to see that universe may be related because of the minimum requirements of both having to be met at the same time or something like that. Refer to: *The Anthropic Cosmological Principle.* A book written by Barrow and Tipler. Publisher, Oxford 1986.

407>Mathicalticeans. Pronounced: math-e-kol-ti-see-ans. This is the British pronunciation, I hope.

CHAPTER GODD

409>Checkered flag. The flag that during a race indicates the winner, but actually it indicates that the race is over. Parallel the thought of whether a glass is half empty or half full. Is then the checkered flag a time to rejoice or mourn? Refer to the Jethro Tull CD, *Too Old to Rock'N' Roll: Too Young To Die!* by Chrysalis records, 1976. Track #10, *The Chequered Flag (Dead or Alive)*.

409>What's in a name? Don't mess with Yahweh or Yahshua. See www.sacredname.org/qna-23.htm, www.rockinauburn.com/columns/name-of-god.html, www.truthofyahweh.org/names.htm. Do an Internet search on the topic, "the book of Israyl".

412>66,451. Yes it's a reference to a movie that has had references slipped in several times throughout the text in this book already. I'll give you one clue. If you figure the date, you're getting hot.

412>*The Right Stuff*. To my knowledge, the words "the right stuff" are never stated by any characters in the movie *The Right Stuff* or in my book. Thus I had thought that I had not mentioned *The Right Stuff* in my book either, creating an association to that movie. But I found that I had mentioned *The Right Stuff*, five times in my book.

413>400,000. I have no reason to believe this number is accurate.

413>Janet Reno was the Attorney General of the United States during the Clinton era. Combined reference to both the handling of the Waco Texas burning of an alleged cult home killing its occupants and the forced breakup of Microsoft because it was a successful company.

413>Molar fillings were once thought to be able to receive radio signals that could then be heard as voices by humans. I believe someone famous made this claim during WWII or whenever, and there's been no going back since then. No documented proof of this was found.

413>Rudes or rude. Ernest T. Bass of *Andy of Mayberry* in episode #133 Oct. 12, 1964, *The education of Ernest T. Bass*, Ernest states; "I got a rude." and was proud of it. Source: UAV Home Video, 1992.

413>Rust spot. Reference to a spiritual vision of Jesus (I believe) on the side of an oil tank when seen at night illuminated by a nearby street light. I can't find exact data of the reporting but I believe it was in Texas during the 1990's. Why do humans believe that the supreme power of the universe would act so stupid?

413>Ultraviolence. Reference word from the movie, *A Clockwork Orange* directed by the late, great Stanley Kubrick, A book written by Anthony Burgess. Used as "ultraviolence horrorshow" by the hero, Alex, in his book.

414>Horrorshow. See the number 413 reference.

414>Refer to St. Catherine of Genoa. Quoting from her Chapter IV, "For man dead in sin merits infinite pain for an infinite time, but God's mercy has allotted infinity to him only in time and has determined the quantity of his pain; in justice God could have given him more pain." Source of quote:
www.ewtn.com/library/spirit/catpur.txt has information about a book published in 1946 by Sheed and Ward, Inc.

415>Volkswagen Fastback. Often pronounced the same in many languages.

415>Zillion. Often used by ordinary humans to denote a number greater than three.

418>Asexual life does not need a "partner" in order to reproduce. This process can occur from spores or budding. Masturbation is not an asexual act.

418>Debbie does "someone." Refers to a series of Porn flicks that started with *Debbie does Dallas* starring Bambi Woods, circa 1978.

420>Concept dress. Trade term used to describe the identifiable traits of a marketable product, maybe.

421>The belief that unsaved humans will have their soul consumed in the fire of hell as opposed to living forever in the fires of Hell. From *The Plain Truth* April 1986, *What the Bible Says About Hell* by Bernard W. Schnippert, quote: "But the Bible plainly says God will destroy - not merely torture - unrepentant souls in hell (Matthew 10:28)."

422>Hell as translated by various editions of the Bible. "Two of these words, *Sheol* in the Hebrew and *Hades* in the Greek, simply mean 'the grave.'" Source: *The Plain Truth* April 1986, *What the Bible Says About Hell* by Bernard W. Schnippert. KJV: 2 Sam 22:6 "The sorrows of hell compassed", NIV: 2 Sam 22:6 "The cords of the grave coiled", NRSV: 2 Sam 22:6 "the cords of Sheol entangled" Source: *QuickVerse*, Parsons Technology, 1992-1994. HG (Hebrew) 2 Sam 22:6 "chebel:H2256 she'owl:H7585 cabab:H5437 cabab:H5437 mowqesh:H4170 maveth:H4194 qadam:H6923."

422>Sex illustrations based on religion. See a *Kama Sutra* Book. For Christians, see Leviticus 18:6-23 for a list of "don'ts."

423>Sheol. "7585. she'owl, sheh-ole'; or she'ol, sheh-ole'; from H7592; hades or the world of the dead (as if a subterranean retreat), includ. its accessories and inmates:--grave, hell, pit." Source: *QuickVerse* for Windows, Parsons Technology 1995. Also see number 508 of this book.

424>Gray matter. A descriptive term for a human brain, usually denoting a level of intelligence. From my remembrance of the brains I have dissected, is that they are pink inside but that could have been the result of the method of my smashing their skulls.

426>Paragraph reveals actual suicidal moments from my life, but I ain't dead yet.

427>Blaise Pascal. "Pascal's Wager." You can't loose the bet, if you bet your soul that there is a god. Or something like that. See reference for 479.

427>Ockham's Razor, Occam's Razor[*sp?*]. Principle proposed by William of Ockham in the 14th century. "Keep it simple" is not exactly it, so you should look up several references. Sources: http://phyun5.ucr.edu/~wudka/Physics7/Notes_www/node10.html and www.penpens.demon.co.uk/books/ockham.html

427>St. Thomas Aquina. Wrote the *Summa Theologiae* in the 13th Century. Check the book: *Extraordinary Popular Delusions & the Madness of Crowds* by Charles MacKay, Andrew Tobias. By Crown Pub. 1995. Originally published in 1841. See the source: www.litrix.com/madraven/madne001.htm by The Litrix Reading Room. Check the heading, *Albertus Magnus and Thomas Aquina*. Quote from topic, "...they never neglected the pursuit of the philosopher's stone and the elixir vitae." Also read, "...it was believed that Albert had seized some portion of the secret of life, and found means to animate a brazen statue,..."

428>Icon. Once thought of as a statue or painting or person of greatness. Popular usage now implies symbols found on computer monitors (CRT's).

429>What many Churches have remained throughout the ages due to being controlled by the corruptible human. 1 John 2:15 "So he made a whip out of cords, and drove all from the temple area, both sheep and cattle; he scattered the coins of the money changers and overturned their tables." Source: NIV. Although I have never seen a painting of such, I can envision Jesus whipping animals and people. I would like to see him walk in during one of our local churches "Casino Night."

430>"Peace on earth" is a misquote from the Bible and it implies all humans will live peaceably, but there is no proof that this was God's intention. NIV: Luke 2:14 "Glory to God in the highest, and on earth peace to men on whom his favor rests." See the same verse in NRSV & KJV. Also a joke of an unknown origin that all beauty contests must wish for "peace on earth" of some type.

431>During Lent most Catholics seem to give up something like chocolate or in-between meal snacks while stating that it will help their diet also. Prior to Lent is "Carnival" in which the orgy of the "self" is taken to an extreme because during Lent you must give up such things. I don't understand it because I have never seen chocolate at "Carnival" but there is a lot of beer. At any rate, "Carnival" did give us one popular activity that usually starts with the phrase,

"Show your teats" followed by women actually showing-off their naked breasts. I would like all of you to submit a 500-word essay on the cause and effect of that behavior in a paper titled: *Genetic behaviors cannot be overpowered by intelligence, even in the 21st century* OR *Bob's ideas concerning "herds" is just dandy*. I submit my book as my essay.

431>E-ride. Archaic: Referring to the best rides at Disneyland or DisneyWorld originally needing an "E" ticket from a ticket book containing "A, B, C, D, & E" labeled tickets.

431>Sans. For you humans under forty, it seems its use is becoming archaic: Sans would mean "without" such as those pants not requiring a belt are called "Sans-a-Belt." Or Groucho Marx once stated that he was "Sans moustache." Middle English>French>Latin, most likely.

432>Catdad. A lame joke on how silly the word dogma appears if you stare at it too long. The opposite of dogma would be catdad.

432>Gas stations used to check your oil, wash your windows, fill your tank, all while using adult male labor, and still the oil companies made profits. The station I used in Lansing Illinois, on the corner of Ridge Rd. and Torrance Ave. in 1973 used to have so many adult males working there that typically two would service your car. They would smile, be very polite, cleaned windows excellently, go inside to make change for you, and you never left your seat, got cold, wet, or gas odors on your hands. The station attendant became your friend, and you would greet him as "Good morning Al, or Sam, or Pete." Please compare this to the "youth in a cage" that sometimes is talking on the Fon to someone else while making change for you.

432>Theory of a cyclic universe has problems in that even if all matter stops its outward motion and slowly starts collapsing onto itself, only to repeat the Big Bang and cycle again and again, unless the universe is "closed" (no type of energy can escape outward) then radiant energy will be lost due to distance traveled and the weak gravity at the peak of expansion could not pull it back. The universe thus looses mass (as energy) with each cycle and will thus end, forever, unless space is truly finite. If that is true, how do you account for the universe, with no end, but finite? I leave this topic before separation anxiety sets in. See the book, *The Big Bang* by Joseph Silk, Publisher, Freeman, 1989. Try pages 102-108 & 388+.

435>Lev 24:20 "fracture for fracture, eye for eye, tooth for tooth; As he has injured the other, so he is to be injured." Lev 24:21 "Whoever kills an animal must make restitution, but whoever kills a man must be put to death." From the NIV translation, I suppose. The ways of the Lord reveal the character of the Lord.

438>Female Beauty contestants would duct tape their breasts "up" because they couldn't have bra straps showing and natural breasts aren't acceptable to societies that believe clothing is natural but the body is not.

438>Liposuction. A recent medical technology of sucking fat cells from a living human body. The use of liposuction on human brains causes death but is only referred to as a partial birth abortion for some reason.

439>Graded school. Archaic, refer to the book *Down the Great River* by Captain Willard Glazier, Publisher, Hubbard Brothers, 1892, Page 246, "It has ....graded public schools,.." Now commonly called "grade schools". The practice of grading began in Germany as early as the 16th century and thence spread worldwide. Source: www.britannica.com.

439>Mormons. As told in the book "Down the Great River" by Captain Willard Glazier, Publisher, Hubbard Brothers, 1892. Pages 286, 287, 288, & 289.

440>NIV: EXO 21:24, "eye for eye, tooth for tooth, hand for hand, foot for foot,..." NIV: MAT 5:39 "But I tell you, Do not resist an evil person. If someone strikes you on the right cheek, turn to him the other also." Nature versus Nurture I guess – gene versus meme.

445> Friedrich Nietzsche, 1844-1900 A German philosopher who wrote about the reality of the physical world as opposed to the distracting thoughts of an "after life." Refer to his writings of *Beyond Good and Evil*, *Overman* and *Thus Spake Zarathistra*. It is possible to perceive relationships between this mindset and Germany before WWII but I haven't found any good source of information to confirm my beliefs. One source stated that his sister was responsible for the using his ideologies as a pro-Nazi (proto-Nazi) validation (against his intentions), but I offer you no documents to confirm this. Check into the mind-set of the 1920's America. Read *A Plan for Peace* by Margaret Sanger and anything else by her, but stay off the Planned Parenthood site, they are running an agenda for genocide (My free speech opinion).

445>"Give a blind man an elbow." I heard this in a Monty Python TV show episode. My source: Monty Python's Flying Circus. A British comedy troupe.

445>From *Thus Spoke Zarathustra* by Friedrich Nietzsche, 1844-1900. Well I suppose this is the story of how mankind and womantype should work to aspire to greatness by not believing in the un-proveable spiritual stuff. Source: www.marilyn-manson.com/overman.htm, *Blueprint for the Antichrist Superstar.*

446>According to the *Holman Bible Dictionary*, Satan of the Old Testament is always portrayed as the adversary of God's people. Source: *Holman Bible Dictionary for Windows*, Version 1.0g 1994 Parsons Technology. I would be inclined to say that our current belief in the devil, his power, and his intentions have been evolved through the faulty logic of the humans and their beliefs being altered with each generation.

447>Driving along, singing a song then boom your on fire and strapped in your car seat no less. One of God's mysterious ways of taking you to Heaven I suppose.

447>"waxed". Also refer to "Waxing roth", Source: *Groucho, Harpo, Chico and sometimes Zeppo* by Joe Adamson, Publisher, Simon and Schuster 1973. Page 191, "The Dean is furious! He's waxing wroth!"

448>There is no direct mention of guardian angels in the Bible. Cherubim have wings, angels take on many forms, and the "whiteness" of angels only appears in the New Testament. Source: *Holman Bible Dictionary* etc. Children are often referred to as angels even though there is no physical or mental similarities. Human women are refereed to angels but there is no biblical reason to do so, and I can't see any behavioral reasons to draw that analogy.

450>See reference for number 453.

453>Why did Eve do it? "Were it not for our transgression we never should have had 'seed'", Source, *Latter Day Saints, Book of Moses*, Chapter 5, June-October 1830, Verse 11. http://scriptures.lds.org/moses/5/. Contrast this belief with NIV Genesis 1:28 (while still in Eden) "God blessed them and said to them, 'Be fruitful and increase in number; fill the earth and subdue it....'" Godd's first command to man and woman was to procreate.

453>Source: NIV Genesis 1:28, 29 "..fill the earth and subdue it. Rule over the fish of the sea ...over every living creature that moves on the ground." "I give you every seed-bearing plant on the face of the whole earth..." Adam, Eve, and all generations were to freely leave and enter Eden and the world would present no attacks against them for all was as in Eden.

455>I have no clue if this is a true title or if I imagined it.

458>After the English botanist Robert Brown. Supposedly everything moves as prescribed by Brownian motion because of unequal forces pushing upon it due to the random motion of molecules around it. These motions may not be perceived by human eyesight. Source: www.math.utah.edu/classes/217/assignment.04.html.

458>*Metamagical Themas*. A book by Douglas Hofstadter, Publisher, Basic Books, Inc. 1985. "Questing for the Essence of Mind and Pattern" is what it is about. One of the most intelligent books ever written.

460>KJV: Isa 14:12 O Lucifer. But does not appear anywhere else or anywhere at all in the NIV or NRSV translations. From Heylel, "The morning Star." Source: *QuickVerse*, Parsons Technology 1992-1994. Lucifer = the devil in modern thought.

460>Pooh-Bah. Quote: "A pompous ostentatious official, especially one who, holding many offices, fulfills none of them." Source: *American Heritage 2000.*

463>Refers to Sherlock Holmes' drug addiction to morphine and cocaine. Refer to *The Sign of Four* by Sir Arthur Conan Doyle, Chapter 1. My source: www.citsoft.com/holmes.3.html.

"For some little time his eyes rested thoughtfully upon the sinewy forearm and wrist, all dotted and scarred with innumerable puncture-marks. Finally, he thrust the sharp point home, pressed down the tiny piston, and sank back into the velvet-lined armchair with a long sigh of satisfaction. Three times a day for many months I had witnessed this performance, ..."

464>I would believe this rate is a direct function of the quality or intelligence of the "therapist" of which the *Homaniakos* visits regularly. Suicide rates as reported in *Scientific American* March 1997, page 20 are as follows: 18% alcoholics, 15% depressed or manic-depressive, and 10% schizophrenics. How many alcoholics are self-medicated manic-depressives? The actual population of the *Homaniakos* species will never be known.

464>*Planet of the Apes*. 1968, 20th Century Fox. "During breaks in filming, actors made up as different ape species tended to hang out together---apes with apes, orangutans with orangutans, chimps with chimps. It wasn't required, it just naturally happened." Source: Quote from www.IMDb.com.

465>She was of a different mind for sure, but anyway the work "Treatise on Purgatory" was written of her life and teachings. Source: www.ewtn.com/library/spirit/catpur.txt has information about a book published in 1946 by Sheed and Ward, Inc.

466>"Pachisi ('Twenty-five') is almost a tradition in India where it is now largely played by children. The Mogul emperor, Akbar the Great, had Pachis boards inlaid in his palaces and used slave girls for pieces." "There are no approved rules for Pachisi,.." Page 14, quote source: *The Family Book of Games* by David Pritchard, Publisher Sceptre Books, Time-Life Books B.V. 1994.

466>Ron Popeil, marketer of this and other products such as; Mr. Microphone and the Pocket Fisherman. Source: http://future.newsday.com/6/fron.htm

467>In the USA, the belly button was considered a sex organ (and for a good reason) until the 1960's and thus was hidden from view in all movies and Television shows. I understand that Alfred Hitchcock didn't have a belly button but I can't find out why. I still personally consider the belly button to be a sex organ; thus sporadic moments of visual arousal are easy to achieve. Seeing female humans pierced belly button satisfies the "Sleeping Beauty Syndrome" that human males go through at puberty.

469>From NIV Genesis 3:6, "When the woman saw that the fruit of the tree was good for food and pleasing to the eye, and also desirable for gaining wisdom, she took some and ate it." In case you've mis-placed your Bible.

470>Nothing has ever been invented. See the source: www.pigeon.psy.tufts.edu/psych26/morgan.htm. Yes, it's the same C. L. Morgan of "Morgan's cannon of interpretation" fame. From his book, *The Animal Mind*, concerning a dog learning to lift a gate's latch in order to exit the yard and if a human happened to see the dog do it after the dog has perfected the trick: "The point here is that observation on one occasion only, no matter how careful and exact that observation may be, does not suffice for the interpretation of this or that instance of animal behavior." Now you would believe that, as humans are only animals, the same logic would apply?

471>This is a misleading notation, I believe "autonomic" is actually the correct word. Internet Source: ©*2002 by Merriam-Webster, Incorporated.* "Occurring involuntarily."

471>Jeremiah denounced the hypocrites who, he said, "had the Lord in their mouths, but not in their kidneys." Source, *Second Book of Wonders*, page 167, Published by The Wonder Book Corporation, 1922. From KJV: "near in their mouth, and far from their reins." Reins are *Kilyah*, a kidney. Source: *QuickVerse*, Parsons Technology, 1992-1994. Yes, the Bible has errors in it, but it remains the divinely written word of Godd. The brain was used to cool the blood.

472>I removed the word that the following definition was placed here to define for you. "A man short in stature." American Heritage fourth edition 2000.

476>Some man was taking photos of *Barbie* dolls in erotic poses. Ultimately the courts decided that he could continue to produce the photographs. I found it on the Internet at ABCnews.com February 23, 2001.

476>Pre-masturbatatorial. At the age before physical sexual activities become thought about. Then, all of a sudden touching yourself is a whole new experience.

477>Hidrosis. Sweating, a disease of the sweat glands. Alt. spelling: Hydrosis. Page 298, source: *Dorland's Pocket Medical Dictionary*, 21st edition. Published by W. B. Saunders Co. 1968 edition.

477>Men as potential rapist. Feminist propaganda spread during the 1990's when in actuality what is more accurate to say, via nature's design, is that all women are potential impregnations.

479>Refer to Edgar Burroughs *Under the Moons of Mars* for the first Star Trek type transportation using technology in place of witchcraft. Source: *Smithsonian* magazine, March 2001, *Tarzan the Eternal* by Bruce Watson. I would have to remark that everybody copies and imitates - hasn't anyone ever thought of something new?

481>From NIV Genesis 3:7 "Then the eyes of both of them were opened, and they realized they were naked; so they sewed fig leaves together and made coverings for themselves." From NIV Genesis 3:11 "And he [God] said, 'Who told you that you were naked?'" Thus as I state elsewhere, it is not your eyes that give you vision in terms of perception and thus the ordinary humans have always had faulty logic as created by God.

482>Ringo Starr's shouted "I've got blisters on me fingers" at the end of the song *Helter Skelter*, from Terry Ott. Source: www.best.com/~abbeyrd/ott.htm. *Helter Skelter* was later associated with the Manson murders, but I don't remember why.

482>In paragraph 480 (I hope) there is a reference to the music of which I am listening, which should be the Korn CD, *Issues*. But it is not until paragraph 482 that I put that CD into my player. The paragraphs were written out of sequence. The illustration is an attempt to get you to understand that your bible also suffers the same occurrences of subjects but it doesn't necessary mean the data is faulty or invalid.

484>Such gods as, Baal, El, Anat (Anath, Athirat, Asherah), Mot (death), Yam (sea, river), and chaos. If I understand this correctly, it would refer to a period during Joshua and the book of Judges. Source: *Holman Bible Dictionary for Windows* Version 1.0g. 1994.

484>Egyptcians. Pronounced, "Egypt-see-ans."

484>Ugaritic Tablets. Tablets discovered in the city of Ugarit, Syria that described the Canaanite religion. Source: *Holman Bible Dictionary for Windows* Version 1.0g. 1994.

485>Concerning Free Will. See NIV Numbers 21:34 & 35. "The Lord said to Moses, "Do not be afraid of him, for I have handed him over to you,..." & "So they struck him down, together with his sons and his whole army, leaving them no survivors....""

487>Refer to the Bible (my source, NIV), Book of Job 1:6, "One day the angels came to present themselves before the Lord, and Satan also came with them." and also Job 2:1. The word "Lucifer" appears in Isaiah 14:12 in the KJV, but not in the NIV or NRSV versions. From Heylel, "The morning Star." Source: *Holman Bible Dictionary for Windows* Version 1.0g. 1994.

488>Devil's Island. A French penal colony off the north East Coast of South America. In operation for about 300 years. It is currently shutdown. Read the book *I escaped from Devil's Island* by Rene Belbenoit, Published by Bantam Books 1949 (paperback).

489>Cherubim have wings and do something for God, but they are not angels. It is common for Euro-Americans to refer to children and women as angels, especially with wings. I do not see how these analogies would have been derived, knowing the nature of children and women. This would fall under the category of "wishful thinking."

490>The movie: *Splash* starring Daryl Hannah's butt, directed by Ronny (Opie) Howard reveals this transformation trait of Mermaids. Mr. Howard is such the nice gentleman, isn't he? Great movies also.

491>Mound of Venus. Poetic reference to a human female's genitalia. Vulgar, AKA "A camel's toe."

492>NIV: Gen 19:24 "Then the LORD rained down burning sulfur on Sodom and Gomorrah - from the LORD out of the heavens." Events are always described within the knowledge of the current technology. Thus the destruction during that era gives the appearance of a volcano in place of a nuclear bomb.

493>The length of the nails used to hold criminals to the crosses in the time of Jesus. I have not verified this information.

493>A cleansing powder for kitchen sinks, etc. Refer to the movie *The Ghost and Mr. Chicken*, starring Don Knots, 1965. Quote source: IMDb. Mrs. Miller, "Well, they say there are still blood stains on the organ keys." Mrs. Hutchinson, "That's right. They've never been able to get them off." Mrs. Cobb, "And they used Bon Ami!"

497>I removed the topic about the King James translation, but the reference data is still interesting. Proper name: King James I, AKA King James VI, commissioned the writing of the Bible according to church/state beliefs of his era in 1611. Some humans believe that only the King James translation is the valid word of God. Also see *Leviathan* from the same era, written by Thomas Hobbes.

497>Though the overall picture of Sheol is grim, the Old Testament nevertheless affirms that God is there (Ps. 139:8;) or that it is impossible to hide from God in Sheol. The Old Testament also affirms that God has power over Sheol and is capable of ransoming souls from its depths (Ps. 30:3; 49:15; 86:13). The question is, is Sheol only for OT Jews? Does everyone else, wait in the grave (the actual ground) until the end of time? I have never heard an elegy that proclaimed, "Well, we lost this one to Hell."

504>See your favorite Video rental store or better still, visit an adult book & novelties store. Naturally, the World Wide Web with proper adult check verification can get you anything you would want to see, or could never imagine seeing, before you see it.

504>Bib-Label Lithiated Lemon-Lime Soda. "You like it, It likes you" Slogan for 7UP. Enriched with Lithium. Source: www.pendulum.org/meds/lithium_wsj.htm. 1994, The Wall Street Journal. "French Wine of Coca: Invigorating Tonic became a popular soft drink because it contained cocaine. It went on to become Coca-Cola and together with other similar drinks like Pepsi-Cola, made the soda fountain a common part of the neighborhood pharmacy." Circa 1870. Source: *Schaffer Library of Drug Policy, 2001*.

504>Sacristan. A person in charge of the sacristy and ceremonial equipment. Internet Source: ©2002 by Merriam-Webster, Incorporated. NIV: Lev 25:44 "Your male and female slaves are to come from the nations around you; from them you may buy slaves." NIV: Lev 25:46 "You can will them to your children as inherited property and can make them slaves for life, but you must not rule over your fellow Israelites ruthlessly."

504>I had used the term "Holy cow" here, but I removed it. "...the slaughter of milk-producing cows was prohibited, and verses of the Rgveda refer to the cow as Devi (goddess), identified with Aditi (mother of the gods)..." *2002 Britannica.com Inc.*

507>Refer to: Saint Catherine of Genoa, *Treatise on Purgatory, The Dialogue*, Source: www.ewtn.com/library/spirit/catpur.txt. Chapter IV, "After death free will can never return, for the will is fixed as it was at the moment of death." I can only reply, "Hmmm." With regards to free will, examine Num 21:34, 35 because apparently there is a lot to be said about God having already planned your fate and you can't change it.

508>phallic phantasticus. A fantasy involving the penis.

510>Well I lost my reference to this one, but if you are handy enough you will find that about the year 1900 the sport of jumping one canoe by another, while both are fully occupied, was very popular. Do you believe me?

513>With regards to Christmas, NIV Gal 4:9, 10: "But now that you know God – or rather are known by God – how is it that you are turning back to those weak and miserable principles? Do you wish to be enslaved by them all over again? You are observing special days and months and seasons and years!"

513>Xmas. NT was written in Greek, Christmas is a created of humans and does not appear in the bible. General knowledge, but usually ignored.

514>666 as the mark of the beast. "al gore" (with space) in ASCII is 666, "Barney" is 666 and "HOLYBIBLE" (no space, all caps) in ASCII is 666. Source: www.greaterthings.com/World-Number/666/index.html. Refer to the Bible, NIV Revelation 13:18 "This calls for wisdom. If anyone has insight, let him calculate the number of the beast, for it is man's number. His number is 666."

515>From the NIV Matthew 2:16, 17, 18. "When Herod realized that he had been outwitted by the Magi, he was furious, and he gave orders to kill all the boys in Bethlehem and its vicinity who were two years old and under, in accordance with the time he had learned from the Magi. Then what was said through the prophet Jeremiah was fulfilled: 'A voice is heard in Ramah, weeping and great mourning, Rachel weeping for her children and refusing to be comforted, because they are no more.'" The exact number of murdered boys is not know.

518>Conversing. NIV: Mat 5:37 Concerning oaths. "Simply let your 'Yes' be 'Yes,' and your 'No,' 'No'; anything beyond this comes from the evil one."

524>Revelation 22:18, NIV, "If anyone adds anything to them, God will add to him the plagues described in this book." (etc.). The earliest copyright statement that I can find.

525>A statement made by the artist Andy Warhol but I can't remember if it is 15 seconds, 15 minutes, or 15 hours of fame? Every human is guaranteed this for some reason.

NOTES

NOTES

NOTES

NOTES

NOTES

NOTES

NOTES

NOTES

NOTES

NOTES

NOTES